IMPLEMENTATION
SCIENCE IN NURSING

···· A Framework for ····
Education and Practice

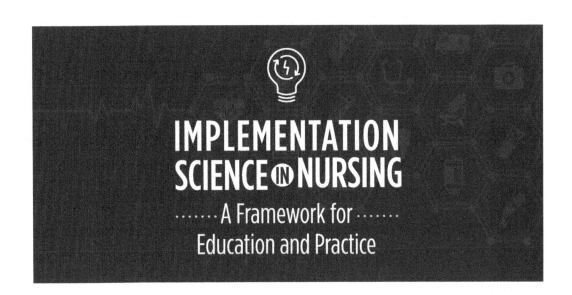

IMPLEMENTATION SCIENCE IN NURSING
······ A Framework for ······
Education and Practice

Editors

Linda A. Roussel, PhD, RN, NEA-BC, CNL, FAAN
Clinical Professor, Graduate Studies
UTHealth Cizik School of Nursing
The University of Texas Health Center at Houston
Houston, Texas

Patricia L. Thomas, PhD, RN, FAAN, FACHE, FNAP, NEA-BC, ACNS-BC, CNL
Associate Dean, Faculty Affairs
Associate Professor
Cohn College of Nursing
Wayne State University
Detroit, Michigan

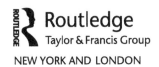

Routledge
Taylor & Francis Group

NEW YORK AND LONDON

First published in 2022 by SLACK Incorporated

Published 2024 by Routledge
605 Third Avenue, New York, NY 10017
4 Park Square, Milton Park, Abingdon, Oxon OX14 4RN

Routledge is an imprint of the Taylor & Francis Group, an informa business

Library of Congress Control Number: 2021952116

ISBN:9781630917388 (pbk)
ISBN:9781003524601 (ebk)

DOI:10.4324/9781003524601

Contents

Acknowledgments . . . . *ix*

About the Editors . . . . *xi*

Contributing Authors . . . . *xiii*

Foreword *by* Sharon Tucker, PhD, APRN-CNS, PMHCNS-BC, NC-BC, FNAP, FAAN . . . .*xvii*

Introduction . . . . *xix*

Chapter 1   Evolution of Evidence-Based Practice: Implications for
             Implementation and Dissemination Sciences
             and Translational Nursing 1
             Clista Clanton, MSLS;
             Patricia L. Thomas, PhD, RN, FAAN, FACHE, FNAP, NEA-BC, ACNS-BC, CNL; and
             Linda A. Roussel, PhD, RN, NEA-BC, CNL, FAAN

Chapter 2   History, Context, and Application of Implementation,
             Decision Sciences, and Evidence-Based
             Practice Uptake 19
             Cynthia Peltier Coviak, PhD, RN, FNAP

Chapter 3   Theories, Frameworks, and Models in
             Implementation and Decision Science 39
             Cynthia Peltier Coviak, PhD, RN, FNAP

Chapter 4   Scholarship for Academic Nursing:
             Alignment With Implementation
             and Dissemination Sciences? 55
             Cynthia Peltier Coviak, PhD, RN, FNAP

             Exemplar 4-1   Knowledge Discovery
                            From Electronic Data 68
                            Cynthia Peltier Coviak, PhD, RN, FNAP

             Exemplar 4-2   Community Health Promotion
                            Project Implementation 70
                            Cynthia Peltier Coviak, PhD, RN, FNAP

Chapter 5   Implementation Science and Practice:
             Implications for Nursing Education
             Through Content, Context, and Projects 73
             Linda A. Roussel, PhD, RN, NEA-BC, CNL, FAAN and
             Patricia L. Thomas, PhD, RN, FAAN, FACHE, FNAP, NEA-BC, ACNS-BC, CNL

Chapter 6   Implementation Science and Practice:
             Entry Level of Practice 89
             Janet E. Winter, DNP, MPA, FNAP, RN

             Exemplar 6-1   Interprofessional Collaboration 106
                            Margaret Moore-Nadler, DNP, RN

Chapter 7   Implementation and Dissemination Sciences
and Practice: Graduate Nursing Education
and Advanced Practice. 107
Cynthia Peltier Coviak, PhD, RN, FNAP

   Exemplar 7-1   Evidence-Based Best Practice for Pediatric
Patient/Family Education in a
Cardiovascular Intensive Care Setting. 130
*Tedra S. Smith, DNP, CRNP, CPNP-PC, CNE, CHSE and
Andrew Loehr, BSN, MSN, CNP*

Chapter 8   Organizational Systems and Leadership:
Impact on Translational Nursing 133
*Linda A. Roussel, PhD, RN, NEA-BC, CNL, FAAN and
Patricia L. Thomas, PhD, RN, FAAN, FACHE, FNAP, NEA-BC, ACNS-BC, CNL*

   Exemplar 8-1   A Strategy for Enhancing Staff Confidence
in De-Escalating a Crisis Situation. 143
Donna Copeland, DNP, RN, NE-BC, CPN, CPON, AE-C

   Exemplar 8-2   Implementation of the Braden Scale for
Predicting Pressure Injury Risk
in the Emergency Department 144
*Tiffany Tscherne, RN, DNP, MBA, FACHE and Donna Copeland,
DNP, RN, NE-BC, CPN, CPON, AE-C*

Chapter 9   The Application of Improvement Science:
Quality Improvement, Change Management,
and Sustainability 145
*David H. James, DNP, MSHQS, RN, CCNS, NPD-BC and
Patricia L. Thomas, PhD, RN, FAAN, FACHE, FNAP, NEA-BC, ACNS-BC, CNL*

   Exemplar 9-1   Application of Run and Control Charts 156
David H. James, DNP, MSHQS, RN, CCNS, NPD-BC

   Exemplar 9-2   Application of Quality Improvement
Concepts: Coin-Spinning Exercise. 159
*David H. James, DNP, MSHQS, RN, CCNS, NPD-BC and
Marti Rice, PhD, RN, FAAN*

Chapter 10   Innovation and Translation: Next Steps in Advancing Health Care
Through Implementation Science 163
*Kristen Noles, DNP, RN, CNL, LSSGB; Rebekah Barber, BSN, MSN, DNP;
Christina Fortugno, MSHA, MBA, BSN, RN, CCRN;
Linda A. Roussel, PhD, RN, NEA-BC, CNL, FAAN; and
Patricia L. Thomas, PhD, RN, FAAN, FACHE, FNAP, NEA-BC, ACNS-BC, CNL*

   Exemplar 10-1   Help Us Support Healing: The Creation of a
Sleep Protocol to Limit Sleep Interruptions
on a Medical-Surgical Unit 172
*Shaun Lampron, DNP, MSN, BSN, RN and
Donna Copeland, DNP, RN, NE-BC, CPN, CPON, AE-C*

   Exemplar 10-2   Using Design Thinking to Guide Innovation:
Innovation in Action 174
Aakansha Gosain, BME and Zena Banker, BME

Chapter 11   Voices From Health Care and Nursing Champions: Implications for Implementation Science and Translational Nursing. 177
Linda A. Roussel, PhD, RN, NEA-BC, CNL, FAAN;
Carolynn Thomas Jones, DNP, MSPH, RN, FAAN; and
Patricia L. Thomas, PhD, RN, FAAN, FACHE, FNAP, NEA-BC, ACNS-BC, CNL

    Exemplar 11-1   Imparting Knowledge and Supporting Evidence-Based Action: The Adult Nonalcoholic Fatty Liver Disease Toolkit. 187
    Kelly Casler, DNP, APRN-CNP, EBP-C, CHSE

    Exemplar 11-2   Nursing Leadership and Evidence-Based Practice Amidst the Pandemic. 191
    Kelli Chovanec, DNP, RN, NE-BC

    Exemplar 11-3   Building a Peer Support System to Mitigate Psychological Trauma in Health Care Workers 194
    Donna Copeland, DNP, RN, NE-BC, CPN, CPON, AE-C

    Exemplar 11-4   Implementing New Informed Consent Practices for Pediatric Coronavirus Disease 2019 Clinical Trials: Innovations, Collaborations, Resilience, and Team Science During a Pandemic. 196
    Carolynn Thomas Jones, DNP, MSPH, RN, FAAN and
    Mallory E. Rowell, MS, BSN, RN

    Exemplar 11-5   Best Practices for Embedding Implementation Science in Doctor of Nursing Practice Projects 200
    Linda A. Roussel, PhD, RN, NEA-BC, CNL, FAAN and
    Jeannie Scruggs Corey, DNP, RN, NEA-BC

    Exemplar 11-6   Evidence-Based Best Practice for Decreasing Inappropriate Referrals to a Comprehensive Vascular Access Team 202
    Somali Nguyen, DNP, CRNP, AGACNP-BC;
    April Garrigan, DNP, APRN, FNP-BC; and
    Shea Polancich, PhD, RN, FAAN

    Exemplar 11-7   Patient Safety Implementation 205
    Jaclyn Castano, MSN, RN, CPPS

    Exemplar 11-8   Interprofessional Evidence-Based Practice Council for Collaborative Practice. 209
    Donna Copeland, DNP, RN, NE-BC, CPN, CPON, AE-C

    Exemplar 11-9   Implementing P6 Acupressure in Conjunction With Pharmacotherapy to Decrease Chemotherapy-Induced Nausea and Vomiting: A Nurse-Led Evidence-Based Practice Initiative to Improve Care and Quality of Life. 211
    Megan Maloney, RN, BSN, DNC;
    Mary L. Schumann, RN, MA, AOCN, OCN;
    and Heather Ugolini, BSN, RN

Exemplar 11-10 Diversity and Inclusion: Bias
              in Perioperative Care 214
              Mercedes Weir, PhD, APRN, CRNA

Exemplar 11-11 Evidence-Based Practice Advocate Program for
              Direct Care Nurses 218
              Paula E. Dunham, DNP, ND, MSA, NPD-BC, EBP-C and
              Debi Sampsel, DNP, RN

Exemplar 11-12 Nursing Academic–Practice Partnerships 222
              Mary G. Carey, PhD, RN, FAHA, FAAN

Financial Disclosures 227
Index 229

ACKNOWLEDGMENTS

We would like to recognize our colleagues, collaborators, students, and mentors who urged us to embark on this textbook. The collective desire has motivated us to step into the next phase of our work guided by the belief that improvement in patient care and care delivery resides in shared commitments across disciplines in education and practice.

The development of this work has helped us to think more deeply and "put to paper" the work and shared insights of those willing to move beyond rote processes to embrace the science in implementation and dissemination. We are grateful for the innovative and pioneering spirit that guided this compilation.

From the earliest discussions through the production of this text, the team at SLACK Incorporated has been unwavering in their support and vision. We owe them a debt of gratitude and appreciation for bringing this book to reality.

Finally, we offer deep and sincere appreciation to our families who continue to encourage us to dream, stretch, and achieve. Their love and encouragement serve to sustain, buoy, and inspire us.

About the Editors

Linda A. Roussel, PhD, RN, NEA-BC, CNL, FAAN is a professor at the University of Texas Houston, Cizik School of Nursing. She is a recognized author and editor of several textbooks focused on nursing administration and management, the clinical nurse leader, project management, and evidence-based practice. She is known for her experience with academic–practice partnerships and curricular innovations including the development of the clinical nurse leader and Doctor of Nursing practice programs. An innovative academician, she regularly presents at national and international conferences and consults with nurse leaders in practice and academe. She is a fellow in the American Academy of Nursing and holds board certification in advanced nursing administration and as a clinical nurse leader.

Patricia L. Thomas, PhD, RN, FAAN, FACHE, FNAP, NEA-BC, ACNS-BC, CNL is the associate dean for Nursing Faculty Affairs and an associate professor at Wayne State University. She is a recognized author and editor of several textbooks focused on nursing administration and management, the clinical nurse leader, project management, and quality improvement. She has been recognized for her mentorship of nurses in operations from the bedside to the board room and in education across undergraduate, graduate, and doctoral programs. She is a fellow in the American Academy of Nursing and a distinguished fellow in the National Academies of Practice. She has board certifications in health care management, advanced nursing administration, adult health clinical nurse specialist, and clinical nurse leader. Dr. Thomas presents and provides consultation nationally and internationally for nursing leadership, curriculum design, and quality and process improvement.

CONTRIBUTING AUTHORS

Zena Banker, BME (Exemplar 10-2)
Executive Assistant, Prescription Care Management
Doctorate of Physical Therapy Program
University of Alabama
Birmingham, Alabama

Rebekah Barber, BSN, MSN, DNP (Chapter 10)
University of Alabama
Birmingham, Alabama

Mary G. Carey, PhD, RN, FAHA, FAAN (Exemplar 11-12)
Director, Clinical Nursing Research Center
Associate Professor, School of Nursing
University of Rochester Medical Center
Rochester, New York

Kelly Casler, DNP, APRN-CNP, EBP-C, CHSE (Exemplar 11-1)
Assistant Professor, Clinical Nursing
Director, Family Nurse Practitioner Program
The Ohio State University College of Nursing
Columbus, Ohio

Jaclyn Castano, MSN, RN, CPPS (Exemplar 11-7)
Tacoma, Washington

Kelli Chovanec, DNP, RN, NE-BC (Exemplar 11-2)
System Director of Care Navigation
ProMedica Health System
Toledo, Ohio

Clista Clanton, MSLS (Chapter 1)
Charles M. Baugh Biomedical Library
University of South Alabama
Mobile, Alabama

Donna Copeland, DNP, RN, NE-BC, CPN, CPON, AE-C (Exemplars 8-1, 8-2, 10-1, 11-3, and 11-8)
Assistant Professor, University of South Alabama
Inservice Specialist, USA Health Children's and Women's Hospital
Mobile, Alabama

Paula E. Dunham, DNP, ND, MSA, NPD-BC, EBP-C (Exemplar 11-11)
Primary Care Quality Outcomes Coordinator
Dayton Veterans Affair Medical Center
Dayton, Ohio

Christina Fortugno, MSHA, MBA, BSN, RN, CCRN (Chapter 10)
Nurse Director
Lakeview Hospital
Bountiful, Utah

April Garrigan, DNP, APRN, FNP-BC (Exemplar 11-6)
Clinical Instructor
University of Alabama School of Nursing
Birmingham, Alabama

Aakansha Gosain, BME (Exemplar 10-2)
Master of Engineering in Bioengineering Program
University of California
Berkeley, California

David H. James, DNP, MSHQS, RN, CCNS, NPD-BC (Chapter 9 and Exemplars 9-1 and 9-2)
Program Development Manager/NICHE Coordinator
Department of Interprofessional Practice and Training
University of Alabama at Birmingham Hospital
Clinical Assistance Professor
University of Alabama School of Nursing
Birmingham, Alabama

Shaun Lampron, DNP, MSN, BSN, RN (Exemplar 10-1)
Chief Nursing Officer, Twin Cities Hospital
Niceville, Florida
Adjunct Professor, University of West Florida
Pensacola, Florida

Andrew Loehr, BSN, MSN, CNP (Exemplar 7-1)
Children's Hospital of Alabama
Birmingham, Alabama

Megan Maloney, RN, BSN, DNC (Exemplar 11-9)
Memorial Sloan Kettering Cancer Center
New York, New York

Margaret Moore-Nadler, DNP, RN (Exemplar 6-1)
Associate Professor
Community Mental Health
University of South Alabama College of Nursing
Mobile, Alabama

Somali Nguyen, DNP, CRNP, AGACNP-BC (Exemplar 11-6)
University of Alabama
Birmingham, Alabama

Kristen Noles, DNP, RN, CNL, LSSGB (Chapter 10)
University of South Alabama Health System
Mobile, Alabama

Cynthia Peltier Coviak, PhD, RN, FNAP (Chapters 2, 3, 4, and 7, Exemplars 4-1 and 4-2)
Professor Emeritus
Kirkhof College of Nursing
Grand Valley State University
Grand Rapids, Michigan

Shea Polancich, PhD, RN, FAAN (Exemplar 11-6)
University of Alabama School of Nursing
Birmingham, Alabama

Marti Rice, PhD, RN, FAAN (Exemplar 9-2)
University of Alabama School of Nursing
Birmingham, Alabama

Mallory E. Rowell, MS, BSN, RN (Exemplar 11-4)
Columbus, Ohio

Debi Sampsel, DNP, RN (Exemplar 11-11)
Director of High Reliable Organization and Evidence-Based Practice
Dayton Veterans Affair Medical Center
Dayton, Ohio

Mary L. Schumann, RN, MA, AOCN, OCN (Exemplar 11-9)
Memorial Sloan Kettering Cancer Center
New York, New York

Jeannie Scruggs Corey, DNP, RN, NEA-BC (Exemplar 11-5)
James Madison University
Harrisonburg, Virginia

Tedra S. Smith, DNP, CRNP, CPNP-PC, CNE, CHSE (Exemplar 7-1)
Associate Professor
Director of Pediatric Partnerships
University of Alabama School of Nursing
Birmingham, Alabama

Carolynn Thomas Jones, DNP, MSPH, RN, FAAN (Chapter 11 and Exemplar 11-4)
Associate Professor of Clinical Nursing
The Ohio State University College of Nursing
Columbus, Ohio

Tiffany Tscherne, RN, DNP, MBA, FACHE (Exemplar 8-2)
Eastern Maine Medical Center
Bangor, Maine

Sharon Tucker, PhD, APRN-CNS, PMHCNS-BC, NC-BC, FNAP, FAAN (Foreword)
Grayce Sills Endowed Professor, College of Nursing
Director, DNP Nurse Executive Track
Director, Translational/Implementation Science Core
Helene Fuld Health Trust National Institute for Evidence-Based Practice
Nurse Scientist, Wexner Medical Center
Certified Meditation and Mindfulness Teacher
Certified Mental Health First Aid Instructor
The Ohio State University
Columbus, Ohio

Heather Ugolini, BSN, RN (Exemplar 11-9)
Memorial Sloan Kettering Cancer Center
New York, New York

Mercedes Weir, PhD, APRN, CRNA (Exemplar 11-10)
Assistant Professor
University of South Florida Nurse Anesthesiology Program
Tampa, Florida

Janet E. Winter, DNP, MPA, FNAP, RN (Chapter 6)
Associate Dean of Undergraduate Programs in Nursing
Associate Professor
Kirkhof College of Nursing
Grand Valley University
Grand Rapids, Michigan

Foreword

It is with great enthusiasm that I provide the foreword for this new, highly needed book, *Implementation Science in Nursing: A Framework for Education and Practice*. Although there have been enormous advances in evidence-based decision making and evidence-based practice (EBP), along with substantial research findings demonstrating the value of EBP for promoting high-quality and safe patient care, the uptake of best evidence by clinicians and organizations remains slow and grossly inadequate. Known and taught widely across disciplines, EBP is a systematic process for providing evidence-based care with generally six or seven steps recognized as key to the process. Educational programs, training workshops, self-learning modules, a host of courses and webinars, textbooks, and articles teach students and health care professionals about EBP and how to apply the steps. Nevertheless, the EBP step that is the most challenging and the primary reason EBP initiatives are not successful is the implementation step, where the practice change is piloted, evaluated, integrated, and sustained. Recognition of this major EBP gap led to the field of implementation science (IS), which is the study of methods and strategies that promote the systematic uptake of research findings and EBPs into routine practices to ultimately improve patient care quality, safety, and outcomes.

This book is a timely resource that guides readers, students, and clinicians to understand how to bring about and sustain change using IS. As a behavioral and organizational change expert, it is clear to me that a solid foundation in understanding change mechanisms and knowledge of factors that influence change is essential for narrowing the research to practice gap. This book brings essential content and experiential learning to key elements of change guided by IS and offers guidance to clinicians and students in the EBP process, specifically for the challenging steps of implementation, sustainability, and dissemination.

As noted by the editors, there are multiple outstanding nursing textbooks on the EBP process and a growing number of foundational textbooks on IS and strategies for accelerating an EBP initiative to change practice. This textbook bridges concepts in EBP and IS for a nursing audience in practice and educational settings. Through an experiential approach, readers learn the elements of implementation and dissemination science, how to use the associated frameworks/models/theories, and how to achieve and sustain desired outcomes through the adoption and implementation of scientific evidence into practice.

The book begins with a discussion of the history of implementation and dissemination science, presents a widely accepted definition, and describes phases of the implementation process, with a strong focus on what is needed to be successful with implementing EBP. Chapter 1 highlights EBP uptake related to population health and precision health care; differentiates evidence, clinical intuition, and clinical judgment; highlights the importance of patient preferences and value; and describes different aspects to knowledge and decision making in health care. A table of definitions is presented that provides a variety of interpretations of IS terminology including EBP, translational, and improvement science. Chapter 2 provides more depth and breadth of definitions and specific models/frameworks and theories to guide implementation processes using real-world examples to illustrate application and provides an overview of scientific methods used to advance IS and its application.

Chapter 3 aligns nursing scholarship with IS and opportunities for nursing to participate in advancing the science and practice. Different ways of knowing are importantly woven into this chapter to help understand change and how nursing knowledge intersects with it. Chapter 4 brings IS to nursing practice and how concepts can be used in nursing and implementing evidence into practice. Chapter 5 narrows the application to entry-level practice and education with expectations, whereas Chapter 6 focuses on advanced nursing practice roles and graduate education. Chapters 7 through 10 direct the use of IS to organizations, systems, and leadership. Content focuses on how the frameworks, tools, and strategies can bring about important and desirable change; how they overlap and augment quality improvement and change management methods; and the integration of innovation and IS. The final chapter brings voices from health care champions to learn from their experiences.

The book, *Implementation Science in Nursing: A Framework for Education and Practice*, is revolutionary and sorely needed for nursing education. In a recent study, our team identified that nurses self-reported not being competent in any of the 24 EBP competencies, and these findings did not differentiate Magnet and non-Magnet designated organizations (Melnyk et al., 2018). We have also repeatedly found that knowledge and beliefs about EBP are associated with implementation competencies. This book can help build these competencies by providing a resource for using IS to guide EBP initiatives. This includes undergraduate and graduate students, practicing nurses, organizational leaders and those charged with change and innovation, and those users interested in further advancing IS. I close with noting the important role of the doctor of nursing practice (DNP) graduate. A key competency of this role is to help lead and inspire EBP and change; thus, IS should be core knowledge in DNP curricula. This book serves as a great resource for DNP-prepared leaders and nurse educators teaching in DNP programs.

— *Sharon Tucker, PhD, APRN-CNS, PMHCNS-BC, NC-BC, FNAP, FAAN*

Reference

Melnyk, B., Gallagher-Ford, L., Zellefrow, C., Tucker, S., Thomas, B., & Sinnott, L. T. (2018). The first U.S. Study on nurses' evidence-based practice competencies indicate major deficits that threaten healthcare quality, safety, and patient outcomes. *Worldviews on Evidence-Based Nursing, 15(1)*, 16-25.

Introduction

Health care providers struggle with the rapid uptake of evidence-based practices (EBPs) evolving from research and scientific knowledge needed for clinical practice, organizational innovations, and advancing policy. We experience an ongoing tension to provide high-quality, value-added practice demonstrated through clinical procedures and technologies to achieve best health care outcomes using the highest levels of research evidence. As educators, we want to provide the tools, techniques, and strategies for our students to advance quality initiatives to improve patient and population health. This is often accomplished through scholarly practice immersion experiences focused on interprofessional implementation projects underpinned by translational science (TS). It is imperative that our students and colleagues are grounded in knowledge translation to reduce the knowledge to action practice gap.

Deimplementation is an even greater challenge, particularly considering the need to identify and remove harmful, non–cost-effective, or ineffective practices based on tradition and often without adequate scientific support (Upvall & Bourgault, 2018). This textbook was conceived to assist educators, practitioners, and students address the long-standing and often recalcitrant approaches used to address patterns and practices in the implementation of change.

Deimplementing inappropriate health interventions is essential for improving population health, maintaining public trust, minimizing patient harm, and reducing unnecessary waste in health care and public health (Norton & Chambers, 2020). Tailored interventions exist in nearly all countries and include financial incentive programs to maximize the performance of health care providers, ongoing professional education, and tools and strategies that actively involve patients in their care through shared decision making.

A variety of names are associated with the growing field of EBP uptake including improvement science, dissemination and implementation, and knowledge transfer or translation (Graham et al., 2006). Chapter 1 provides a table of definitions that gives context to the various ways TS has been described and advanced. Knowledge may take many forms including EBP guidelines, technologies, wearable patient monitoring devices, or health care delivery models that have been deemed value added. Through knowledge translation and transfer, a change of practice and behaviors are required; however, resisting change is also evident, particularly when evidence is limited or negative. This is the ongoing push and pull that thwarts the spread and sustainability of outcomes.

Eccles and Mittman (2006) described implementation science (IS) as the scientific study of methods that facilitate the systematic uptake of research findings and other EBPs into routine practices with the outcomes of improved quality and effectiveness of health care services and systems administration. Knowledge translation is a related field whose focus is to enhance the utility of research and includes the design and conduct of studies, as well as the dissemination and implementation of findings (Graham et al., 2006). Improvement science (quality and safety management) consists of a set of activities that aim to improve health care quality and safety facilitated by measurement, feedback to decision makers, and organizational change (Dixon-Woods, 2019). The "know-do" gap in health care requires that nurse educators and practitioners continue to incorporate TS and practice into their educational and clinical practices. This provides important content and context for experiential learning and project development.

The authors of this textbook have more than 50 years of clinical, administration, and educational practice experience and have incorporated their knowledge, skills, and abilities in EBP in working with undergraduate and graduate nursing students. They have been steadfast in their pursuit of integrating TS into practice as the science has evolved and advanced over time. This has advanced their work in enhancing academic–clinical–community partnerships to further the spread and sustainability of positive health care population and systems-level outcomes. TS and practice have also informed scholarly projects at all educational levels that are underpinned with theories, models, and frameworks for improvement, IS, and dissemination science (DS). This textbook provides the authors' ongoing work in bringing the best of TS and practice through the presentation of rigorous content and exemplars that illustrate real-world examples for educators, practitioners, and students. Each chapter provides a thoughtful work in the integration of the best evidence in TS and practice.

Outline of the Textbook and Relevance to Nurse Educators and Practitioners

Chapter 1 provides a historical look and the evolution of EBP, emphasizing the implications for IS and DS. The chapter describes the EBP process as having largely been driven by academic clinical researchers and educators who have always relied on journal publications and meeting presentations to disseminate or spread the word on effective interventions, practices, and policies. Defined by the National Institutes of Health (NIH), dissemination is "the targeted distribution of information and intervention materials to a specific public health or clinical practice audience. The intent is to spread knowledge and the associated evidence-based intervention" (Glasgow et al., 2012, p. 1275). There has been a noted "know-do" (knowledge translation) gap because research findings translated into improving public health or changing practice have not always been the concern of traditional health care researchers (Bauer et al., 2015). It is evident that more diverse and rigorous dissemination efforts are needed to increase the number of evidence-based interventions that are successfully and sustainably implemented in practice settings to lower the often-quoted 17-year gap of when research evidence makes an impact on clinical practice (Morris et al., 2011). Chapter 1 defines the terms that the reader will be using throughout the textbook.

Dissemination and implementation outcomes are introduced in Chapter 1. Through their research efforts, Brownson et al. (2012) provided a taxonomy of dissemination and implementation outcomes. These outcomes provide definitions, level of analysis, theoretical basis, other terms used in the literature, the stage of dissemination and implementation, and examples of methods of measurement. This beginning work assists the translational scientist and practitioner in developing a frame of reference in which to tailor strategies with outcomes for successful project management. A taxonomy offers a language that the interprofessional team can focus on when working on improvement plans outlining implementation and dissemination outcomes. Building consensus can be attained using a common language, which also can maximize limited resources in decision making and strategic planning. Nine dissemination and implementation outcomes are identified by Brownson et al. (2012) and include the following: acceptability, reach, adoption, appropriateness, feasibility, fidelity, cost, prevention, and sustainability. Knowing these outcomes can provide an excellent framework for designing implementation strategies grounded in research and development. For example, *acceptability* is defined as agreeable, palatable, or satisfactory to stakeholders and those involved in the process. Considering acceptability (what is acceptable), the researcher or practitioner focuses on a specific intervention, practice, technology, or service within a setting of care. The level of analysis is the individual with a theoretical basis stemming from diffusion theory and complexity for the relative advantage of dissemination and implementation of outcomes. The literature includes other terms that define acceptability such as satisfaction with the innovation and systems readiness. The dissemination and implementation acceptability outcome is best used for early adoption and ongoing penetration. Methods of measurement include surveys, key informant interviews, and administrative data. Fidelity of implementation and dissemination is included with factors that influence the process of successful follow-through. Deimplementation is also included and described as important to the appropriate use of evidence-based strategies. This is an evolving component of TS and practice.

Chapter 2 content enhances the application of TS to advance decision science. The author describes the need for nursing involvement with IS and DS, particularly considering the long-standing concerns for improving quality and safety in health care. The unique expertise of nurse scientists is also of significance. Notably, several staff members from the NIH identified gaps in the translational research completed to date. Discussing what they considered "late-stage" translation, which brings basic research to the real world, they observed a needed focus on the *context* in which a therapy would be used. This was, they asserted, a realm of study for which physicians were insufficiently skilled and that bore "really difficult dynamic, adaptive, and multiscale issues" while "establishing access to health systems, addressing health disparities, economics, poverty, and behavior change" (Sampson et al., 2016, p. 155). The areas of challenge identified have long been the focus of nursing science as well as nursing practice. Nursing engagement in translational nursing that will address these issues, as well as the identification of methods for implementation success in working with high-risk populations and in settings where resources are scarce, can be a major contribution to the field (DeVon et al., 2016; Tinkle et al., 2013). Chapter 2 also underscores the importance of IS and DS for nursing science. More nurse scientists are involved in Clinical and Translational Science Awards in areas of basic science such as genomics. Also, guidance for submitting NIH pragmatic trial grant applications (Littleton-Kearney, 2018) as well as for publishing findings of pragmatic trials (Pickler & Kearney, 2018) are now available. In addition, the work that nurse scientists have done to make research accessible to nursing professionals and to maximize the benefits of basic science for clients and organizations is becoming more evident and visible to health care consumers. The author also describes implementation and dissemination strategies for research testing to enhance translation.

Chapter 3 provides the theories, models, and frameworks that underpin TS and practice. Six frameworks are introduced to the reader, some specific to implementations, others to dissemination, and some that have implications for both implementation and dissemination. Each of the frameworks is described, and application examples of utility for a broader translation are provided. Additionally, instruments, checklists, and methods associated with dissemination frameworks are included in the chapter. Critical measurement issues are addressed and their impact on translational research offered. Martinez et al. (2014) provided guidance regarding measurement issues to those who may embark on DS or IS investigations. These measurement issues are outlined and include a growing number of frameworks, theories, and models and a need to establish instrument psychometric properties, the use of "homegrown" and adapted instruments, choosing the most appropriate evaluation method and approach, the practicality of the instrument for use in real-world settings, and a need for decision-making tools (Martinez et al., 2014, pp. 2-6). For each of the identified issues, a discussion of the problems created by the issue and recommendations for resolution are provided. For example, the growth in frameworks, theories, and models creates the problems of homonymy and synonymy. *Homonymy* is a situation in which a concept's definition is represented by different items in different instruments, whereas *synonymy* is a circumstance when measures for different concepts have overlapping or the same items representing them (Lewis et al., 2015; Martinez et al., 2014). To combat these problems, Martinez et al. (2014) recommended a process among translational scientists to develop consensus definitions of major concepts in the field so that psychometric testing on instruments representing the concepts could commence in a systematic manner. Chapter 3 also provides identification of measurement problems by Martinez et al. (2014) and others, which has been fruitful in stimulating action to address them. The Society for Implementation Research Collaboration created an instrument review project, and the National Institute for Mental Health at NIH has provided funding to members of the Society for Implementation Research Collaboration to review, synthesize, and rate the psychometric properties and practicality of instruments designed to measure DS and IS outcomes (Lewis et al., 2015; Society for Implementation Research Instrument Review Project, 2019; Zoellner & Porter, 2017). As a result of that work, a repository has been created wherein instruments for concepts from the CFIR are reviewed, and data summarizing their psychometric characteristics are available for a society membership fee (Society for Implementation Research Instrument Review Project, 2019).

Chapter 4 focuses on scholarship for academic nursing and describes the alignment with IS and DS. The author describes successive position statements by the American Association of Colleges of Nursing (AACN) visions of the future of academic nursing (AACN, 2016) and the qualifications and skills of nursing faculty (AACN, 2019). These documents created the foundations for a revised definition of scholarship for nursing (AACN, 2018), encompassing all four of the domains of scholarship identified in Boyer's (1996) famous report to the Carnegie Foundation. The consensus position statement *Defining Scholarship for Academic Nursing* (AACN, 2018) and a document contributing to the statement, *Advancing Healthcare Transformation: A New Era for Academic Nursing* (AACN, 2016), presented expectations that nursing faculty would "demonstrate a commitment to inquiry, generate new knowledge for the discipline, connect practice with education, and lead scholarly pursuits that improve health and health care" (AACN, 2016, as cited in AACN, 2018, p. 1). Chapter 4 includes positions of AACN regarding the nature of research, practice, and education in nursing as interprofessional, as well as being multidisciplinary, interdisciplinary, and transdisciplinary (AACN, 2018, p. 2), specifically the intersections among the interests of health system improvement, interprofessional and multidisciplinary scholarship, knowledge transfer, and connections to practice engender logical connections to the major concerns that DS and IS address and that are appropriate emphases for the practice and scientific bases of nursing. AACN's (2018) statement on scholarship "calls out" Boyer's (1996) views, including the scholarship of integration, application, and teaching, as well as discovery. Chapter 4 describes the scholarship of application as being associated with practice and integration as an activity that can occur in concert with practice and teaching; empirics, the major roles, and responsibilities of nursing faculty also fit Boyer's observations well. Practice and teaching are pursuits complementary to the ethical, esthetic, and personal patterns of knowing described by Carper (1978). Their inclusion in the academic scholarship of nursing augment and harmonize with the scholarship of discovery, which has been the traditional scholarly emphasis of the nursing professionals. In addition, AACN (2018) advocates for scholarship expectations that place value on "all scholarly contributions" that are "inclusive and supports multiple ways of knowing" (p. 2). The position statement thereby promotes Carper's (1978) view of knowing in nursing united with Boyer's (1996) views and illustrates the scholarship for academic nursing.

Chapter 5 integrates basic principles and concepts from IS and DS and practice centered on translational nursing. Specifically, this chapter serves as an overview of the chapters that follow, with the focus on nursing education and systems. The authors describe IS and DS at the various levels in nursing education including entry-level, graduate nursing, and advanced nursing practice. Content related to evidence-based implementation from the teaching–learning perspective are included. Selected IS content is introduced, and context is offered related to planning, development, and implementation of relevant assignments that culminate in scholarly projects. Frameworks are provided (i.e., University of Iowa Hospital and Clinics and Registered Nurses' Association of Ontario) that illustrate examples that can be applied to experiential learning and scholarly projects. Chapter 5 outlines evidence-based implementation teaching strategies describing best practices for teaching–learning at the entry and graduate advanced nursing practice levels. Armed with a basic understanding of implementation models, specifically evidence-based nursing implementation models, the authors provide a foundational understanding to educate students about this phase of EBP uptake. In Chapter 5, the authors discuss Dolansky et al.'s (2017) excellent review using IS to better integrate Quality and Safety Education for Nurses competencies in nursing education. The authors give a historical perspective of IS and describe the Expert Recommendations for Implementation Change project's consensus document, which outlines terms and definitions for 73 discrete implementation strategies. The reader can refer to the work of Powell et al. (2015) for more information on how the team arrived at these implementation strategies. Additionally, in Chapter 5, the reader will note that Waltz et al. (2015) evaluated and refined the strategies based on the critical nature of intervention and the feasibility of the implementation. Seven categories were identified: (a) evaluative strategies such as audit and feedback, (b) interactive assistance strategies such as facilitation, (c) strategies for adapting and tailoring implementation to the local context such as with tailored strategy selection, (d) strategies for developing stakeholder interrelationships such as with the use of champions and coalition building, (e) training and education strategies, (f) strategies for supporting clinicians/educators, and (g) engagement strategies for consumers/students. Example assignments are if nurse educators can incorporate these into their evidence-based and translational courses.

Chapter 6 provides content on IS and practice focused on entry-level practice for nursing. Specifically, the author describes the undergraduate curriculum perspective for content and context and integrating IS and practice into clinical rotations and simulation experiences. Additionally, the author illustrates the implications for preceptorships and residencies for entry-level nursing students and explores the principles of IS and DS in undergraduate student projects. Curriculum and accreditation issues are included in the chapter, with well-developed tables that provide excellent examples at the didactic, clinical, and simulated experiential levels. Didactic nursing education formulated on research and EBP as well as interprofessional education is applied into the practice setting through experiential clinical assignments. The author has an intensive focus on academic–clinical partnerships. Specifically, shared implementation practices between academic and practice partners can optimize learning among BS/BSN students while ensuring high-quality, safe, person-centered outcomes within an array of practice settings where students are placed. Furthermore, strategies to ensure that the nursing intervention is delivered as intended brings consistency to student learning through simulated experiences and guided reflective prompting that explore the factors affecting implementation.

Chapter 7 emphasizes IS and DS and practice at the graduate nursing education and advanced practice levels. Specifically, the author outlines key differences between the doctor of philosophy (PhD)/doctor of nursing science (DNS)/doctor of the science of nursing (DSN) and practice-focused degrees at the doctoral or master's level in nursing and relates this to the understanding and use of research and the roles that graduates will undertake in relation to research. Additional content includes the exploration of practice-focused graduate students' differentiation between TS and EBP and how this advanced knowledge prepares them to lead change in clinical areas. Chapter 7 outlines experiences that foster the development of knowledge and skills in TS and EBP for research-focused doctoral and doctor of nursing practice (DNP) students. The author identifies the importance of PhD and DNP collaboration in education for TS and the impact on population health and health care system change. Chapter 7 offers application of master of science in nursing (MSN) student competencies and application for TS and EBP. The author describes a PhD–DNP student partnership that can be created to enable engagement in TS and EBP as a team; assignments and experiences that can be completed together include (a) identifying a practice issue that would improve practice and/or efficiency in a setting; (b) completing an exhaustive literature review; (c) proposing a TS project; (d) completing a limited project or the initial phase of a project using DS or IS frameworks and procedures; and (e) conducting the evaluation, including evaluation research methods where applicable. These activities can include areas of practice in which an evidence gap exists, requiring original research by the PhD student.

Chapter 8 describes organizational systems and leadership and the impact on translational nursing. The authors delineate change management responses on a continuum and the effectiveness of using a framework to enhance successful implementation. Implications for team and engagement science concepts that facilitate exemplar work with interprofessional teams are explored. The authors outline a variety of research strategies (qualitative, quantitative, mixed methods, and community action research) supporting leadership and organizational systems assessments. The impact of influence and messaging enhancing implementation, dissemination, and sustainability are addressed using organizational assessment tools and strategies to improve health system outcomes. We know that context and frameworks are pivotal to successful implementation practice and are strengthened in translational nursing practice with implications for academic–clinical–community partnership. Understanding systems thinking and health systems thinking provides a foundation for a deeper reflection on IS and DS. With a system thinking perspective guiding health systems thinking, Powell and Stone (2015) offered excellent insights from a patient safety lens. Chapter 8 describes the work of Powell and Stone (2015), who report on a working model/framework of Emanuel et al. (2008) on patient safety as a system. This well-thought-out model considers recipients of care, systems for therapeutic action, and workers (teams trained to rescue from or manage failure). Methods such as continuous quality improvement including technology (hardware), the physical environment (plant), and advocacy (policy), as well as competence, communication, and teamwork, provide ways to intervene within the components of the patient safety system (Powell & Stone, 2015). In addition to the model described, Powell and Stone (2015) also considered multiteams, including a coordinating team, core team, and ancillary and support services. Microsystems thinking as the basic building block is also discussed in relationship to mesosystems and macrosystems. Patient safety and high-reliability organizations are also included from a health system thinking perspective. Leadership, culture, and dynamic process improvement are key principles of high-reliability organizations (Chassin & Loeb, 2013). These principles are incorporated into the health care system's organizational culture and consider strategies such as just culture (Marx, 2001), staff engagement, coaching and mentoring, and well-designed data systems that capture patient harm and near misses. Contextualizing organizational systems and how leaders can access these tools and strategies are key to successful implementation and dissemination of critical health systems and population outcomes (Powell & Stone, 2015). These concepts are foundational to translational nursing practice and have implications for academic–clinical–community partnerships.

Chapter 9 focuses on the application of improvement science and includes quality improvement, change management, and sustainability. The authors provide content and context that enables the reader to appreciate continuous quality improvement as an essential part of the daily work of all health care professionals. Chapter 9 analyzes the strengths and limitations of common quality improvement methods, including the design, implementation, and evaluation of tests of change in daily work using an experiential learning method such as Plan-Do-Study-Act. The alignment of improvement science and IS is explored. Principles of change management are outlined to successfully lead teams. Quality improvement tools are described with specific application and how best to use appropriate tools when engaging in process improvement work. There are excellent exemplars and assignments that can be implied with teaching TS and in project planning and development. The authors discuss the work of Granger (2018) on the science of improvement, which is often considered to be synonymous with quality improvement. Although the science of improvement does encompass what has traditionally been thought of as quality improvement, the use of data to drive process changes that add value (Perla et al., 2013). The science of improvement encompasses a broader framework that consistently addresses three components. The three foundational questions that the science of improvement seeks to address are as follows: (a) What is the goal? (b) Is the change an actual improvement? and (c) What can we change to see an improvement? (Granger, 2018). To help health care professionals address these questions, various theories, models, and frameworks have been developed including the Institute for Healthcare Improvement model for improvement, the lean six sigma model, and Shewhart's theory of variation.

Chapter 10 provides content on innovation, translation, and next steps in advancing health care through IS. The authors outline the alignment of innovation science and IS that brings health care to the next level of improvement. The authors describe curiosity and inquiry and implication for state-of-the-art improvement. Chapter 10 outlines IS and DS and their impacts on population health and achieving the quadruple aim. Innovation and the "next big idea" for improvement and sustainability through the exemplar models are described. Chapter 10 discusses the science of improvement, which includes innovation, rapid cycle testing, and dissemination to generate an understanding about what changes produce improvements (Institute for Healthcare Improvement, n.d.). The goal of improvement science is to ensure that improvement efforts are based on supportive evidence and best practices planned for implementation (Shojania & Grimshaw, 2005). Innovation and creativity greatly support enhanced nursing practice. Innovation is the essential component of nursing practice that permits response and adaptation to the variation presented in health care delivery (Rundio et al., 2016). To successfully implement changes at the point of care, a nurturing environment, the ability to function independently, and a willingness to take risks are all warranted (Fasnacht, 2003).

Chapter 11 includes voices from the field and provides excellent exemplars that integrate content and context to TS and practice. Nurse educators and practitioners apply models, theories, and frameworks to conceptualizing experiential learning, project planning, and development. Using the various concepts threaded throughout the chapters, the authors help faculty and students connect the dots and make sense of the many components and factors integrated into dissemination and implementation concepts.

Conclusion

Eccles and Mittman (2006) delineated three major aims of IS as they relate to health care and include generating reliable strategies for improving health-related processes and outcomes and to facilitate the widespread adoption of these strategies, producing insights and generalizable knowledge regarding implementation processes, barriers, facilitators, and strategies and developing, testing, and refining implementation theories and hypotheses, methods, and measures. It is "how" the strategy works that provides guidance in adapting, modifying, and customizing it by facilitating an understanding of its mechanisms of action so that the strategy can be made to work more effectively. Strengthening organizational leadership or modifying culture or mindset is critical to TS and practice. Being mindful and intentional in how chapters are outlined and build on each other is important to building content and applying context to advance nursing education and practice.

— Linda A. Roussel, PhD, RN, NEA-BC, CNL, FAAN
— Patricia L. Thomas, PhD, RN, FAAN, FACHE, FNAP, NEA-BC, ACNS-BC, CNL

References

American Association of Colleges of Nursing. (2016). *Advancing healthcare transformation: A new era for academic nursing*. https://www.aacnnursing.org/Portals/42/Publications/AACN-New-Era-Report.pdf

American Association of Colleges of Nursing. (2018). *Defining scholarship for academic nursing.* https://www.aacnnursing.org/News-Information/Position-Statements-White-Papers/Defining-Scholarship-Nursing

American Association of Colleges of Nursing (2019). *Academic Progression in Nursing: Moving Together Toward a Highly Educated Nursing Workforce.* Position Statement. Washington, DC: Author.

Bauer, M., Damschroder, L., Hagedorn, H., Smith, J., & Kilbourne, A. (2015). An introduction to implementation science for the non-specialist. *BMC Psychology, 3*, 32. https://doi.org/10.1186/s40359-015-0089-9

Boyer, E. L. (1996). The scholarship of engagement. *Journal of Public Service & Outreach, 1*(1), 11-20.

Brownson, R. C., Colditz, G. A., & Proctor, E. K. (2012). *Dissemination and implementation research in health, Translating science to practice.* Oxford University Press.

Carper, B. (1978). Fundamental patterns of knowing in nursing. *Advances in Nursing Science, 1*(1), 13-23.

Chassin, M. R., & Loeb, J. M. (2013). High-reliability health care: Getting there from here. *The Milbank Quarterly, 91*(3), 459-490. https://doi.org/10.1111/1468-0009.12023

DeVon, H. A., Rice, M., Pickler, R. H., Krause-Parello, C. A., Eckart, P., Corwin, E., & Richmond, T. S. (2016). Engaging members and partner organizations in translating a nursing science agenda. *Nursing Outlook, 64*, 516-519. https://doi.org/10.1016/j.outlook.2016.07.010

Dixon-Woods, M. (2019). Harveian Oration 2018. Improving quality and safety in healthcare. *Clinical Medicine: Journal of the Royal College of Physicians of London, 19*(1), 47-56. https://doi.org/10.7861/clinmedicine.19-1-47

Dolansky, M. A., Schexnayder, J., Patrician, P. A., & Sales, A. (2017). Implementation science: New approaches to integrating quality and safety education for nurses' competencies in nursing education. *Nurse Educator, 42*(5S, Suppl. 1), S12-S17. https://doi.org/10.1097/NNE.0000000000000422

Eccles, M. P., & Mittman, B. S. (2006). Welcome to implementation science. *Implementation Science, 1*, 1. https://doi.org/10.1186/1748-5908-1-1

Emanuel, L., Berwick, D., Conway, J, Conway, J., Combes, J., Hatlie, M., Leape, L., Reason, J., Schyve, P., Vincent, C., Walton, M., Henriksen, K., Battles, J. B., Keyes, M. A., & Grady, M. L. (2008). What exactly is patient safety? In K. Henriksen, J. B. Battles, & M A. Keyes (Eds.), *Advances in patient safety: New directions and alternative approaches* (Vol. 1: Assessment). Agency for Healthcare Research and Quality.

Fasnacht, P. H. (2003). Creativity: A refinement of the concept for nursing practice. *Journal of Advanced Nursing,* 41(2), 195-202. https://doi.org/10.1046/j.1365-2648.2003.02516.x

Glasgow, R. E., Vinson C., Chambers, D., Khoury, M. J., Kaplan, R. M., & Hunter, C. (2012). National Institutes of Health approaches to dissemination and implementation science: Current and future directions. *American Journal of Public Health, 102*(7), 1274-1281. https://doi.org/10.2105/AJPH.2012.300755

Graham, I. D., Logan, J., Harrison, M. B., Straus, S. E., Tetroe, J., Caswell, W., & Robinson, N. (2006). Lost in knowledge translation: Time for a map? *Journal of Continuing Education Health Professions, 26*, 13-24.

Granger, B. B. (2018). Science of improvement versus science of implementation: Integrating both into clinical inquiry. *AACN Advanced Critical Care, 29*(2), 208-212. https://doi.org/10.4037/aacnacc2018757

Institute for Healthcare Improvement (n.d.). Science of improvement. http://www.ihi.org/about/Pages/ScienceofImprovement.aspx

Lewis, C. C., Weiner, B. J., Stanick, C., & Fischer, S. M. (2015). Advancing implementation science through measure development and evaluation: A study protocol. *Implementation Science, 10*, 102. https://doi.org/10.1186/s13012-015-0287-0

Littleton-Kearney, M. (2018). Pragmatic clinical trials at the National Institute of Nursing Research. *Nursing Outlook, 66*, 470-472. https://doi.org/10.1016/j.outlook.2018.02.001

Martinez, R. G., Lewis, C. C., & Weiner B. J. (2014). Instrumentation issues in implementation science. *Implementation Science, 9*, 1-9. https://doi.org/10.1186/s13012-014-0118-8

Marx, D. (2001). *Patient Safety and the "Just Culture": A Primer for Health Care Executives.* New York, NY: Columbia University.

Morris, Z. S., Wooding, S., & Grant, J. (2011). The answer is 17 years, what is the question: Understanding time lags in translational research. *Journal of the Royal Society of Medicine, 104*(12), 510-520. https://doi.org/10.1258/jrsm.2011.110180

Norton, W. E., & Chambers, D. A. (2020). Unpacking the complexities of de-implementing inappropriate health interventions. *Implementation Science, 15*, 2. https://doi.org/10.1186/s13012-019-0960-9

Perla, R. J., Provost, L. P., & Parry, G. J. (2013). Seven propositions of the science of improvement: exploring foundations. *Quality Management in Healthcare, 22*(3), 170-186.

Pickler, R. H., & Kearney, M. H. (2018). Publishing pragmatic trials. *Nursing Outlook, 66*, 464-469.

Powell, B. J., Waltz, T. J., Chinman, M. J., Damschroder, L. J., Smith, J. L., Matthieu, M. M., Proctor, E. K., & Kirchner, J. E. (2015). A refined compilation of implementation strategies: Results from the Expert Recommendations for Implementing Change (ERIC) project. *Implementation Science, 10*, 21. https://doi.org/10.1186/s13012-015-0209-1

Powell, S., & Stone, R. (2015). *The patient survival handbook: Avoid being the next victim of medical error.* Book Logix Publishing Services.

Rundio, A., Wilson, V., & Meloy, F. A. (2016). *Nurse executive: Review and resource manual.* American Nurses Association.

Sampson, U. K. A., Chambers, D., Riley, W., Glass, R. I., Engelgau, M. M., & Mensah, G. A. (2016). Implementation research: The fourth movement of the unfinished translation research symphony. *Global Heart, 11*, 153-158.

Shojania, K. G., & Grimshaw, J. M. (2005). Evidence-based quality improvement: The state of the science. *Health Affairs, 24*(1), 138-150.

Society for Implementation Research Instrument Review Project. (2019). The SIRC instrument review project (IRP): A systematic review and synthesis of implementation science instruments. https://societyforimplementationresearchcollaboration.org/sirc-instrument-project/

Tinkle, M., Kimball, R., Haozous, E. A., Shuster, G., & Meize-Grochowski, R. (2013). Dissemination and implementation research funded by the US National Institutes of Health, 2005-2012. *Nursing Research and Practice, 2013*, 909606. https://doi.org/10.1155/2013/909606

Upvall, M. J., & Bourgault, A. M. (2018). De-implementation: A concept analysis. *Nursing Forum.* Advance online publication. https://doi.org/10.1111/nuf.12256

Waltz, T. P., Powell, B. J., & Matthieu, M. M., Damschroder, L. J., Chinman, M. J., Smith, J. L., Proctor, E. K., & Kirchner, J. E. (2015). Use of concept mapping to characterize relationships among implementation strategies and assess their feasibility and importance: Results from the Expert Recommendations for Implementing Change (ERIC) study. *Implementation Science, 10*, 109. https://doi.org/10.1186/s13012-015-0295-0

Zoellner, J. M., & Porter, K. J. (2017). Translational research: Concepts and methods in dissemination and implementation research. In A.M. Coulston, C. J. Boushey, M. G. Ferruzzi, & L. M. Delahanty (Eds.), *Nutrition in the prevention and treatment of disease* (4th ed., pp. 125-143) [Digital Edition version]. Elsevier.

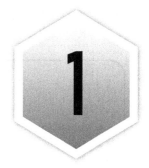

EVOLUTION OF
EVIDENCE-BASED PRACTICE
Implications for Implementation and Dissemination Sciences and Translational Nursing

Clista Clanton, MSLS
Patricia L. Thomas, PhD, RN, FAAN, FACHE, FNAP, NEA-BC, ACNS-BC, CNL
Linda A. Roussel, PhD, RN, NEA-BC, CNL, FAAN

CHAPTER OBJECTIVES

- Provide a brief overview of implementation and dissemination sciences including defining terms, phases, and the evolution of evidence-based practice
- Describe seminal documents in transforming health systems through translational sciences
- Identify challenges to sustained outcomes and why complex problems require systematic approaches to spreading evidence-based practice initiatives within the health care system
- Describe concepts of adoption, adaption, and integration in dissemination and implementation sciences and implications for translational nursing
- Outline characteristics that influence fidelity and its relationship to implementation and dissemination
- Describe deimplementation and its importance to translational nursing and effective health care outcomes

Roussel, L. A., & Thomas, P. L. (Eds.). *Implementation Science in Nursing:*
A Framework for Education and Practice (pp. 1-18).
© 2022 Taylor & Francis Group.

KEY WORDS

- Adaptation
- Adoption
- Deimplementation
- Evidence-based practice
- Fidelity
- Implementation and dissemination sciences
- Implementation and dissemination science research
- Integration
- Knowledge translation
- Population health
- Precision medicine
- Translational nursing

Nursing, as a practice profession, brings an action-oriented approach to care delivery that resides in both art and science. As such, continuous learning and continuous improvement are foundational drivers. The proximity of nurses to patients, families, and members of the health care team positions them to serve as the coordinator and action-oriented enactor. Yet, what can be overlooked is the role of science behind those actions. This chapter provides an overview of evidence-based practice (EBP), outlining the impact of translational sciences (TS) on nursing practice. Understanding the evolution of EBP gives context to the essential work that nurses have in improving patient care, population, and health systems outcomes.

TRANSFORMING HEALTH SYSTEMS: EVIDENCE-BASED PRACTICE UPTAKE

Landmark studies by the Institute of Medicine including *To Err Is Human: Building a Safer Health System* (1999), *Crossing the Quality Chasm: A New Health System for the 21st Century* (2001), and *Health Professions Education: A Bridge to Quality* (2003) created the platform to radically transform care delivery with the expectation that improvements are sustained. Across disciplines and settings, commitment and tremendous investments have been made to produce these changes, but the sustainability of improvements, replication, and outcomes have been elusive. TS offers hope for long-term gains backed by models, theories, frameworks, and evidence-based strategies that consider health systems thinking, organizational context, and leadership. This textbook provides educators, students, and practitioners a dynamic resource for using principles and concepts from this evolving field that can be integrated into interprofessional collaborative team projects, assignments, and discussions that improve the outcomes of population health and the delivery of services within health care systems. Although there are continued challenges with the clarity of concepts and terms in this growing field, the authors offer several definitions and concepts of TS that are integrated throughout the chapters. Table 1-1 provides definitions that are used throughout this textbook. Additionally, when using the various terms, the authors also define their specific meaning(s) as it relates to the content covered within the chapters. This chapter begins a historical perspective providing the backdrop for the ongoing development of EBP uptake focused on the many factors critical to true translation, application, spread, and sustainability.

Bauer et al. (2015) identified that, on average, it takes 17 years to incorporate evidence-based interventions into routine care while noting that half of the evidence never reaches widespread clinical application. From a historical perspective, this was not viewed as problematic based on the artificial and widely accepted divide between clinicians and researchers. Recently, biomedical research funders have become concerned about the lack of public health impacts of the research. With fewer

TABLE 1-1

Definitions

Implementation science	Scientific study of methods that facilitate the systematic uptake of research findings and other evidence-based practices into routine practices with the outcomes of improved quality and effectiveness of health care services and systems administration (Eccles & Mittman, 2006)
	"Scientific study of the use of strategies to adopt and integrate evidence-based health interventions into clinical and community settings in order to improve patient outcomes and benefit population health" (National Institutes of Health, 2016, para. 7)
	Examines the barriers and facilitators influencing the successful implementation of the best evidence into practice and described as the promotion of methods that facilitate adoption and integration of evidence-based practices, interventions, practices, and policies (Fogarty International Center, 2017)
	Reinforces innovative approaches to evidence-based interventions, tools, policies, protocols, and guidelines by understanding and overcoming barriers to the adoption, adaptation, integration, scale-up, and sustainability (National Institutes of Health, 2016)
	Study of methods to promote the integration of research findings and evidence into health care policy and practice; it seeks to understand the behavior of health care professionals and other stakeholders as a key variable in the sustainable uptake, adoption, and implementation of evidence-based interventions (Fogarty International Center, 2017)
	Study of "how and how well systems adopt existing evidence into practice" (Granger, 2018)
Implementation practice	Tailors and applies evidence for the types of implementation strategies (implementation research) in different context and settings to meet the needs of different communities and people and to achieve positive outcomes (Metz, 2019)
Knowledge translation	A related field of translational science with the focus of enhancing the utility of research and including the design and conduct of studies as well as the dissemination and implementation of findings (Graham et al., 2006)
	"Dynamic and iterative process that involves synthesis, dissemination, exchange and ethically-sound application of knowledge to improve the health of Canadians, provide more effective health services and products and strengthen the health care system" (Canadian Institutes of Health Research, 2018, 2019, para. 1)

(continued)

TABLE 1-1 (CONTINUED)

Definitions

Improvement science	Consists of a set of activities that aim to improve health care quality and safety facilitated by measurement, feedback to decision makers, and organizational change (Dixon-Woods, 2019)
	The goal of improvement science is to ensure that improvement efforts are based on supportive evidence and best practices planned for implementation (Shojania & Grimshaw, 2005)
	Study of which processes are best suited to achieve quality outcomes in complex health care systems (Granger, 2018)
Translational science	Form of scientific inquiry that provides health professionals with data that can inform and substantiate the approaches taken to facilitate knowledge transfer, document the processes and outcomes of the knowledge transfer, and ensure the ongoing use of the evidence-based practices that are introduced (Titler, 2018)
	Testing implementation interventions to foster uptake and use of evidence to improve patient outcomes and population health, and identify what implementation strategies work for whom, in what settings, and why (Titler, 2018)
Translational nursing	Incorporates translational science including implementation and dissemination sciences and practices in evidence-based practice uptake to improve patient care and health systems outcomes through professional nursing practice (Titler, 2018)
Dissemination science	Systematic examination of the ways that information about innovative interventions is transmitted to appropriate professional audiences or organizations for the purposes of fostering adoption in clinical or public health practice (Glasgow et al., 2012; Greenhalgh et al., 2004; Titler, 2018)
Dissemination practice	"Targeted distribution of information and intervention materials to a specific public health or clinical practice audience. The intent is to spread knowledge and the associated evidence-based intervention" (Glasgow et al., 2012, p. 1275)
Evidence-based practice	"Clinical decision making that considers the best available evidence; the context in which the care is delivered; client preference; and the professional judgment of the health professional" (Pearson et al., 2012, p. 2)
	"Evidence may include information from evidence-based theories, opinion leaders, and expert panels" (Melnyk & Fineout-Overholt, 2015, p. 4)
	"Application of evidence in practice (the 'doing of' EBP), whereas translational science is the study of implementation interventions, factors, and contextual variables that effect knowledge uptake and use in practices and communities" (Titler, 2018, p. 3)

(continued)

TABLE 1-1 (CONTINUED)
Definitions

Team science	Involves scientific collaboration (i.e., research carried out by more than one individual in an interdependent fashion, including research conducted by small teams and larger groups [Cooke et al., 2015]) Collaborative intention to address a scientific challenge that considers the strengths and expertise of professionals prepared in different fields (Cooke et al., 2015)
Quality improvement	Framework used to systematically improve the ways care is delivered to patients; involves processes that can be measured, analyzed, improved, and controlled; continuous efforts to achieve stable and predictable process results to reduce process variation and improve the outcomes of these processes, both for patients and the health care organization and system (Agency for Healthcare Research and Quality, 2021)
Implementation research	Addresses a persistent gap in how we spread evidence through an understanding of the behaviors of clinicians, support staff, organizations, policy makers, and consumers that influence the adoption, implementation, and sustainability of evidence-based practice guidelines and intervention (Bauer et al., 2015)
Dissemination research	"Scientific study of targeted distribution of information and intervention materials to a specific public health or clinical practice audience. The intent is to understand how best to spread and sustain knowledge and the associated evidence-based interventions" (National Institutes of Health, 2016, para. 5)
Deimplementation	Process of identifying and removing harmful, non–cost-effective, or ineffective practices based on tradition and often without adequate scientific support (Upvall & Bourgault, 2018)

dollars globally for research, debates over the trade-offs between investing in projects with predictable results vs. more innovative research involving real-world samples for public health impact have developed. A paradigmatic shift has ensued, with less focus on efficacy studies and an emergence of a range of generalizable effectiveness trials with overlapping names and conceptual structures. They include effectiveness trials, pragmatic clinical trials, practical clinical trials, and large simple trials (discussed in Chapter 3). While addressing generalizability, these trials do not ensure public health impact (Bauer et al., 2015).

Implementation science (IS) is defined as the "scientific study of the use of strategies to adopt and integrate evidence-based health interventions into clinical and community settings in order to improve patient outcomes and benefit population health" (National Institutes of Health [NIH], 2016, para. 7). Therefore, IS serves as a vehicle to address concerns centered on the sustainability of EBP interventions in general practice by providing support in the development of institutional memory, technology transfer, and factors that impede EBP uptake (e.g., competing demands on providers; misaligned research evidence in operational priorities; and limited knowledge, skill, and resources). Implementation research addresses a persistent gap in how we spread evidence through an understanding of the behaviors of clinicians, support staff, organizations, policy makers, and consumers that influence the adoption, implementation, and sustainability of EBP guidelines and intervention (Bauer et al., 2015).

Dissemination research "is the scientific study of targeted distribution of information and intervention materials to a specific public health or clinical practice audience. The intent is to understand how best to spread and sustain knowledge and the associated evidence-based interventions" (NIH, 2016, para. 5). In light of this, dissemination research is a prerequisite for how information needs to be packaged for health care organizations, administrators, clinicians, policy makers, and consumers so practice change occurs across constituencies (NIH, 2016, para. 6) and addresses how we provide information to those individuals and groups we expect to make and sustain change. Table 1-1 provides definitions that are used throughout this chapter and will help with the consistency of TS language.

Although it is important to bring best evidence consistently into current practice, it will also be necessary to integrate implementation and dissemination science into nursing education to adequately prepare future nurses. The American Association of Colleges of Nursing (AACN) recognized this need and embraced the challenge as evidenced in publications including the AACN's nursing essentials (2006, 2008, 2011), *Defining Scholarship for Academic Nursing* (2018), *Advancing Healthcare Transformation: A New Era for Academic Nursing* (2016), *AACN's Vision for Academic Nursing* (2019), and *The Doctor of Nursing Practice: Current Issues and Clarifying Recommendations* (2015). These will be discussed more fully in Chapters 2, 3, and 4. The focus of this chapter is to establish the historical perspective of EBP as the foundation of implementation and dissemination science as cornerstones for nursing education and practice. We identify challenges to sustained outcomes and why complex problems require systematic approaches to spreading EBP initiatives within the health care system. We also address the "know-do" gap in health care, with an emphasis on nursing education, implication for practice immersion experiences, and scholarly project development.

EVIDENCE-BASED PRACTICE AND THE PATH TO IMPLEMENTATION AND DISSEMINATION SCIENCE

It has been almost 35 years now that the tenets of evidence-based medicine (EBM) entered the vernacular of the health care environment (Eddy, 2011). The impassioned call by early EBM champions to train physicians to base their patient care decisions on a combination of clinical expertise, research evidence, and patient values and preferences (Sackett et al., 1996) led to far-reaching changes in not only how health care is practiced but also in how research is conducted, disseminated, and implemented. As nursing and allied health disciplines adopted those early EBM tenets and developed EBP models to suit their practice settings and roles on health care teams, waves of graduating health sciences students have entered ambulatory clinics and hospitals with at least a basic familiarity of the following terminology used in EBP: best evidence, well-built clinical questions (PICO [Population, Intervention, Comparison, Outcome], PICOT [Population, Intervention, Comparison, Outcome, Time], and PICOS [Population, Intervention, Comparison, Outcome, Study Type]), hierarchy/levels of evidence, practice guidelines, randomized controlled trials (RCTs), systematic reviews, and meta-analyses/meta-syntheses. Whether or not these earlier waves of health care professionals prepared with this new knowledge base were able to practice these concepts depended on multiple factors including if senior-level physicians, nurses, or administrators were supportive of them and/or implementing EBP themselves (Boström et al., 2009; Ramos et al., 2003); time factors (Guyatt et al., 2000); and if access was available to the research evidence and in formats useful in the clinical setting (Del Fiol et al., 2014; Sadeghi-Bazargani et al., 2014).

The development of accreditation standards for EBP/EBM across the health sciences educational spectrum was largely driven by the Institute of Medicine's goal that by 2020 most health care decisions would be based on accurate, timely, and current information informed by the best available evidence. McGinnis et al. (2009) posited that this should produce a growing base of health care providers who are prepared to put evidence into practice. The double-edged sword of externally driven requirements and standards by government agencies and insurers for reimbursement rates based on patient outcomes indicates that EBP in health care is not only well established but is also one of the drivers influencing the economic viability of our health care systems (Holmes et al., 2013; Padula et al., 2016).

However, both old and new challenges to the effective implementation of evidence to improve patient care remain, including a wide variation in the implementation of EBP and increased questioning of the quality of research evidence because drug and medical device industries have a growing influence over research agendas (Angell, 2008; Kung et al., 2012). Specific issues outlined by EBM leader Trisha Greenhalgh and colleagues (2014) include increasingly subtle biases in industry-sponsored studies, the unmanageable number of clinical guidelines, a shift from investigating and managing established disease to detecting and intervening in nondiseases, an overemphasis on following algorithmic rules to the detriment of individualized and patient-initiated aspects of clinical consultations, and the poor fit of studies that focused on specific conditions when applied to patients with particular comorbidities.

Although the challenges are real and can often seem like a many-headed Hydra monster, there is also a growing acknowledgment that complex problems require more thoughtful and systematic approaches than were perhaps initially envisioned in earlier attempts to spread EBP initiatives within health care organizations. IS examines the barriers and facilitators influencing the successful implementation of the best evidence into practice and is described as the promotion of methods that facilitate the adoption and integration of EBPs, interventions, practices, and policies (Fogarty International Center, 2017). The EBP process has largely been driven by academic clinical researchers and educators who have always relied on journal publications and meeting presentations to disseminate or spread the word on effective interventions, practices, and policies.

As defined by the NIH, dissemination is "the targeted distribution of information and intervention materials to a specific public health or clinical practice audience. The intent is to spread knowledge and the associated evidence-based intervention" (Glasgow et al., 2012, p. 1275). However, whether research findings translated into improving public health or changing practice has not always been the concern of traditional health care researchers (Bauer et al., 2015). More diverse and rigorous dissemination efforts are needed in order to increase the number of evidence-based interventions that are successfully and sustainably implemented in practice settings and subsequently lower the often-quoted 17-year gap of when research evidence makes an impact on clinical practice (Morris et al., 2011).

How research is being conducted is also under increasing scrutiny. One issue is decreased research funding coupled with decisions about which research to fund being based on issues relevant to the users of that research (Kleinert & Horton, 2014). Another is the growing awareness of waste or duplication in research efforts, resulting in an estimated 85% of research investment being wasted (Macleod et al., 2014). More innovative research approaches designed to potentially have a greater public health impact are resulting in the use of study designs with a focal point more on effectiveness as opposed to efficacy. Efficacy trials focus on the performance of an intervention under ideal and controlled circumstances, whereas effectiveness trials focus on the intervention's performance under "real-world" conditions. Although the distinction between the two types of studies functions on a continuum and any one study will likely contain aspects of both designs, efficacy studies may overestimate an intervention's effect when implemented in clinical practice settings. Effectiveness studies are designed to better account for the external system-level factors that may impact an intervention's effect, such as patient, provider, and practice setting variables (Singal et al., 2014).

Even when slicing into more focused segments of evidence-based implementation research, such as the uptake of nursing guidelines into clinical practice and the sustainability of guideline implementation, the need for the development of additional frameworks and the ability to apply the right framework during different phases of implementation are apparent. The gap in understanding what processes contribute to successful implementation is at least partially due to a reliance on research designs, such as RCTs and systematic reviews, that do not take into account the complexity of human social interaction or contextual aspects that impact uptake and practice change. Consequently, new frameworks are being developed that answer the call for more circular, inclusive, and process-oriented knowledge translation theories. One such framework looks at the role that individual factors play in practice guideline uptake, as well as offering specific leadership strategies to facilitate transformative change (Matthew-Maich et al., 2013). When moving beyond guideline uptake and then looking at sustainability in resulting practice changes, the need to address a multiplicity of factors demonstrated that a single intervention would be insufficient, and a multi-level sustainability action plan for staff, leaders, and the organization was needed instead (Higuchi et al., 2017).

Another factor contributing to the necessity for more successful implementation of EBP initiatives is the need for a comprehensive approach for improving the health of populations and the patient experience of health care, including both quality and safety, while also reducing costs of care (Berwick et al., 2008). In the decade since the Institute for Healthcare Improvement (IHI) introduced this Triple Aim framework, published studies indicated major differences on how Triple Aim dimensions have been defined and operationalized. A current systematic review suggested that the majority of studies in a primary care setting were unable to implement the Triple Aim and demonstrated a need for more consistent measurement tools and definitions (Obucina et al., 2018), whereas another study indicated that the framework is not a one size fits all, and that the United States health care system as a whole may not be suitable to pursuing the Triple Aim due to the lack of a dominant national integrator with the ability to focus and coordinate services to help the population on all three dimensions at once (Mery et al., 2017). After working with over 100 institutions in six phases of pilot testing, the IHI recommended a change process that includes "identification of target populations; definition of system aims and measures; development of a portfolio of project work that is sufficiently strong to move system-level results, and rapid testing and scale up that is adapted to local needs and conditions" (IHI, n.d.).

Although the United States spends almost 18% of its gross domestic product on health care expenditures ($3.3 trillion in 2016 dollars, with a projected $5.7 trillion per year by 2026), this has not translated into better health outcomes or health care because almost two thirds of U.S. adults suffer from largely preventable chronic diseases (Randall et al., 2019). Because of the combination of an aging population with the chronic disease burden, the need for earlier and better interventions that are less costly is glaringly apparent. Precision medicine is one suggested approach to address these issues. Instead of a population-based, top-down approach that uses pathology to define disease, precision medicine uses a bottom-up approach that identifies predisease states using genetics, biomarkers, and modeling to prevent the disease from developing and/or becoming irreversible.

> Western medicine (allopathic medicine) is based on the premise that *one predominant and strong agent* causes disease in people who are otherwise *normal*. Precision medicine is the alternative system based on the premise that *one or more weak agents* cause disease in a person because one or more of their specialized cells are *abnormal*. Thus, the approach, methods, analysis, and results are expected to be very different—but not mutually exclusive. (Whitcomb, 2019, p. e00067)

The two different models will also have different evidence bases. The randomized clinical trials, along with the systematic reviews and meta-analyses that synthesize the RCTs on a specific clinical question, will not suffice when evaluating the effectiveness of precision medicine interventions. Because each patient is different, new approaches will be needed, such as N-of-1 trial designs or "basket" studies (a group of small adaptive RCTs) focused on targeting the disease mechanism (Whitcomb, 2019). Emerging technologies, such as genomic testing and sequencing, digital health tracking, digital therapeutics, telemedicine, and cloud-based technologies, can help facilitate the transition to a more proactive care model like precision medicine, but the barriers to successful implementation are still significant. The development and standardization of precision health tools are needed to foster adoption by clinicians, along with validated assessment metrics that capture useful human data that can be integrated into medical systems. Specialized data platforms that facilitate data sharing among stakeholders are required to encourage collaboration and analyses, including increasing the interoperability of electronic health records and the ability for researchers to extract information from patient records. Research that explores the cost-effectiveness and benefits of precision medicine, along with an organization that can focus exclusively on precision medicine and help coordinate related initiatives in education, advocacy, research efforts, and patient input, are also priority areas (Randall et al., 2019).

The amount of U.S. federal funding dollars that is spent on research relevant to health quality, dissemination, and outcomes was about $270 million in 2010, which represents mere pennies compared to each dollar spent in new discoveries in basic biomedical and behavioral research. Researchers from the NIH went on record in 2012 stating the following:

> We believe that effectiveness research and dissemination and implementation research are much stronger in tandem than as separate areas of inquiry. Effectiveness research is stronger if it anticipates and includes issues related to dissemination and implementation processes such as adoption decisions and implementation questions within intervention testing, and dissemination or implementation research is stronger if it assesses continued effectiveness as interventions or prevention approaches spread to and are adopted by large, diverse populations. (Glasgow et al., 2012)

In 2019, the NIH R01 Research Project Grant funding opportunity announcement expanded on the increasing importance of research to support innovative approaches to implementation strategies for the adoption, adaptation, integration, scale-up, and sustainability of evidence-based interventions, as well as the importance of understanding circumstances in which interventions need to be stopped or reduced ("deimplementation").

As the call for improvements in implementation and dissemination sciences continues to grow, the need for nurse scientists and other health care providers, researchers, and educators trained in knowledge translation processes will be increasingly important. Understanding the role of outcomes in research and practice can provide a framework for building relevant dissemination and implementation outcomes.

DISSEMINATION AND IMPLEMENTATION OUTCOMES: IMPLICATIONS FOR EDUCATION, PRACTICE, AND CRITICAL DECISION MAKING

A number of national and international agencies are advancing the science of dissemination and implementation. Specifically, the NIH, the Agency for Healthcare Research and Quality, the National Cancer Institute, and the Centers for Disease Control and Prevention are agencies that support funding for TS moving from bench research to community spread of effective evidence-based strategies. From an international perspective, there are also organizations and agencies vested in dissemination and implementation research and outcomes including the U.K. Centre for Reviews and Dissemination, the U.K. Medical Research Council, and the Canadian Institutes of Health Research. According to Brownson et al. (2012), before researchers can test dissemination and implementation strategies for effectiveness, comparative effectiveness, and cost-effectiveness, these interventions must be identified and described in a way that fosters their control, manipulation, and measurement. The researchers further note that although there has been some work on the acute care side, this body of knowledge is underdeveloped in population- and community-based care. "A variety of tools are needed to capture health care access and quality, and no measurement issues are more pressing that those of dissemination and implementation science" (Brownson et al., 2012, p. 274).

Individual Provider, Organization, and Policy Impact

Through their research efforts, Brownson et al. (2012) provided a taxonomy of dissemination and implementation outcomes. These outcomes provide definitions, level of analysis, theoretical basis, other terms used in the literature, the stage of dissemination and implementation, and examples of methods of measurement. This beginning work assists the translational scientist and practitioner in developing a frame of reference in which to tailor strategies with outcomes for successful project management. A taxonomy offers a language that the interprofessional team can focus on when working on improvement plans outlining implementation and dissemination outcomes. Building consensus can be attained using a common language that also can maximize limited resources in decision making and strategic planning.

The following nine dissemination and implementation outcomes are identified by Brownson et al. (2012): acceptability, reach, adoption, appropriateness, feasibility, fidelity, cost, prevention, and sustainability. Knowing these outcomes can provide an excellent framework for designing implementation strategies grounded in research and development. For example, acceptability is defined as agreeable, palatable, or satisfactory to stakeholders and those involved in the process. Considering acceptability (what is acceptable), the researcher or practitioner focuses on a specific intervention, practice, technology, or service within a setting of care. The level of analysis is the individual with a theoretical basis stemming from diffusion theory and complexity for the relative advantage of dissemination and implementation of outcomes. The literature includes other terms that define acceptability, such as satisfaction with the innovation and system readiness. The dissemination and implementation acceptability outcome is best used for early adoption and ongoing penetration. Methods of measurement include surveys, key informant interviews, and administrative data.

Another example of a dissemination and implementation outcome is feasibility, which can occur at the individual, organization, and policy levels. Feasibility can be described as the extent to which a new program or policy can be successfully used or performed within an agency, in a setting, or in a certain population. Theoretical underpinnings of feasibility include diffusion theory, trialability, compatibility, and observability. Other terms that describe feasibility include actual fit or utility, suitability, practicability, and community readiness. Feasibility as a dissemination and implementation outcome needs to be introduced in the early adoption phase using surveys and administrative data as methods of measurement.

Adoption, penetration, and sustainability are three dissemination and implementation outcomes at the individual, organization, and policy levels. The theoretical basis for these outcomes comes from the RE-AIM (Reach, Effectiveness, Adoption, Implementation, Maintenance) theory, specifically necessary for reach and maintenance. Adoption can be described as the intention, initial decision, or action to undertake an EBP. Adoption also includes the engagement or disengagement with the innovation throughout the implementation. Terms for adoption in the literature include uptake, utilization, intention to try, use of the innovation, and knowledge transfer. The theoretical basis for adoption is diffusion theory, trialability, observability, and RE-AIM. Proctor et al. (2011) identified the RE-AIM framework and adoption and trialability from Rogers' diffusion of innovation theory. Diffusion of innovation is one of the oldest social science theories and was developed to explain how, over time, an idea or product gains momentum and diffuses (or spreads) through a specific population or social system.

Other terms in the literature for penetration include spread, access to services, and level of utilization. Sustainability terms include maintenance, continuation, durability, incorporation, integration, institutionalization, sustained use, and routinization. The phases of dissemination and implementation for adoption and penetration are early and mid to late in the process; sustainability occurs late in the dissemination and implementation phase. There are several methods recommended for the measurement of adoption, including surveys, observation, key informant interviews, focus groups, and administrative data. Methods of measurement for penetration and sustainability include surveys, case studies, and key informant interviews. Record and policy reviews are also useful methods of measurement for the sustainability of dissemination and implementation outcomes.

Considering the interrelationships among dissemination and implementation outcomes, Brownson et al. (2012) described the ways that this can be accomplished. This has implications for education, practice, and critical decision making. The authors described the Dingfelder and Mandell (2010) model that identified dissemination as a contributor to successful implementation outcomes, emphasizing the complex ways this occurs. Specifically, as noted by Brownson et al., (2012) "... the perceived appropriateness, feasibility, and implementation costs associated with an intervention will likely bear upon ratings of the intervention acceptability. Acceptability, in turn, will likely affect adoption, penetration, and sustainability" (p. 271). Using Rogers's diffusion of innovations (1995) as a theoretical underpinning, the ability to adopt or adapt an innovation for local use may increase its acceptability.

Using their taxonomy, Brownson et al. (2012) suggested that the team models the outcomes using interesting and useful formulas. An example is as follows:

Implementation success = f of effectiveness (= high) + awareness (= low)

The authors describe this example as "An evidence-based intervention may be highly effective, but it may be largely unknown to potential adopters; this poor dissemination outcome (low awareness) would likely undermine the likelihood of its implementation" (p. 272).

Following is another example that notes that the program (intervention) may be only mildly acceptable to key stakeholders because it is seen as too costly to sustain. The authors model this by the following formula:

Implementation success = f of effectiveness (= high) + acceptability
(= moderate) + cost (= high) + sustainability (low)

A final example notes that an intervention might be moderately effective but highly acceptable to stakeholders because current care is poor, the intervention is inexpensive, and current training protocols ensure high penetration through providers. The team models this as follows (p. 272):

Implementation success = f of intervention effectiveness (= moderate) + acceptability
(= high) + potential to improve care (feasibility) (= high) + penetration (= high)

Using the implementation outcomes as described previously (acceptability, feasibility, penetration, sustainability, etc.) and modeling with your team can provide valuable information as you "forecast" your project plan strategies and outcomes. There are many tools available when working on EBP, program evaluation, and improvement initiatives. As nurse educators and practitioners, we challenge our students and clinical partners to incorporate new tools and techniques in their team's work for enhancing engagement and developing a common language that improves communication and efficient team building. This can assist the team with tailoring evidence-based implementation strategies and outcomes that best "fit" with their organizational and health care delivery systems.

ADAPTATION

Adaptation is a key concept in IS. When we apply adaptation to implementation, we engage in a process of thoughtful and deliberate alteration to the design or delivery of an intervention. The goal of adaptation is improving the fit or effectiveness in any given context (Stirman et al., 2014, 2015). As a form of modification, for a broader concept of adaption, the focus is to integrate any changes made to the intervention whether it is deliberate and proactive or as a reaction to unanticipated changes or challenges that may emerge in the process (Barrera et al., 2017; Cooper et al., 2016). Because they are often not documented (process, nature, and outcomes of modification), adaptation and modifications have not been fully evaluated, although they are of keen interest in the field of IS (Sundell et al., 2016; von Thiele Schwarz et al., 2018).

To better understand adaptations and modifications, implementation scientists have developed frameworks. Specifically, Wiltsey Stirman et al. (2019) created the Framework for Reporting Adaptations and Modifications–Enhanced (FRAME), which includes eight aspects to consider. These aspects are aligned and consider (a) when and how in the implementation process the modification was made; (b) whether the modification was planned/proactive or unplanned/reactive; (c) who determined that the modification should be made; (d) what is modified; (e) at what level of delivery the modification is made; (f) the type or nature of context or content-level modifications; (g) the extent to which the modification is fidelity consistent; and (h) the reasons for the modification, including the intent or goal of the modification (e.g., improve fit, adapt to a different culture, reduce costs) and contextual factors that influenced the decision. The authors suggested that the updated FRAME tool be used to support research on the timing, nature, goals, and reasons for and impact of modifications to EBP interventions. The updated FRAME includes consideration of when and how modifications occurred, whether it was planned or unplanned, relationship to fidelity, and reasons and goals for modification.

Using tools, such as FRAME, gives educators and practitioners resources for their tool kit in successful implementation. For example, working with graduate nurses in developing improvement projects can be strengthened by using models that can be tested through the process. It is often in the adaptation of our implementation strategy that we immerse our interprofessional teams into the contextual features of the system. Specifically, doing a deep dive into the organization's culture, the dynamics of how the system makes changes, leadership's engagement, and strategic decision making offers valuable internal data that provide essential information in delineating implementation strategies. The organizational climate and culture provide the context to understanding the inner workings of the health care system. Specifically, the organizational climate and culture relate to the meanings people attach to interrelated bundles of experiences when working in the system. Leading system change involves understanding the action of leading a group of people or an organization and knowing the characteristics important for facilitating change processes in organizations. The IHI notes that when doing small tests of change to determine the success of outcomes, the team decides if the implementation strategies should be adopted, adapted, or abandoned. Adaptation and modifying the context in which the evidence is implemented can be challenging and an art and a science in project development and management. Educating students and practitioners of the nuances also takes qualitative and quantitative approaches to the processes. This can be challenging given the importance of maintaining fidelity in the implementation process.

Fidelity is described as the extent to which a program was delivered as intended. Adherence to a protocol is an example of fidelity. Using mixed methods provides a more comprehensive approach to addressing modifications that may be required to continue iterative cycles of small tests of change. Allen et al. (2012) described characteristics that influence fidelity including implementer characteristics; characteristics of the intervention, organization, or setting; and the population for whom the intervention is intended for use. Considering the implementer characteristics, the authors noted that a novice researcher or practitioner may be new to evidence-based intervention strategies and thus may have limited ability to anticipate, problem solve, or make decisions regarding implementation challenges. Therefore, fidelity may be compromised when the implementer's skills, knowledge, training, and confidence are insubstantial, resulting in a reduced amount, type, or quality of intervention delivered. Conversely, highly trained and educated implementers may be "too quick" to modify from the proposed plan because of their confidence in past successful project outcomes. There can be much variation here.

The characteristics of the intervention can also influence fidelity, particularly when considering complexity, trialability, and the overall advantage of implementing a new strategy over a current practice. The authors noted that interventions that allow for greater flexibility and are amenable to adaptation may be less cumbersome (less complex) for practitioners to implement without eliminating or changing the core components of the intervention. Interventions that are clearly stated and well described for replication are also considered more likely to be implemented with fidelity because of the detail and possibly the resources provided.

The context (i.e., the organization or setting) also has an impact on fidelity. "Organization resources, including availability of trained staff, financial capital, and existence of a program 'champion' exert a strong impact on the way programs can be implemented" (Allen et al., 2012, p. 286). Furthermore, organizational dynamics, such as the structure, communication channels, and decision-making processes, that can be made on the front line can also facilitate readiness for change and fidelity.

The end user (population) of the implementation strategy also influences fidelity. The consideration of demographics (age, sex, socioeconomic status, and education levels), sociocultural norms, and literacy levels influence "participant responsiveness" to the intervention and are critical population factors aligned with the appropriateness and feasibility of implementing core elements. It is important to consider cultural and ethical/moral issues that influence health equity and justice when analyzing the population characteristics (Allen et al., 2012).

DEIMPLEMENTATION: IMPLICATIONS FOR TRANSLATIONAL NURSING

Deimplementation has been described as the process of identifying and removing harmful, non–cost-effective, or ineffective practices based on tradition and often without adequate scientific support (Upvall & Bourgault, 2018). It is a significant concept for ongoing theory development in IS and clinical practice. Deimplementing inappropriate health interventions is essential for improving population health, maintaining public trust, minimizing patient harm, and reducing unnecessary waste in health care and public health (Norton & Chambers, 2020). There is ongoing discussion of deimplementation of ineffective, contradicted, mixed, and untested health interventions. These interventions may also be referred to as "inappropriate" and are increasingly prominent in the published literature (Norton & Chambers, 2020).

Norton and Chambers (2020) cited a scoping review that identified 43 different terms for deadoption, such as deprescribe, decrease use, reassess, withdraw, and abandon, with the most frequently cited being disinvest. Niven et al. (2015) described a substantial body of literature that identified current approaches and challenges to de-adoption of low-value clinical practices. The researchers noted that there is a greater need to determine an optimal strategy for delineating low-value practices and facilitating and sustaining deadoption. The researchers also proposed that a model be used by providers and decision makers to facilitate efforts to deadopt ineffective and harmful practices (Niven et al., 2015).

In their systematic review, Colla et al. (2017) reported that multicomponent interventions integrating both patient and clinician roles in overuse have the most significant potential to reduce low-value care. Strategies with a sound evidence base and that appear useful include clinical decision support and performance feedback. Provider education by itself supports changes and when coupled with promising strategies has a greater impact. More research is required on other variables including the effectiveness of pay for performance, insurer restrictions, and risk-sharing contracts to reduce the use of low-value care. The researcher concluded that more research is needed to reduce the gaps, and greater experimentation coupled with rigorous evaluation and publication is essential to further develop the body of knowledge.

Morgan et al. (2017) described a framework for conceptualizing, understanding, and guiding deimplementation. The authors incorporated drivers of overuse into domains and related them to the patient–clinician interaction. The Choosing Wisely campaign served to inform how a framework could be useful in deimplementation work (Horvath et al. 2016; Perry Undum Research/Communication, 2014). The framework for understanding and reducing use included several domains, such as the culture of health care consumption, patient factors and experiences, the practice environment, the culture of professional medicine, and clinicians' attitudes and beliefs. For each domain, the authors outlined a number of concepts to consider, such as factors (values, demographics, influence, and past experiences), the level of evidence supporting the concepts (weak to moderate, strong, or absent to moderate), the specific impact (variable and continuity of care), and the likely magnitude of the effect on overuse (moderate, moderate to high, or high). According to the authors, the framework illustrates drivers of overuse, which can enhance the understanding of overuse and assist with contextualizing change, prioritizing research goals, and advancing specific interventions.

From the policy makers' perspective, the framework can inform efforts to reduce overuse by underscoring the need for complex interventions and by being clear about the influence of interventions targeting specific domains. Quality improvement professionals and practitioners can apply the framework when doing root cause analyses of overuse-related problems and consider the allocation of limited resources. Furthermore, weak evidence informing the role of the most recognized drivers of overuse can advance an important research agenda (i.e., pressing needs can be delineated such as relevant physician and patient cultural factors, exploring interventions that influence culture, identifying features of the practice environment that maximize care appropriateness, and aligning specific practices during the patient–clinician interaction that minimize overuse while continuing to provide needed care; Morgan et al., 2017).

Norton and Chambers (2020) illuminated opportunities for ongoing ways to advance research on the deimplementation of inappropriate interventions in health care and public health. In their article, they described unique aspects of deimplementing inappropriate interventions that demonstrate the differences from implementing evidence-based interventions, including multilevel factors, types of action, strategies for deimplementation, outcomes, and unintended negative consequences. In describing multilevel factors, the authors specifically addressed health intervention characteristics, patient characteristics, health professional characteristics, and organizational characteristics. The authors also delineated types of action and tailored strategies for deimplementation.

Relating health intervention characteristics, Norton and Chambers (2020) described features first delineated by Rogers (2010), which include relative advantage, compatibility, complexity, triability, and observability, as well as costs, adaptability, form, risks, and interdependence. There is still work to be done regarding which intervention characteristics affected deimplementation with the same magnitude and in the same direction. Strength of evidence and level of complexity are two characteristics of an inappropriate intervention that are tailored to deimplementation. Patient characteristics include attitudes, behavioral skills, social norms, and demographic characteristics. Characteristics of health professionals that affect deimplementation again overlap with some of those for implementation, such as behavioral skills, self-efficacy, and knowledge. Health professionals' characteristics may include experience of negative events, cognitive dissonance, and fear of medical malpractice. Organizational characteristics that influence deimplementation include organizational culture and climate, leadership, resources, and structure.

Deimplementation may also include removing, replacing, reducing, or restricting the delivery of an inappropriate intervention. Specifically, removing an intervention is the process of eliminating the delivery of an inappropriate intervention, which can include removal of a drug from the market or recall of a device. When replacing an intervention, this includes not only eliminating the inappropriate intervention but also starting a new, evidence-based intervention that focuses on the same or similar proximal or distal patient-level health behaviors or health outcomes. For example, when the provider is replacing an intervention, this involves changing the opioid prescriptions as first-line therapy for the treatment of acute lower back pain with a stepwise approach, beginning with physical therapy. When reducing interventions, the provider changes the frequency and/or intensity with which that intervention is administered. This may include reducing the frequency with which screening tests are delivered (every 3 months vs. every month), reducing the intensity of medication dosage (250 mg to 50 mg), or a combination of both.

Lastly, when restricting an intervention, this means that the scope of an intervention is narrowly focused by the target population, health professional, and/or delivery setting. For example, restricting may include initiating a change from universal to high-risk screening for patients or restricting treatment provided in both general and specialty clinics to only specialty clinics.

Norton and Chambers (2020) described a data-driven approach that allows for testing theory-based hypotheses, identifying longitudinal moderators, single and multilevel mediators, and mechanisms of deimplementation and assessing how the relationship between barriers and strategies changes over time. Rapid, state-of-the-art qualitative methods would complement these quantitative data and provide a more in-depth understanding of context and process. Deimplementation is an essential concept to consider from the dissemination and implementation outcomes perspectives.

CONCLUSION

This chapter provided a historical perspective of TS, the evolution of EBP, and implications for implementation and dissemination sciences and translational nursing. Considering deimplementation in overall IS was also addressed. Understanding how far we have come and exploring future needs are important to strengthening the field and providing practical tools, strategies, and techniques for effective, sustainable implementation and dissemination.

REFLECTIVE QUESTIONS

1. Using the Brownson et al. (2012) taxonomy of dissemination and implementation outcomes, select two outcomes and describe how you will apply specific methods of measurement to a project you are currently working on. Describe the level of analysis and theoretical basis for your dissemination and implementation outcomes and the methods of measurement you would use.

2. Understanding fidelity is critical to implementation and dissemination, using the four characteristics described by Allen et al. (2012), recall a recent project and describe how considering each of these characteristics would strengthen your project plan.

3. Identify a nursing intervention that should be deimplemented. Describe how a framework would be useful in the deimplementation process.

REFERENCES

Agency for Healthcare Research and Quality. (2021). Module 4: Approaches to quality improvement. https://https://www.ahrq.gov/ncepcr/tools/pf-handbook/mod4.html

Allen, J. D., Linnan, L. A., & Emmons, K. M. (2012). Fidelity and its relationship to implementation effectiveness, adaptation, and dissemination. In R. C. Brownson, G. A. Colditz, & E. K. Proctor (Eds.), *Dissemination and implementation research in health, Translating science to practice* (pp. 281-304). Oxford University Press.

American Association of Colleges of Nursing. (2006). *The essentials of doctoral education for advanced nursing practice.* https://www.aacnnursing.org/Portals/42/Publications/DNPEssentials.pdf

American Association of Colleges of Nursing. (2008). *The essentials of baccalaureate education for professional nursing practice.* http://www.aacnnursing.org/Portals/42/Publications/BaccEssentials08.pdf

American Association of Colleges of Nursing. (2011). *The essentials of master's education in nursing.* https://www.aacnnursing.org/Portals/42/Publications/MastersEssentials11.pdf

American Association of Colleges of Nursing. (2015). *The doctor of nursing practice: Current issues and clarifying recommendations.* https://www.pncb.org/sites/default/files/2017-02/AACN_DNP_Recommendations.pdf

American Association of Colleges of Nursing. (2016). *Advancing healthcare transformation: A new era for academic nursing.* http://www.aacnnursing.org/Portals/42/AACN-New-Era-Report.pdf?ver=201707-06-120430557

American Association of Colleges of Nursing. (2018). Defining scholarship for academic nursing. https://www.aacnnursing.org/News-Information/Position-Statements-White-Papers/Defining-Scholarship-Nursing

American Association of Colleges of Nursing. (2019). AACN's vision for academic nursing. https://www.aacnnursing.org/Portals/42/News/White-Papers/Vision-Academic-Nursing.pdf

Angell, M. (2008). Industry-sponsored clinical research: A broken system. *JAMA. 300*(9), 1069-1071. https://doi.org/10.1001/jama.300.9.1069

Barrera, M., Berkel, C., & Castro, F. G. (2017). Directions for the advancement of culturally adapted preventive interventions: Local adaptations, engagement, and sustainability. *Prevention Science, 18*(6), 640-648.

Bauer, M., Damschroder, L., Hagedorn, H., Smith, J., & Kilbourne, A. (2015). An introduction to implementation science for the non-specialist. *BMC Psychology, 3,* 32. https://doi.org/10.1186/s40359-015-0089-9

Berwick, D. M., Nolan, T. W., & Whittington, J. (2008). The triple aim: Care, health, and cost. *Health Affairs, 27*(3). https://doi.org/10.1377/hlthaff.27.3.759

Boström, A. M., Ehrenberg, A., Gustavsson, J. P., & Wallin, L. (2009). Registered nurses' application of evidence-based practice: A national survey. *Journal of Evaluation in Clinical Practice, 15*(6), 1159-1163. https://doi.org/10.1111/j.1365-2753.2009.01316.x

Brownson, R. C., Colditz, G. A., & Proctor, E. K. (2012). *Dissemination and implementation research in health: Translating science to practice.* Oxford University Press.

Canadian Institutes of Health Research. (2018). About us- CIHR. http://www.cihr-irsc.gc.ca/e/37792.html

Canadian Institutes of Health Research. (2019). Knowledge translation. http://www.cihr-irsc.gc.ca/e/29529.html

Colla, C. H., Mainor, A. J., Hargreaves, C., Sequist, T., & Morden, N. (2017). Interventions aimed at reducing use of low-value health services: A systematic review. *Medical Care Research and Review: MCRR, 74*(5), 507-550. https://doi.org/10.1177/1077558716656970

Cooke, N. J., Hilton, M. L., Committee on the Science of Team Science, Board on Behavioral, Cognitive, and Sensory Sciences, Division of Behavioral and Social Sciences and Education, National Research Council. (2015). *Enhancing the effectiveness of team science.* National Academies Press.

Cooper, B. R., Shrestha, G., Hyman, L., & Hill, L. (2016). Adaptations in a community-based family intervention: Replication of two coding schemes. *Journal of Primary Prevention, 37*(1), 33-52.

Del Fiol, G., Workman, T. E., & Gorman, P. N. (2014). Clinical questions raised by clinicians at the point of care a systematic review. *JAMA Internal Medicine, 174*(5), 710-718. https://doi.org/10.1001/jamainternmed.2014.368

Dingfelder, H.E., & Mandell, D.S. (2010). Bridging the research-to-practice gap in autism intervention: An application of diffusion of innovation theory. *J Autism Dev Disord, 41,* 597–609. https://doi.org/10.1007/s10803-010-1081-0

Dixon-Woods, M. (2019). How to improve healthcare improvement-an essay by Mary Dixon-Woods. *BMJ, 367,* l5514. https://doi.org/10.1136/bmj.l5514

Eccles, M. P., & Mittman, B. S. (2006). Welcome to *Implementation Science* [Editorial]. *Implementation Science, 1,* 1-3. https://doi.org/10.1186/1748-5908-1-1

Eddy, D. M. (2011). The origins of evidence-based medicine: A personal perspective. *Virtual Mentor, 13*(1), 55-60. https://doi.org/10.1001/virtualmentor.2011.13.1.mhst1-1101

Fogarty International Center. (2017, July 27). Implementation science news, resources and funding for global health researchers. July 27, 2017. Retrieved October 19, 2017, from https://www.fic.nih.gov/researchtopics/pages/implementationscience.aspx

Glasgow, R. E., Vinson C., Chambers, D., Khoury, M. J., Kaplan, R. M., & Hunter, C. (2012). National Institutes of Health approaches to dissemination and implementation science: current and future directions. *American Journal of Public Health, 102*(7), 1274-1281. https://doi.org/10.2105/AJPH.2012.300755.

Graham, I. D., Logan, J., Harrison, M. B., Straus, S. E., Tetroe, J., Caswell, W., & Robinson, N. (2006). Lost in knowledge translation: Time for a map? *The Journal of Continuing Education in the Health Professions, 26*(1), 13-24. https://doi.org/10.1002/chp.47

Granger, B. B. (2018). Science of improvement versus science of implementation: Integrating both into clinical inquiry. *AACN Advanced Critical Care, 29*(2), 208-212. https://doi.org/10.4037/aacnacc2018757.

Greenhalgh, T., Howick, J., & Maskrey, N. (2014). Evidence based medicine: A movement in crisis? *BMJ, 348,* g3725. https://doi.org/10.1136/bmj.g3725

Greenhalgh, T., Robert, G., Macfarlane, F., Bate, P., & Kyriakidou, O. (2004). Diffusion of innovations in service organizations: A systematic review and recommendations. *The Milbank Quarterly, 82,* 581-629. https://doi.org/10.1111/j.0887-378X.2004.00325.x

Guyatt, G. H., Haynes, R. B., Jaeschke, R. Z., et al. (2000). Users' Guides to the Medical Literature: XXV. Evidence-based medicine: principles for applying the Users' Guides to patient care. Evidence-Based Medicine Working Group. *JAMA, 284*(10), 1290-1296. https://doi.org/10.1001/jama.284.10.1290

Higuchi, K. S., Davies, B., & Ploeg, J. (2017). Sustaining guideline implementation: A multisite perspective on activities, challenges and supports. *Journal of Clinical Nursing, 26*(23-24), 4413-4424. https://doi.org/10.1111/jocn.13770

Holmes, R., Moschetti, W., Martin, B., Tomek, I., & Finlayson, S. (2013). Effect of evidence and changes in reimbursement on the rate of arthroscopy for osteoarthritis. *American Journal of Sports Medicine, 41*(5), 1039-1043. https://doi.org/10.1177/0363546513479771

Horvath, K., Semlitsch, T., Jeitler, K., Paier-Abuzahra, M., Posch, N., Domke, A.& Siebenhofer, A. (2016). Choosing wisely: Assessment of current US top five list recommendations' trustworthiness using a pragmatic approach. *BMJ Open, 6.* https://doi.org/10.1136/bmjopen-2016-012366

Institute of Medicine. (2001). *Crossing the quality chasm: A new health system for the 21st century.* National Academy Press.

Institute of Medicine. (2003). *Health professions education: A bridge to quality.* The National Academies Press. https://doi.org/10.17226/10681

Institute of Medicine. (1999). *To err is human: Building a safer health system.* National Academy Press.

Institute for Healthcare Improvement. (n.d). IHI Triple Aim Initiative. The IHI Triple Aim. http://www.ihi.org/engage/initiatives/TripleAim/Pages/default.aspx

Kleinert, S., & Horton, R. (2014). How should medical science change? *The Lancet, 383*(9913), 197-198. https://doi.org/10.1016/S0140-6736(13)62678-1

Kung, J., Miller, R. R., & Mackowiak, P. A. (2012). Failure of clinical practice guidelines to meet Institute of Medicine Standards: Two more decades of little, if any, progress. *Archives of Internal Medicine, 172*(21), 1628-1633. https://doi.org/10.1001/2013.jamainternmed.56

Macleod, M., Michie, S., Roberts, I., Dirnagl, U., Chalmers, I., Ioannidis, J., Al-Shahi Salman, R., Chan, A., Glasziou, P. (2014). Biomedical research: increasing value, reducing waste. *The Lancet, 383*(9912), 101-104. https://doi.org/10.1016/S0140-6736(13)62329-6

Matthew-Maich, N., Ploeg, J., Dobbins, M., & Jack, S. (2013). Supporting the uptake of nursing guidelines: What you really need to know to move nursing guidelines into practice. *Worldviews on Evidence Based Nursing, 10*(2), 104-115. https://doi.org/10.1111/j.1741-6787.2012.00259.x

McGinnis, J. M., Goolsby, W. A., & Olsen, L. (2009). *Leadership commitments to improve value in health care: Finding common ground: Workshop summary.* National Academies Press.

Melnyk, B. M., & Fineout-Overholt, E. (2015). *Evidence-based practice in nursing & healthcare: A guide to best practice* (3rd ed.). Wolters Kluwer.

Mery, G., Majumder, S., Brown, A., & Dobrow, M. J. (2017). What do we mean when we talk about the Triple Aim? A systematic review of evolving definitions and adaptations of the framework at the health system level. *Health Policy, 121*(6), 629-636. https://doi.org/10.1016/j.healthpol.2017.03.014

Metz, A. (2019). Implementation practice. National Implementation Research Network. University of North Carolina. https://nirn.fpg.unc.edu/practicing-implementation/implementation-practice

Morgan, D. J., Leppin, A., Smith, C. D., & Korenstein, D. (2017). A practical framework for understanding and reducing medical overuse. *Journal of Hospital Medicine, 12*(5), 346-351. https://doi.org/10.12788/jhm.2738

Morris, Z. S., Wooding, S., Grant, J. (2011). The answer is 17 years, what is the question: Understanding time lags in translational research. *Journal of the Royal Society of Medicine, 104*(12), 510-520. https://doi.org/10.1258/jrsm.2011.110180

National Institutes of Health. (2016). Program announcement for Dissemination and Implementation Research in Health. National Institutes of Health website. Published May 10, 2016. https://grants.nih.gov/grants/guide/pa-files/PAR-16-238.html

Niven, D. J., Mrklas, K. J., Holodinsky, J. K., Straus, S. E., Hemmelgarn, B. R., Jeffs, L. P., & Stelfox, H. T. (2015). Towards understanding the de-adoption of low-value clinical practices: A scoping review. *BMC Medicine, 13*, 255. https://doi.org/10.1186/s12916-015-0488-z

Norton, W. E., Chambers, D. A. (2020). Unpacking the complexities of de-implementing inappropriate health interventions. *Implementation Science, 15*, 2. https://doi.org/10.1186/s13012-019-0960-9

Obucina, M., Harris, N., Fitzgerald, J. A., Chai, A., Radford, K., Ross, A., Carr, L., & Vecchio, N. (2018). The application of triple aim framework in the context of primary healthcare: A systematic literature review. *Health Policy, 122*, 900-907.

Padula, W. V., Gibbons, R. D., Valuck, R. J., Makic, M. B. F., Mishra, M. K., Pronovost, P. J., & Meltzer, D. O. (2016). Are evidence-based practices associated with effective prevention of hospital-acquired pressure ulcers in US academic medical centers? *Medical Care, 54*(5), 512-518. https://doi.org/10.1097/MLR.0000000000000516

Pearson, A., Jordan, Z., & Munn, Z. (2012). Translational science and evidence-based healthcare: A clarification and reconceptualization of how knowledge is generated and used in healthcare. *Nursing Research and Practice, 2012*, 1-6. https://doi.org/10.1155/2012/792519

Perry Undum Research/Communication. (2014). Unnecessary tests and procedures in the health care system: The ABIM Foundation. https://www.choosingwisely.org/wp-content/uploads/2015/04/Final-Choosing-Wisely-Survey-Report.pdf

Proctor, E., Silmere, H., Raghavan, R., Hovmand, P., Aarons, G., Bunger, R., Griffey, R., & Hensley, M. (2011). Outcomes for implementation research: Conceptual distinctions, measurement challenges, and research agenda. *Administration and Policy in Mental Health, 38*, 65-76. https://doi.org/10.1007/s10488-010-0319-7

Ramos, K., Linscheid, R., & Schafer, S. (2003). Real-time information-seeking behavior of residency physicians. *Family Medicine, 35*(4), 257-260.

Randall, J. A., Altimus, C. M., Hsiao, Y. L., & Briggs, L. (2019). Next generation prevention—A giving smarter guide. Milken Institute. Accessed August 24, 2019. https://www.milkeninstitute.org/reports/next-generation-prevention-giving-smarter-guide

Rogers, E. M. (1995). *Diffusion of innovations* (4th ed). Free Press.

Rogers, E.M. (2010). *Diffusion of Innovations*. Simon and Schuster.

Sackett, D. I., Rosenberg, W. M., Gray, J. A., Haynes, R. B., & Richardson, W. S. (1996). Evidence based medicine: What it is and what it isn't. *British Medical Journal, 312*(7023), 71-72. https://doi.org/10.1136/bmj.312.7023.71

Sadeghi-Bazargani, H., Tabrizi, J. S., & Azami-Aghdash, A. (2014). Barriers to evidence-based medicine: A systematic review. *Journal of Evaluation Clinical Practice, 20*(6), 793-802. https://doi.org/10.1111/jep.12222

Shojania, K. G., & Grimshaw, J. M. (2005). Evidence-based quality improvement: The state of the science. *Health Affairs, 24*(1), 138-150.

Singal, A., Higgins, P., & Waljee, A. (2014). A primer on effectiveness and efficacy trials. *Clinical Translational Gastroenterologist, 5*(1), e45.

Stirman, S. W., Gamarra, J. M., Bartlett, B. A., Calloway, A., & Gutner, C. A. (2014). Empirical examinations of modifications and adaptations to evidence-based psychotherapies: Methodologies, impact, and future directions. *Clinical Psychology, 24*(4), 396-420.

Stirman, S.W., Gutner, C., Edmunds, J., Evans, A. C., & Beidas, R. (2015). Relationships between clinician-level attributes and fidelity-consistent and fidelity-inconsistent modifications to an evidence-based psychotherapy. *Implementation Science, 10*(1), 115.

Sundell, K., Beelmann, A., Hasson, H., & von Thiele Schwarz, U. (2016). Novel programs, international adoptions, or contextual adaptations? Meta-analytical results from German and Swedish intervention research. *Journal of Clinical Child Adolescent Psychology, 45*(6), 784-796.

Titler, M. G. (2018). Translation research in practice: An introduction. *Online Journal of Issues in Nursing, 23*, 1-15.

Upvall, M. J., & Bourgault, A. M. (2018). De-implementation: A concept analysis. *Nursing Forum, 53*(3), 376-382. https://doi.org/10.1111/nuf.12256.

von Thiele Schwarz, U., Förberg, U., Sundell, K., & Hasson, H. (2018). Colliding ideals–An interview study of how intervention researchers address adherence and adaptations in replication studies. *BMC Medical Research Methodology, 18*(1), 36.

Whitcomb, D. (2019). Primer on precision medicine for complex chronic disorders. *Clinical Translational Gastroenterologist, 10*(7), e00067. https://doi.org/10.14309/ctg.0000000000000067

Wiltsey Stirman, S., Baumann, A. A., & Miller, C. J. (2019). The FRAME: An expanded framework for reporting adaptations and modifications to evidence-based interventions. *Implementation Science, 4*, 58. https://doi.org/10.1186/s13012-019-0898-y

HISTORY, CONTEXT, AND APPLICATION OF IMPLEMENTATION, DECISION SCIENCES, AND EVIDENCE-BASED PRACTICE UPTAKE

Cynthia Peltier Coviak, PhD, RN, FNAP

CHAPTER OBJECTIVES

- Provide a historical perspective of translational science
- Distinguish dissemination, implementation, and translation research and their implications for nursing practice
- Describe evidence-based practice, implementation science, and dissemination science and their application to nursing practice
- Outline testing methods for implementation and dissemination strategies
- Identify tools for planning dissemination and implementation research

KEY WORDS

- Carper's way of knowing
- Dissemination science
- Effectiveness trials
- Efficacy trials
- Evidence-based practice
- Fidelity
- Implementation and dissemination strategies
- Implementation science
- Pragmatic clinical trial
- Translational science

Roussel, L. A., & Thomas, P. L. (Eds.). *Implementation Science in Nursing: A Framework for Education and Practice* (pp. 19-37).
© 2022 Taylor & Francis Group.

Implementation science (IS) and dissemination science (DS), subcategories of translational science (TS), have developed in the last 2 decades as a response to concerns that the advances in health care research were not evident in practice. This chapter provides a historical overview of the origins of DS and IS in nursing. Traditional methods for developing and testing nursing interventions are described, and tools for planning dissemination research are provided.

Historical Perspective

As a discipline and a profession, nursing's concern with using the findings of research to improve care can be traced to Nightingale (1859/1992; Titler et al., 2001) but more formally to scholarly work completed in the 1970s (Beyea & Slattery, 2013). During that decade, major endeavors, such as the Conduct and Utilization of Research in Nursing Project (Haller et al., 1979) and Nursing Child Assessment Satellite Training (Barnard & Eyres, 1979), were undertaken to advance nursing's capacity to effect change in care processes. These projects coincided with a period when physicians were challenged by Dr. Archie Cochrane, in his 1972 monograph *Effectiveness and Efficiency: Random Reflections on Health Services*, to base their medical practices on findings from randomized controlled trials. He initiated a call for evidence-based medicine, which he advocated as a means of reducing morbidity (Shah & Chung, 2009). As major contributors to the health care system, nurses recognized the applicability of Dr. Cochrane's criticisms for their practice as well. How much Cochrane's writings influenced Carper (1978) in her essay on "Fundamental Patterns of Knowing in Nursing" is not known, but she considered empirics as the source of one "pattern of knowing" for informing nursing actions. This prompted efforts to increase practicing nurses' valuing of research-based evidence, including the creation of models and pilot projects to encourage their use of research on a wider scale (Funk et al., 1989a, 1989b).

Almost 3 decades after Cochrane's monograph and the earliest nursing efforts, the landmark Institute of Medicine (IOM) report *To Err Is Human: Building a Safer Health System* (2000) emphasized concerns that patient safety was endangered when research findings were not applied. Further tension was produced by the acknowledgment that the rewards of public and private investments in health care were often not apparent in practice environments (Cabana et al., 1999; Farquhar et al., 2002; Sung et al., 2003). Various nurse leaders developed strategies to address these disquieting circumstances (Fineout-Overholt et al., 2004; Melnyk et al., 2004; Rosswurm & Larrabee, 1999; Stetler, 2001; Titler et al., 1994). Evidence-based practice (EBP) for nursing, as well as for other health professions, was becoming a professional mandate and a standard expectation for nurses' performance as care providers.

Apprehensions about the mismatches between what was discovered through disciplinary science and what was observed in professional practice also created momentum for major shifts in funding priorities of federal and private sponsoring bodies. Although discovery and experimental trials remained a central emphasis for the scientific agencies of the U.S. Department of Health and Human Services, by the late 1990s and early 2000s, significant alterations in policies resulted in grant programs from the Department of Health and Human Services' Agency for Healthcare Research and Quality that were focused on research translation. The Translating Research into Practice Awards funded 27 investigations in 1999 and 2000 that studied these phenomena (Farquhar et al., 2002). At the National Institutes of Health (NIH), a "roadmap" was envisioned and put into place in 2004 that addressed the need to move research to practice more rapidly (NIH Office of Strategic Coordination–The Common Fund, 2014; Zerhouni, 2003). Similar modifications in research priorities were simultaneously occurring in Canada, the United Kingdom, Australia, and other countries around the world (Canadian Institutes of Health Research, 2018; Greenhalgh et al., 2004). From this convergence of forces, the field of TS arose.

With the emergence of this new field, a new language and conceptualizations of scientific activities also developed. *Translation* and *research translation* were already common terms among health care scientists because of the previous efforts to use research findings to promote EBP (Rubio et al., 2010). The terms signified a process or activities carried out in phases that would make research findings clinically useful. In 2006, when the NIH started the Clinical and Translational Science Awards (CTSAs) to further its roadmap initiatives and the open access journal *Implementation Science* was launched (Eccles & Mittman, 2006), widespread discussions of phases of the translation research progression began. A spectrum of activities ranging from laboratory or "bench" experiments and systematic application of therapies or interventions to the community or public health domains were initially categorized to phases labeled *T1, T2,* or *T3,* denoting Translation Level 1, 2, or 3 (Drolet & Lorenzi, 2011; Glasgow, Vinson et al., 2012; Rubio et al., 2010).

In the original taxonomies of translation levels, the first phase, T1 research, was basic or laboratory research in which discoveries related to physiologic and pathophysiologic mechanisms occur (Drolet & Lorenzi, 2011; Glasgow, Vinson et al., 2012; Rubio et al., 2010). T2 was considered to be "patient oriented," encompassing epidemiology, health services research, and community-based participatory research (Rubio et al., 2010, p. 5), but when applied to populations was also proposed to be focused on initial trials or the first level of application of basic research findings to humans (Glasgow, Vinson et al., 2012). Arising from the disagreements in definitions of T2 research, classifications T3 and, eventually, a fourth level, T4, were applied to further distinguish a set of highly variable research activities. In 2013, a new IOM report, *The CTSA Program at NIH: Opportunities for Advancing Clinical and Translational Research,* adapted a framework proposed by Blumberg et al. (2012) that is now recognizable in the 2015 National Center for Advancing Translational Sciences' (NCATS) translational science spectrum framework (n.d.). Basic and laboratory science was designated by Blumberg et al. (2012) and the IOM as a T0 phase, and T1 to T4 activities ranged from Phase 1 clinical trials (T1) to community and population-level translation (T4). The T0 to T4 terminologies were abandoned by NCATS, and instead the NIH spectrum uses the descriptive names of basic science, preclinical and clinical research, clinical implementation, and public health phases.

The NCATS spectrum model illustrates the NIH's view that dissemination of findings from preclinical and clinical research occurs in the clinical implementation phase, and it clarified that implementation research also is included in that phase. In the public health phase, population health outcomes from prevention and treatment efforts are studied. Thus, although there is not an exact alignment of the NCATS spectrum to the T0 through T4 phases, the activities of dissemination and implementation research occur in each typology roughly at the third stage of a treatment's testing, after it has progressed from the basic research phase and has had limited clinical testing. However, because of ongoing debates concerning the research translation phases, definitions of IS and DS or research and activities that occur within these study types have not been consistent in the literature (Chesla, 2008; Fort et al., 2017; Rubio et al., 2010).

With the previous discussion as a background, IS and DS will now be defined, as well as other terms that will be used in this text. First, for the purposes of our discussions, in many cases the terms *research* and *science* will be used as synonyms when activities or actions are described. When one "does" research or science, the activities are part of a process of systematically gathering information about objects or events in the world and the actions or perceptions of others (Merriam-Webster, Inc., 2019). As ideas, subjects, or objects (nouns), the two terms may have somewhat different meanings. When science is a noun, it represents the body of knowledge of a discipline or profession, which may include theories or philosophical beliefs, as well as information gained from systematic observations and experimentation (Merriam-Webster, Inc., 2019). Research as a noun refers to individual investigations or periods of study of phenomena or the outcomes of the investigations (e.g., scientists refer to "their" research). Research contributes to and becomes part of the science of a discipline; science encompasses research and other forms of knowledge pertinent to a field and is a broader term.

Because science and research are regarded as similar terms when used as verbs, translation or translational research and translation or translational science should be similar when discussing activities. Building on our earlier discussions of how basic science is moved to everyday use, it can now be asserted that TS or research in nursing examines dissemination and widespread implementation of interventions and treatments that have previously been tested for usefulness in addressing client health concerns. Titler (2018) maintained that TS and IS are interchangeable terms, defining both as efforts of "testing implementation interventions to promote uptake and use of evidence to improve patient outcomes and population health, and explicate what implementation strategies work for whom, in what settings, and why" (p. 3). However, in most interprofessional discussions of TS, IS and DS are differentiated, referring to subcategories of TS that have overlapping but distinct purposes. IS has been described as the "scientific study of methods to promote systematic uptake of research findings and other evidence-based practices into routine practice" (Eccles & Mittman, 2006, p. 1). In addition to examining whether interventions are still effective when removed from highly controlled conditions, IS may focus on the effects of the implementation on health professionals and organizations (Eccles & Mittman, 2006). Data obtained through IS are collected and analyzed to discern the practicality, usefulness, and effectiveness of the interventions in providing care in the everyday world. DS is usually considered to be a systematic examination of the ways that information about innovative interventions is transmitted to appropriate professional audiences or organizations for the purposes of fostering adoption in clinical or public health practice (Glasgow, Vinson et al., 2012; Greenhalgh et al., 2004; Titler, 2018). From these definitions, researchers may include examination of dissemination efforts in their IS investigations, but DS is uniquely concerned with information transmission. In contrast, IS addresses the activities surrounding the actual execution of innovations in a real-world context.

EBP, IS, and DS have become confusing terms for many nurses. The confusion is unsurprising because all have a place in the processes of research translation in nursing practice, and all are concerned with evidence, but what each has as a goal in relation to evidence is what differentiates them. For EBP, the focus is to use the evidence to address practice issues. The aims of IS and DS include the creation of additional evidence and contributing to the discipline's body of knowledge through the conduct of research. The specific focus of IS and DS is the process of introducing evidence into practice. IS and DS activities are concerned with discovery, engaging in, and furthering disciplinary science. It is true that a discipline's science (body of knowledge) may be expanded on during the processes of EBP, but that is not the intention of the activities unless IS and DS are added as additional emphases to an EBP project. Also, actions that have been discovered or tested through IS and DS that foster successful implementation of EBP can be applied in new EBP efforts.

With these considerations in mind, a definition of EBP can now be added to those provided for IS and DS. EBP is defined by the Joanna Briggs Institute as "clinical decision making that considers the best available evidence; the context in which the care is delivered; client preference; and the professional judgment of the health professional" (Pearson et al., 2012, p. 2). Melnyk and Fineout-Overholt (2015), major experts in EBP in nursing, add that the evidence may include information from evidence-based theories, opinion leaders, and expert panels (p. 4). Differentiated from research utilization, EBP incorporates multiple sources of evidence, whereas research utilization is usually the application of information from single investigations (Melnyk & Fineout-Overholt, 2015).

Various strategies for accomplishing EBP have been described in numerous articles and texts. Table 2-1 provides a brief description of several well-known frameworks developed for fostering EBP among nurses. Major publications in which they are explained are identified. In order to maintain the focus of this chapter on the frameworks and models specific to IS and DS, readers seeking more information on the various EBP frameworks in order to use them in their practices are encouraged to consult the sources cited in the table. The remainder of this chapter focuses on topics central to engagement in DS and IS.

TABLE 2-1

Nursing Frameworks, Theories, and Models for Promoting Evidence-Based Practice

NAME OF FRAMEWORK	AUTHORS, DATE OF PUBLICATION	MODEL PRINCIPLES
ACE Star Model of Knowledge Transformation	Stevens, 2012, 2013, 2015	Interdisciplinary; designed for quality improvement. Emphasizes the various *forms* of knowledge and five stages of knowledge transformation represented by points of a star: 1. Discovery research 2. Evidence summary 3. Translation to guidelines 4. Practice integration 5. Process, outcome evaluation The use of the Star Model allowed for identification of competencies required for using evidence-based practice in clinical role.
ARCC: Advancing Research and Clinical Practice Through Close Collaboration	Melnyk et al., 2017	Key to successful implementation of evidence-based practice is a cadre of clinical EBP mentors for nursing staff. Steps in the process of initiating an EBP innovation in a health care system are: 1. Assess potential organizational barriers and strengths for the EBP implementation 2. Develop and use EBP mentors and other strategies (journal clubs, workshops, etc.) 3. Implement EBP process while using mentors to increase staff confidence in ability 4. Assess outcomes of EBP process: nurse satisfaction, cohesion, intent to leave; patient outcomes; organizational outcomes, including reduced costs
Iowa Model of Evidence-Based Practice	Titler et al., 1994, 2001	*Triggers*, problem-focused or knowledge-focused starts the process. Whether addressing the trigger is a priority for organization is assessed. A team is formed that collects, critiques, and synthesizes evidence. If evidence is sufficient, practice change is piloted; if not, research is proposed or other evidence (e.g., case reports) is considered. If pilot is successful, change in practice guidelines and overall adoption are implemented.

(continued)

TABLE 2-1 (CONTINUED)

Nursing Frameworks, Theories, and Models for Promoting Evidence-Based Practice

NAME OF FRAMEWORK	AUTHORS, DATE OF PUBLICATION	MODEL PRINCIPLES
		Practice change effects on patients and families, costs, staff workload, etc. are monitored. Activities are disseminated.
Johns Hopkins Nursing Evidence-Based Practice Model	Dearholt & Dang, 2012	Three cornerstones of practice, education, and research create environment to foster EBP. Process phases in three main categories: 1. Practice question phase Interprofessional team is created, the question is refined, stakeholders identified, and leadership and team meetings identified 2. Evidence phase A search is conducted; evidence is appraised, summarized, and synthesized; and recommendations for change developed 3. Translation phase Feasibility, fit, appropriateness of recommendation determined, action plan created and implemented, actions evaluated, report delivered to stakeholders, next steps determined, dissemination
Rosswurm and Larrabee Model for Evidence-Based Practice Change	Rosswurm & Larrabee, 1999	Six steps in process: 1. Assess need for practice change 2. Link problem interventions and outcomes 3. Synthesize best evidence 4. Design practice change 5. Implement and evaluate practice change 6. Integrate and maintain practice change
Stetler Model of Research Utilization to Facilitate Evidence-Based Practice	Stetler & Marram, 1976 Stetler, 2001	Five phases of activity: 1. Preparation: priorities for change identified, work of finding evidence, and organization of process 2. Validation: evidence is critiqued systematically, evaluated for usefulness, and summarized 3. Comparative evaluation: evaluation of synthesized evidence against need 4. Translation/application: planning for and carrying out change in practice; development of plan for ongoing process 5. Evaluation: evaluating extent of implementation and whether goals were met

IMPLEMENTATION SCIENCE, DISSEMINATION SCIENCE, AND TRANSLATIONAL NURSING SCIENCE

As we noted previously, discussions of TS, IS, and DS appeared in published literature just before the inauguration of the NIH Roadmap initiative (Zerhouni, 2003), making the translation research field barely 20 years old. In the writings published around the time when TS emerged, most authors represented the disciplines of medicine and public health. To a degree, the dominance of medicine's literature is not unexpected because of the early conceptualizations of TS as being investigations to move "bench" research to clinical practice. The contention that epidemiological research was also a form of "basic" science (Woolf, 2008) also makes the higher representation of authors from public health understandable. In fact, some early translation models (e.g., RE-AIM [Reach, Effectiveness, Adoption, Implementation, Maintenance] from Glasgow et al., 1999; and Society for Prevention Science Framework from Kellam and Langevin, 2003) were proposed and used in community settings, thereby stimulating a body of work in IS from that field. However, what was absent was a body of literature contributed by nurse scientists. This is even though nurses had a long-standing involvement in research utilization and efforts to promote EBP.

The disparity in the literature between nursing and other disciplines may also be attributed to the confusion about the differences between TS, IS, DS, and EBP that have already been discussed. The confusion was and remains prominent even among nursing's foremost leaders. In a 2018 editorial in *Nursing Science Quarterly*, Parse (2018) described the deliberations of an international conference that took place in the fall of 2017, at which active questioning about definitions of IS and TS occurred. In her account, conferees could identify little difference between the terms denoting the new sciences and the more established expressions of research utilization and EBP.

With the confusion about these terms, it is unsurprising that nursing's voice is less prominent among the scientists engaged in TS, and that published nursing investigations recognized as IS or DS studies have been scarce and are relatively recent. Although nurses were concerned with EBP, and, in fact, some DS and IS models were derived from those developed for EBP, few nurse scientists were engaged in the study of dissemination and implementation processes. A promising development is that nurses were members of funded interdisciplinary research teams when the NIH launched the CTSAs and Roadmap initiatives (Knafl & Grey, 2008). However, between 2005 and 2012, nursing faculty or schools of nursing held only three NIH R01 grants (the category allowing the largest amount of funding for a single study) through program announcements dedicated to dissemination and implementation research (Tinkle et al., 2013).

Irrespective of historical trends, the need for nursing involvement with DS and IS is great. Certainly, the long-standing concerns for improving quality and safety in health care are important reasons. The unique expertise of nurse scientists is also of significance. Recently, several staff members from the NIH identified gaps in the translational research completed to date. Discussing what they considered "late-stage" translation, which brings basic research to the real world, they noted a needed focus on the *context* in which a therapy would be used. This was, they asserted, a realm of study for which physicians were insufficiently skilled and that bore "really difficult dynamic, adaptive, and multiscale issues" while "establishing access to health systems, addressing health disparities, economics, poverty, and behavior change" (Sampson et al., 2016, p. 155). The areas of challenge identified in this essay are certainly matters that have long been the focus of nursing science as well as of nursing practice. Nursing engagement in TS that will address these issues, as well as the identification of methods for implementation success in working with high-risk populations and in settings where resources are scarce, can be a major contribution to the field (DeVon et al., 2016; Tinkle et al., 2013).

The importance of IS and DS for nursing science is now being recognized. A new investigative approach known as a *pragmatic trial* has resulted in great interest in TS among nurse researchers

(Finnegan & Polivka, 2018) because this method can hasten the movement of an efficacious intervention to standard nursing practice. More nurse scientists are involved in CTSAs in areas of basic science, such as genomics. These activities have occupied greater attention in prominent nursing research societies and journals (Broome, 2013; Genomic Nursing State of the Science Advisory Panel, 2013; Knafl & Grey, 2008; Wyman, 2014). Also, guidance for submitting NIH pragmatic trial grant applications (Littleton-Kearney, 2018) as well as for publishing findings of pragmatic trials (Pickler & Kearney, 2018) are now available. In addition, the work that nurse scientists have done to make research accessible to nursing professionals and to maximize the benefits of basic science for clients and organizations is becoming more evident and visible to health care consumers.

CLINICAL INTERVENTION, DISSEMINATION SCIENCE, AND IMPLEMENTATION SCIENCE

We have discussed how DS and IS are defined. Now we must consider how they are executed, and how they differ from traditional research activities. Nursing interventions or nursing therapies are the foundations of nursing care, and strong evidence to support the safe, effective use of a new intervention is generated first through the conduct of clinical trials (Whittemore & Grey, 2002). The NIH created a classification of clinical trials for the development of health interventions that follow a phasic progression in which various degrees of experimental control are exerted. Higher degrees of control allow the nurse researcher to have confidence that the intervention is responsible for observed changes in a client's status rather than extraneous factors also present that can make the intervention successful (Ferguson, 2004; Whittemore & Grey, 2002). The carefully controlled procedures of a trial that maximize researchers' confidence in its conclusions contribute to the internal validity of the investigation (Ferguson, 2004; Singal et al., 2014). However, the efforts to amplify the internal validity of a trial also contribute to a context that is artificial and unlike a usual clinical practice setting (Marchand et al., 2011). Overemphasis on internal validity in clinical trials that have been the mainstay of health care research was a major impetus for the emergence of TS.

Testing Interventions: From Basic Research to Pragmatic Investigations

To further understand the goals of TS, an additional explanation of the usual procedures for developing interventions is needed. Whittemore and Grey (2002) outlined adaptations of the NIH clinical trial stages that could be used for the development of nursing interventions. These stages parallel the T0 to T4 TS phases that were discussed previously. The first phase, basic research, allows a nurse researcher to use theories and extant literature to design the intervention. In Phase II, pilot testing of the intervention is completed, which allows for a power analysis to be calculated in preparation for Phase III, efficacy clinical trials. In Phase III, the intervention is tested in ideal conditions, and in Phase IV, effectiveness trials, the realities of usual clinical practice are incorporated into the testing. The fifth phase in their classification moves the development process beyond the steps usually recognized by the NIH. In Phase V, the public health effects of the intervention would be determined.

Whittemore and Grey's (2002) classification scheme includes three intervention development phases of great importance to TS. Efficacy trials, effectiveness trials, and the evaluation of public health effects represent key stages of intervention development that require rigor and meticulous procedures. Efficacy trials are experimental approaches that are used to test interventions under highly controlled conditions and are considered the "gold standard" for determining the worth of a specific approach. Efficacy trials emphasize procedures that maximize internal validity of the experiment so that evidence of the value and utility of an intervention is strong. Participants are carefully selected to be as similar to the other participants as possible and are randomized to the new intervention or the control condition, and the intervention is delivered in highly standardized procedures to minimize unevenness in factors that could mask or boost the effects of the new therapy (Marchand et al., 2011; Singal et al., 2014; Whittemore & Grey, 2002). These trials are usually called *randomized controlled trials*. Efficacy trials are most often conducted with individuals, although other client groups or organizations may also be involved, such as families or schools. Along with determining whether an intervention is successful, efficacy trials are designed to obtain information that the intervention is safe or at least poses similar or fewer risks than a current, standard practice. This information obtained in efficacy trials substantiates the progression to the next phase of intervention development in effectiveness trials.

Effectiveness trials, on the other hand, are designed to determine how well an intervention addresses an issue of concern in real-world conditions (Singal et al., 2014; Whittemore & Grey, 2002). In effectiveness trials, many of the controls that are used in efficacy trials, such as the control of procedures for delivering the intervention, are relaxed. External validity (also known as *generalizability*) is emphasized (Singal et al., 2014), meaning the intervention yields outcomes similar to those from efficacy studies when enacted in usual clinical settings with usual staff, a setting's usual clients, and when other usual resources are available (Ferguson, 2004). A key issue in an effectiveness study is determining the appropriate degree of fidelity (faithfulness) to the original experimental procedures that is needed to obtain the intervention's desired outcomes in a real clinical environment (DiNapoli, 2016; Marchand et al., 2011). At this phase, although effectiveness trials of the intervention are being completed and the next step is to incorporate the new intervention into routine practice, TS becomes a central focus. Depending on the frameworks from which a researcher functions, completion of effectiveness testing of the intervention may be desired before full-scale translation efforts, or a new experimental strategy may be used. This new design, the pragmatic clinical trial (PCT), is becoming a significant research approach among nurses engaged in TS.

The characteristics of a PCT are being described in nursing and other health literature (Battaglia & Glasgow, 2018; Finnegan & Polivka, 2018; Gaglio et al., 2014; Singal et al., 2014). In many cases, PCTs are indistinguishable from effectiveness trials. However, these trials are considered by many scientists to be a "hybrid" of efficacy and effectiveness trials (Marchand et al., 2011). As "hybrids," they are defined as follows:

> . . . randomized trials that seek to compare the effectiveness of two or more interventions in real-world settings. Generally, PCTs are closely integrated with clinical practice, incorporate outcomes that are relevant to patients and other relevant stakeholders, include a broad range of clinical settings, and have minimal exclusion criteria so that the patients reflect those receiving care outside of the trial. (Whicher et al., 2015, p. 442)

This definition implies that PCTs include elements of efficacy trials (randomization and comparisons of interventions) and effectiveness trials (a broad range of clinical settings). However, one area that may differentiate PCTs from effectiveness trials is an added examination of the outcomes that may be of concern to "relevant stakeholders." Not only might researchers examine the intervention's effects on clients, staff, and settings, but they also could involve perspectives from individuals outside of the trial site. These individuals could include health care funders or policy makers. This additional dimension of evaluation of the intervention in relation to the context of its use is one that provides a bridge to the concerns of TS.

Because of the broader view of outcomes that may be associated with PCTs, they are being promoted as a means of testing interventions in a manner that would allow the therapies to be moved to general practice more rapidly; therefore, PCTs are very relevant to IS and DS (Battaglia & Glasgow, 2018). In PCTs, there may still be various methods of control used, such as randomization of participants to the new intervention or to a usual care condition, but as described earlier, other forms of experimental control can be lessened (Battaglia & Glasgow, 2018; Finnegan & Polivka, 2018). It should be recognized that the degree of control in any of the dimensions of the experimental design (i.e., eligibility, exposure to the treatment, and fidelity or faithfulness to the new procedures) can vary (Battaglia & Glasgow, 2018; DiNapoli, 2016). Therefore, the nurse scientist conducting a PCT is not only interested in the outcomes of the intervention but also in how the processes of implementation of the intervention are impacted in the shifts from efficacy to effectiveness trials. The outcomes in a setting that has few resources or very diverse clients may not be comparable with those of a setting where these characteristics have been controlled in efficacy trials. These differences have implications for the feasibility of the spread of a particular therapeutic approach in general practice. Thus, PCTs are valuable designs for building science around the dissemination and implementation of innovative nursing therapies.

Conducting Implementation Science Investigations

Effectiveness trials and PCTs are being developed as intermediate steps in readying nursing interventions for widespread use in practice. As noted by Whittemore and Grey (2002), widespread implementation of an intervention eventually should precede the evaluation of its effect on public health. Although effectiveness and PCTs place some importance on methods for assessing factors surrounding the success or failure of an intervention in a particular context, they do not place as much emphasis on these elements as investigations directed toward examining the phenomena of dissemination and implementation of research. Part of the reason may be the outright complexity of a study that includes manipulation and monitoring of both a new intervention and interventions targeted toward staff and other stakeholders of a care setting or community (Glasgow, 2009). Methods that foster implementation and dissemination of well-designed and efficacious interventions are of primary interest to a nurse translational scientist in order to build a body of knowledge for IS and DS that is sound.

Implementation Strategies: Testing Methods of Implementation (Research)

Numerous theories and frameworks have been created that can guide implementation research. Some of these are dedicated to the study of the organizational context in which change will occur. Others address the way change is introduced and the change facilitator's characteristics and activities. Several of these frameworks are discussed in greater detail in Chapter 3. In this chapter, attention is given to general issues of concern for implementation and dissemination research that are important to all IS and DS investigations.

In their discussion of the methods for rigorous development of nursing interventions, Whittemore and Grey (2002) noted that the examination of concepts and theories relevant to a problem is an important first step. An implementation scientist should proceed in a similar manner. A framework, theory, or model and research approach should be chosen that fit with the focus of the innovation effort and context in which a new practice will be implemented. Simultaneously, fidelity of an intervention to the theoretical foundations that underlie its original development should be maintained while it is being delivered in the new setting (Glasgow, 2009; Hanafin & O'Reilly, 2015).

Many of the procedures originally used in early efficacy trials must be modified in the settings for implementation research. The knowledge and skills of interveners, the participants in the intervention, and the timing and "dose" of the intervention (which includes the length of time devoted to the intervention delivery in one session and the number of interventions to achieve the desired effect) are all alterations of methods that will occur when it is executed in a real-world setting. Because of the changes from the efficacy trial, it should be assumed that the delivery of the intervention will be altered; however, to yield outcomes similar to those of the efficacy trials, adequate fidelity to the theoretical foundations of the intervention must be maintained (Glasgow, 2009; Hanafin & O'Reilly, 2015). If the central premises of a theory are lost or misrepresented during the research translation effort, the true effectiveness of the intervention in the new setting cannot be determined because something else—not the theory-based intervention—has been put into place. In translation literature, this has been called a *Type III* error (Basch et al., 1985).

An example of this problem can be seen if we consider an intervention that uses the concept of self-efficacy as its foundation. Bandura (1997) maintained that self-efficacy develops through mastery experiences, vicarious learning (modeling), social persuasion, and physiological and emotional responses to situations. If an intervention was designed to use all of these influences on self-efficacy by operationalizing each concept in a particular way and one of the influences is omitted at the new implementation setting, there is a risk that the therapeutic approach will no longer result in outcomes comparable with those obtained in the efficacy trials. Certainly, some of the reduction in effectiveness may be due to the changes the different interveners and organizational properties brought to the situation, but because the intervention was too far removed from its original theoretical premises, it will not be possible for the researcher to ascertain the relative contributions of each of these alterations to the reduction of efficacy and effectiveness in the setting. The implementation scientist's ability to discern how contextual factors contribute to implementation success or failure and to add this information to the field of IS is impaired.

This discussion brings to the forefront the need for rigor in IS that is as important as it is in other scientific endeavors. IS requires careful planning for ensuring rigor in a study's design. Many variations of both quantitative and qualitative designs can be used. A researcher's training and skills in executing various methodologies as well as the feasibility of conducting IS settings will be concerns in planning an implementation study and will impact design decisions.

Factors that have been identified as either fostering or posing barriers to innovation should be considered to judge the feasibility of implementing a study in a particular setting. Several authors have observed that there are characteristics of the organization, its staff, the intended intervention "targets" (staff or clients), and other stakeholders such as the community, policy makers, or funders that should be balanced in relation to the complexity and resource intensity of the intervention in deciding on how to embark on an implementation study in a particular site (Battaglia & Glasgow, 2018; DiNapoli, 2016; Glasgow, 2009; Marchand et al., 2011; Stirman et al., 2004). Some authors (Madon et al., 2007; Newhouse et al., 2013) have suggested that a strong experimental design for an IS study might use cluster randomization, which entails randomization of several sites to either the implementation of the new therapy or to the control in order to avoid "contamination" of treatment effects within a site's staff or clients—a situation much more likely with the simultaneous relaxation of other procedural controls that were used during efficacy trials. However, Newhouse et al. (2013) noted that insufficient power may be a threat to statistical validity of a trial when clustering is used because researchers may fail to use analyses that account for the groupings and individuals within them.

Cluster randomization designs may not be feasible if there is too much variability in organizational characteristics among available research sites or if there is only one organization willing to consent to the IS investigation. Therefore, one setting may be the only available option and a different design such as comparative effectiveness research may be considered (Glasgow, Green et al., 2012). In comparative effectiveness research, the new intervention would be implemented in one set of staff and clients and compared with existing standard therapies in terms of safety, effectiveness, and cost (Williams et al., 2016). Another possible remedy could be a variation of a within-subjects repeated measures study. In this type of study, all staff and clients would be included in the innovation but not simultaneously. The assessment of important knowledge or attitudinal variables before the implementation would allow researchers to determine whether change occurred afterward. To avoid assignment of the more enthusiastic staff and clients to the innovation early in the study, the order in which each participant group would be included could be randomized (Zoellner & Porter, 2017). Although many threats to internal validity would still be present, some of the effects of introducing a novel intervention could be reduced. These types of design alteration are acceptable when it is remembered that the focus of IS is not solely the evaluation of an intervention in a real-world setting but rather uniquely concerned with exploration of the factors that were impacted within the setting when the intervention was introduced.

Some qualitative research traditions, such as phenomenology, would be ill suited for the usual aims of an IS investigation because of incompatible philosophical foundations. The focus of IS on determining activities that are effective in introducing change does not fit with phenomenology's emphasis on experience and existence as a human being (Rodriguez & Smith, 2018). However, methods such as open-ended, targeted interviews and focus groups are becoming mainstays of IS, and mixed methods studies are considered to be of great value in IS investigations (Glasgow, 2009; Holtrop et al., 2018; Newhouse et al., 2013; Palinkas et al., 2011). In planning IS that includes qualitative methods, Carper's (1978) discussions about personal knowledge as a pattern of knowing apply to nurse scientists. Nurse researchers' skills in conducting various types of investigations and their training in quantitative and/or qualitative methods are always relevant, but particularly when collecting unstructured data. Personal knowledge about one's own capabilities to conduct effective interviews and enact focus group leadership will be necessary. A research team comprised of experts in both qualitative and quantitative methods is highly desirable to maintain rigor, particularly since the inclusion of qualitative methods within an IS study is an emerging approach (Battaglia & Glasgow, 2018; Glasgow, 2009). In addition, expertise in interpreting open-ended responses through content analysis or other appropriate qualitative data analysis techniques will also be required, and a team with diverse qualifications provides great advantages for completing a project.

Despite the challenges of qualitative or mixed method designs for nurse scientists and their teams, these methods have many benefits for IS. Whittemore and Grey (2002) noted that information about client experiences with an intervention can be valuable for the initial design of the therapy. Qualitative interviews could uncover these experiences as the new approach emerges from effectiveness trials and testing commences in usual clinical or community settings. Interviews could also be extended to the evaluation of an intervention in a setting with very diverse clients (Newhouse et al., 2013; Palinkas et al., 2011). Both the clients and the staff who deliver the intervention could provide opinions about its worth, ease of implementation, effects on the well-being of the clients, and other important outcomes (Stirman et al., 2004). Focus groups could be held before and after an intervention is implemented to obtain input about the ways the intervention should or could be introduced, modified, or expanded to further its helpfulness or ease burdens of its use.

In summary, to effectively choose a design for an IS investigation, researchers must consider various characteristics of the intended organization and staff and client participants. These must be balanced against the complexity, intensity, cost, and potential benefits of a new intervention for the context of its use. Table 2-2 presents some of the possible differences in characteristics among these three audiences from the participants of efficacy trials that may affect design decisions, with possible design adaptations that could mitigate the effects of differences on implementation success.

Dissemination Strategies: Testing Methods of Dissemination (Research)

Earlier in this chapter, it was noted that goals of dissemination research may be incorporated into IS investigations but that DS focuses more keenly on the way innovations are effectively communicated to a particular audience. To address concerns that too little research is used in practice, nurse leaders need to know more about the factors that support the introduction of changes in practice and those that address barriers to this. Processes and participant perceptions associated with the introduction and spread of the practice change will be the phenomena explored in a DS investigation.

To choose a design for a DS study, questions to consider are whether the research focus will be determining from two or more potential approaches the *best* way to promote dissemination or whether it will be describing *how* a dissemination process occurred. In studying how the processes occurred, a wide range of designs could be used, including experimental to purely descriptive or qualitative. However, for the first question of what is the best way to promote dissemination, an experimental, quasi-experimental, or similar design will be the strongest. Varying degrees of

TABLE 2-2

Potential Differences in Participant Characteristics From Efficacy Trial Samples and Potential Design Adaptations

PARTICIPANT GROUP	POTENTIAL PARTICIPANT DIFFERENCES	POSSIBLE DESIGN ADAPTATIONS
Clients	Lower levels of education Fewer resources/support for participation Higher number of risk factors Heterogeneity in age, race, ethnicity, and income	Evaluate intervention complexity and adapt intervention while maintaining reasonable fidelity Monitor safety concerns related to risk factors Larger sample size and randomization to control vs. intervention groups to distribute demographic differences May need to revisit efficacy trials with different demographic groups
Staff	Lower levels of education Greater training needs Higher or lower motivation for change and favorable attitudes toward intervention and its success Overall high or low satisfaction with job and unease regarding current situation vs. what is desirable Workload differences and job expectation differences	Evaluate intervention complexity and adapt intervention while maintaining reasonable fidelity Ongoing monitoring of fidelity to procedures Provide testimonials from early trials Provide incentives within policies of the intervention site Provide outline of expected improvements in current situation, such as cost/benefit gains, changes in intensity of usual interventions following change, etc. Monitor degree of involvement and workload shares of staff; provide support and coaching during implementation and evaluation
Organization	Greater/fewer resources available for intervention implementation: funding, staffing, skill mix of staff, and appropriate mentors Perceptions of cost/benefit balance	Plan to provide needed resources to introduce intervention, consider external funding and staff positions, and provide adequate resources for paid time for training mentors and future intervention specialists

(continued)

TABLE 2-2 (CONTINUED)

Potential Differences in Participant Characteristics From Efficacy Trial Samples and Potential Design Adaptations

PARTICIPANT GROUP	POTENTIAL PARTICIPANT DIFFERENCES	POSSIBLE DESIGN ADAPTATIONS
	Competing demands, such as visits from regulating and accrediting bodies, major funding drives, large numbers of orientees or staff departures, etc. Overall concerns about long-term sustainability: commitment, costs, stakeholder buy-in, and legal/regulatory incentives or constraints for new practice	Provide estimates of costs from early trials; keep detailed records of expenditures for all costs, direct and indirect; provide full account of implementation trial costs and costs mitigated because of initial investment. Quantify, to best of ability, the savings from interventions no longer needed after implementation Plan start-up and end dates of implementation trials to avoid anticipated stressful times or adjust staffing of project to account for the other demands Obtain rigorous evaluation of client and staff perceptions and buy-in; intervention impact on safety, quality issues, and client experiences; regulatory concerns; and cost projections for 2- to 5-year periods

Data sources for potential participant differences and design adaptations: Battaglia & Glasgow, 2018; Glasgow, 2009; Marchand et al., 2011; and Stirman et al., 2004.

internal validity will result from the types of control embedded in the procedures. Comparisons can be made between groups that experienced different types of communication about an innovation, received messages about the innovation from different sources, were provided different reinforcements for the use of an intervention in practice, and experienced other variations in the dissemination procedures. Groups of participants could be randomized to these conditions or not. The key point in the relation to experimental procedures for DS investigations is that the focus is on determining the impact of the ways the change in practice was introduced and reinforced in relation to the uptake of the innovation.

Data collection for DS has much less of a focus on the consequences from the use of an intervention in a setting than on the assessment of how a practice change is promoted, the speed of adoption, staff characteristics fostering change, organizational activities that improve uptake, and other similar factors. In addition, concern for the sustainability of a practice change has saliency for a DS investigation. Multiple researchers have linked ongoing sustainability and further dissemination of an intervention to the staff and organization dissemination factors noted previously (Stirman et al., 2004). The measures used for a DS investigation will focus on capturing organizational characteristics and staff members' knowledge, skills, and attitudes to a greater extent than may occur in IS.

The question of how dissemination occurred is a process question. To examine a how question, qualitative methods can be very valuable (Newhouse et al., 2013; Palinkas et al., 2011). Processes are difficult to study through intermittent data collection methods that reflect one point in time. However, many qualitative methods such as interviews, journals, and focus groups can capture stories of what occurred, what participants felt, how they adapted to the change, and how they perceive the efforts can continue. Questions or prompts can guide respondents through the chronology of the dissemination events, or these methods can be started at the study's outset, maintained during the implementation, and continued afterward. They can also be used to encourage rich descriptions of the events and the context surrounding the dissemination efforts. As the implementation period concludes, staff and organizational input into the best ways to foster sustainability and further expansion of the new practice to other departments, organizations, or communities can be obtained.

Adaptations of various traditional research designs and methods that are appropriate approaches to IS and DS have been presented. The unique foci of DS and IS on contexts and processes surrounding the adoption of innovative practice interventions must guide the decisions about design adaptations to fit the emphases of DS and IS. Table 2-3 provides examples of ways that traditional experimental and descriptive designs may be applied or adapted using quantitative and qualitative methods to address the aims of IS and DS.

Tools for Planning Dissemination and Implementation Research

Usual concerns in designing IS and DS investigations have been discussed that account for the general aims of a study and the likely settings of the research. These investigations must be designed to include rigorous methods that allow a researcher to generate valuable conclusions for the field of TS. Nurse scientists engaged in IS and DS will also use the distinctive models, frameworks, and theories of TS to guide their designs, methods, and data collection. A variety of tools and checklists have been created for planning TS studies and measuring various concepts of the frameworks. In Chapter 3, major frameworks developed for the IS and DS fields are summarized. The associated checklists and other instruments are discussed after those descriptions.

CONCLUSION

In this chapter, nursing's involvement with TS from its evolution to the present day was summarized. TS, DS, IS, and EBP were differentiated, and adaptations of the usual procedures for the development of practice interventions that can be extended to TS were explained, as well as appropriate designs for DS and IS studies.

REFLECTIVE QUESTIONS

1. Describe the NCATS spectrum model and the NIH's perspective on dissemination related to TS and EBP uptake.
2. Define EBP, IS, and DS in context to TS and implications for practice and education.
3. Provide examples of how interventions can be tested from basic research to pragmatic investigations related to TS.
4. Explore the challenges and benefits of qualitative or mixed methods designs for IS for nurse scientists and their teams.

TABLE 2-3

Potential Design Applications and Adaptations for Dissemination and Implementation Research

STUDY DESIGNS	DISSEMINATION RESEARCH	IMPLEMENTATION RESEARCH
Experimental	Randomize participants to two or more different messages, sources of messages, and/or methods of dissemination Randomize settings (cluster design) to different messages and/or methods of dissemination	Randomize participants to two or more interventions or various adaptations of efficacious intervention Randomize settings (cluster design) to implementation/nonimplementation conditions
Comparative effectiveness	Randomize participants to usual method of innovation dissemination or to new dissemination message/method Randomize settings to usual or to novel messages and/or methods of dissemination	Randomize participants to usual intervention condition or to new intervention condition Randomize settings to usual intervention condition or to new intervention condition
Descriptive	Obtain predissemination and/or postdissemination perceptions of clients, staff, organizational leaders, via surveys, interviews, and focus groups Collect quantitative data regarding the length of time for recent implementations of new practice after the introduction of intervention information	Obtain preimplementation and/or postimplementation perceptions of clients, staff, organizational leaders, via surveys, interviews, and focus groups Collect quantitative data regarding the length of time for recent implementations of new practice after start-up of the intervention trial Obtain data to measure outcomes of implementation of new intervention for clients, staff, organization
Qualitative	Interviews/focus groups with clients and staff concerning helpful/unhelpful messages, helpful/unhelpful methods of information receipt, and recommended revisions in dissemination messages and methods	Interviews/focus groups with clients and staff concerning intervention acceptability; training methods; effects on clients, staff, and client-staff relationships; change facilitator; organizational supports; and methods of change Diaries of thoughts, feelings, and insights during implementation

REFERENCES

Bandura, A. (1997). Sources of self-efficacy. In A. Bandura (Ed.), *Self-efficacy: The exercise of control* (pp. 79-115). W. H. Freeman.

Barnard, K. E., & Eyres, S. J. (Eds.). (1979). *Child health assessment: Part 2. The first year of life* (DHEW Publication No. HRA 79-25). U.S. Government Printing Office. https://hdl.handle.net/2027/umn.31951000066877g

Basch, C. E., Sliepcevich, E. M., Gold, R. S., Duncan, D. F., & Kolbe, L. J. (1985). Avoiding Type III errors in health education program evaluations: A case study. *Health Education Quarterly, 12*(4), 315-331.

Battaglia, C., & Glasgow, R. E. (2018). Pragmatic dissemination and implementation research models, methods and measures and their relevance for nursing research. *Nursing Outlook, 66,* 430-445.

Beyea, S. C., & Slattery, M. J. (2013). Historical perspectives on evidence-based nursing. *Nursing Science Quarterly, 26,* 152-155.

Blumberg, R. S., Dittel, B., Hafler, D., Von Herrath, M., & Nestle, F. O. (2012). Unraveling the autoimmune translational research process layer by layer. *Nature Medicine, 18*(1), 35-41. https://doi.org/10.1038/nm.2632

Broome, M. E. (2013). The continuum of translational research: Special issue from the Council for the Advancement of Nursing Science [Editorial]. *Nursing Outlook, 61,* 193-194

Cabana, M. D., Rand, C. S., Powe, N. R., Wu, A. W., Wilson, M. H., Abboud, P. C., & Rubin, H. R. (1999). Why don't physicians follow clinical practice guidelines? A framework for improvement. *JAMA, 282,* 1458-1465.

Canadian Institutes of Health Research. (2018). About us- CIHR. http://www.cihr-irsc.gc.ca/e/37792.html

Carper, B. (1978). Fundamental patterns of knowing in nursing. *Advances in Nursing Science, 1*(1), 13-23.

Chesla, C. A. (2008). Translational research: Essential contributions from interpretive nursing science. *Research in Nursing & Health, 31,* 381-390.

Cochrane, A. (1972). Effectiveness and efficiency: Random reflections on health services. Nuffield Trust.

Dearholt, S.L., & Dang, D. (2012). *Johns Hopkins Nursing evidence-based practice: Models and guidelines* (2nd ed.). Sigma Theta Tau International.

DeVon, H. A., Rice, M., Pickler, R. H., Krause-Parello, C. A., Eckart, P., Corwin, E., & Richmond, T. S. (2016). Engaging members and partner organizations in translating a nursing science agenda. *Nursing Outlook, 64,* 516-519. https://doi.org/10.1016/j.outlook.2016.07.010

DiNapoli, P. P. (2016). Implementation science: A framework for integrating evidence-based practice. *American Nurse Today, 13*(7), 40-41.

Drolet, B. C., & Lorenzi, N. M. (2011). Translational research: understanding the continuum from bench to bedside. *Translational Research, 157,* 1-5.

Eccles, M. P., & Mittman, B. S. (2006). Welcome to *Implementation Science* [Editorial]. *Implementation Science, 1,* 1-3. https://doi.org/10.1186/1748-5908-1-1

Farquhar, C. M., Stryer, D., & Slutsky, J. (2002). Translating research into practice: The future ahead. *International Journal for Quality in Health Care, 14,* 233-249.

Ferguson, L. (2004). External validity, generalizability, and knowledge utilization. *Journal of Nursing Scholarship, 36,* 16-22.

Fineout-Overholt, E., Levin, R., & Melnyk, B. M. (2004). Strategies for advancing evidence-based practice in clinical settings. *Journal of the New York State Nurses Association, 35*(2), 28-32.

Finnegan, L., & Polivka, B. (2018). Advancing nursing science through pragmatic trials [Editorial]. *Nursing Outlook, 66,* 425-427.

Fort, D. G., Herr, T. M., Shaw, P. L., Gutzman, K. E., & Starren, J. B. (2017). Mapping the evolving definitions of translational research. *Journal of Clinical and Translational Science, 1,* 60-66. doi:10.1017/cts.2016.10

Funk, S. G., Tornquist, E. M., & Champagne, M. T. (1989a). A model for improving the dissemination of nursing research. *Western Journal of Nursing Research, 11,* 359-365.

Funk, S. G., Tornquist, E. M., & Champagne, M. T. (1989b). Application and evaluation of the dissemination model. *Western Journal of Nursing Research, 11,* 486-491.

Gaglio, B., Phillips, S. M., Heurtin-Roberts, S., Sanchez, M. A., & Glasgow, R. E. (2014). How pragmatic is it? Lessons learned using PRECIS and RE-AIM for determining pragmatic characteristics of research. *Implementation Science, 9,* 1-11. https://doi.org/10.1186/s13012-014-0096-x

Genomic Nursing State of the Science Advisory Panel. (2013). A blueprint for genomic nursing science. *Journal of Nursing Scholarship, 45,* 96-104.

Glasgow, R. E. (2009). Critical measurement issues in translational research. *Research on Social Work Practice, 19,* 560-568. https://doi.org/10.1177/1049731509335497

Glasgow, R. E., Green, L. W., Taylor, M. V., & Stange, K. C. (2012). An evidence integration triangle for aligning science with policy and practice. *American Journal of Preventive Medicine, 42*(6), 646-654. https://doi.org/10.1016/j.amepre.2012.02.016

Glasgow, R. E., Vinson, C., Chambers, D., Khoury, M. J., Kaplan, R. M., & Hunter, C. (2012). National institutes of health approaches to dissemination and implementation science: Current and future directions. *American Journal of Public Health, 102,* 1274-1281. doi:10.2105/AJPH.2012.300755

Glasgow, R. E., Vogt, T. M., & Boles, S. M. (1999). Evaluating the public health impact of health promotion interventions: The RE-AIM framework. *American Journal of Public Health, 89,* 1322-1327.

Greenhalgh, T., Robert, G., Macfarlane, F., Bate, P., & Kyriakidou, O. (2004). Diffusion of innovations in service organizations: A systematic review and recommendations. *The Milbank Quarterly, 82,* 581-629. https://doi.org/10.1111/j.0887-378X.2004.00325.x

Haller, K. B., Reynolds, M. A., & Horsley, J. A. (1979). Developing research-based innovation protocols: Process, criteria, and issues. *Research in Nursing and Health, 2,* 45-51. https://doi.org/10.1002/nur.4770020202

Hanafin, S., & O'Reilly, E. D. (2015). Implementation science: Issues of fidelity to consider in community nursing. *British Journal of Community Nursing, 20,* 437-443.

Holtrop, J. S., Rabin, B. A., & Glasgow, R. E. (2018). Qualitative approaches to use of the RE-AIM framework: Rationale and methods. *BMC Health Services Research, 18,* 177. https://doi.org/10.1186/s12913-018-2938-8

Institute of Medicine. (2000). *To err is human: Building a safer health system.* National Academies Press. https://doi.org/10.17226/9728

Kellam, S. G., & Langevin, D. J. (2003). A framework for understanding "evidence" in prevention research and programs. *Prevention Science, 4,* 137-153.

Knafl, K., & Grey, M. (2008). Clinical translational science awards: Opportunities and challenges for nurse scientists. *Nursing Outlook, 56,* 132-137. https://doi.org/10.1016/j.outlook.2008.03.006

Littleton-Kearney, M. (2018). Pragmatic clinical trials at the National Institute of Nursing Research. *Nursing Outlook, 66,* 470-472. https://doi.org/10.1016/j.outlook.2018.02.001

Madon, T., Hofman, K. J., Kupfer, L., & Glass, R. I. (2007). Implementation science. *Science, 318*(5857), 1728-1729.

Marchand, E., Stice, E., Rohde, P., & Becker, C. B. (2011). Moving from efficacy to effectiveness trials in prevention research. *Behaviour Research and Therapy, 49,* 32-41. https://doi.org/10.1016/j.brat.2010.10.008

Melnyk, B. M., & Fineout-Overholt, E. (2015). *Evidence-based practice in nursing & healthcare: A guide to best practice* (3rd ed.). Wolters Kluwer.

Melnyk, B. M., Fineout-Overholt, E., Feinstein, N. F., Li, H., Small, L., Wilcox, L., & Kraus, R. (2004). Nurses' perceived knowledge, beliefs, skills, and needs regarding evidence-based practice: Implications for accelerating the paradigm shift. *Worldviews on Evidence-Based Nursing, 1*(3), 185–193.

Melnyk, B. M., Fineout-Overholt, E., Giggleman, M., & Choy, K. (2017). A test of the ARCC© model improves implementation of evidence-based practice, healthcare culture, and patient outcomes. *Worldviews on Evidence-Based Nursing, 14*(1), 5-9. https://doi.org/10.1111/wvn.12188WVN 2017

Merriam-Webster, Inc. (2019). Research and science. https://www.merriam-webster.com/dictionary/

National Center for Advancing Translational Sciences. (n.d.). Translational science spectrum. https://ncats.nih.gov/files/translation-factsheet.pdf

National Institutes of Health Office of Strategic Coordination–The Common Fund. (2014). *A decade of discovery: The NIH Roadmap and Common Fund 2004-2014.* NIH Pub No. 14-8013. https://commonfund.nih.gov/sites/default/files/ADecadeofDiscoveryNIHRoadmapCF.pdf

Newhouse, R., Bobay, K., Dykes, P. C., Stevens, K. R., & Titler, M. (2013). Methodology issues in implementation science. *Medical Care, 51,* S32-S40.

Nightingale, F. (1859/1992). *Notes on nursing: What it is and what it is not.* J.B. Lippincott.

Palinkas, L. A., Aarons, G. A., Horwitz, S., Chamberlain, P., Hurlburt, M., & Landsverk, J. (2011). Mixed method designs in implementation research. *Administration and Policy in Mental Health, 38,* 44-53. https://doi.org/10.1007/s10488-010-0314-z

Parse, R. R. (2018). Everything old is new again: Implementation science [Editorial]. *Nursing Science Quarterly, 31,* 213-214.

Pearson, A., Jordan, Z., & Munn, Z. (2012). Translational science and evidence-based healthcare: A clarification and reconceptualization of how knowledge is generated and used in healthcare. *Nursing Research and Practice, 2012,* 1-6. https://doi.org/10.1155/2012/792519

Pickler, R. H., & Kearney, M. H. (2018). Publishing pragmatic trials. *Nursing Outlook, 66,* 464-469.

Rodriguez, A. & Smith, J. (2018). Phenomenology as a healthcare research method. *Evidence-Based Nursing, 21*(4):96-98. https://doi.org/10.1136/eb-2018-102990

Rosswurm, M. A., & Larrabee, J. H. (1999). A model for change to evidence-based practice. *Image—the Journal of Nursing Scholarship, 31,* 317-322.

Rubio, D. M., Schoenbaum, E. E., Lee, L. S., Schteingart, D. E., Marantz, D. E., Anderson, K. E., Dewey Platt, L., Baez, A., & Esposito, K. (2010). Defining translational research: Implications for training. *Academic Medicine, 85*(3), 470-475. https://doi.org/10.1097/ACM.0b013e3181ccd618

Sampson, U. K. A., Chambers, D., Riley, W., Glass, R. I., Engelgau, M. M., & Mensah, G. A. (2016). Implementation research: The fourth movement of the unfinished translation research symphony. *Global Heart, 11*, 153-158.

Shah, H. M., & Chung, K. C. (2009). Archie Cochrane and his vision for evidence-based medicine. *Plastic and Reconstructive Surgery, 124*, 982-988. https://doi.org/10.1097/PRS.0b013e3181b03928

Singal, A. G., Higgins, P. D. R., & Waljee, A. K. (2014). A primer on effectiveness and efficacy trials. *Clinical and Translational Gastroenterology, 5*(1), e45-e48. https://doi.org/10.1038/ctg.2013.13

Stetler, C. B. (2001). Updating the Stetler model of research utilization to facilitate evidence-based practice. *Nursing Outlook, 49*, 272-279.

Stetler, C. B., & Marram, G. (1976). Evaluating research findings for applicability in practice. *Nursing Outlook, 24*, 559-563.

Stevens, K. R. (2012). Delivering on the promise of EBP. *Nursing Management, 19*(1), 19-21. https://doi.org/10.1097/01.NUMA.0000413102.48500.1f

Stevens, K. R. (2013). The impact of evidence-based practice in nursing and the next big ideas. *Online Journal of Issues in Nursing, 18*(2), 4. https://doi.org/10.3912/OJIN.Vol18No02Man04

Stevens, K. R. (2015). *Star Model of EBP: Knowledge transformation.* Academic Center for Evidence-based Practice, The University of Texas Health Science Center at San Antonio. https://doi.org/10.1097/01.NUMA.0000413102.48500.1f

Stirman, S. W., Crits-Christoph, P., & DeRubeis, R. J. (2004). Achieving successful dissemination of empirically supported psychotherapies: A synthesis of dissemination theory. *Clinical Psychology: Science and Practice, 11*, 343-359. https://doi.org/10.1093/clinsy/bph091

Sung, N. S., Crowley, W. F., Genel, M., Salber, P., Sandy, L., Sherwood, L. M., Johnson, S. B., Catanese, V., Tilson, H., Getz, K., Larson, E. L., Scheinberg, D., Reece, E. A., Slavkin, H., Dobs, A., Grebb, J., Martinez, R. A., Korn, A., & Rimion, D. (2003). Central challenges facing the national clinical research enterprise. *JAMA, 289*(10), 1278-1287. https://doi.org/10.1001/jama.289.10.1278

Tinkle, M., Kimball, R., Haozous, E. A., Shuster, G., & Meize-Grochowski, R. (2013). Dissemination and implementation research funded by the US National Institutes of Health, 2005-2012. *Nursing Research and Practice, 2013*, 1-15. https://doi.org/10.1155/2013/909606

Titler, M. G. (2018). Translation research in practice: An introduction. *Online Journal of Issues in Nursing, 23*, 1-15.

Titler, M. G., Kleiber, C., Steelman, V. J., & Goode, C. (1994). Infusing research into practice to promote quality care. *Nursing Research, 43*(5), 307-313.

Titler, M. G., Kleiber, C., Steelman, V. J., Rakel, B. A., Budreau, G., Everett, L. Q., Buckwalter, K. C., Tripp-Reimer, T., & Goode, C. J. (2001). The Iowa model of evidence-based practice to promote quality care. *Critical Care Nursing Clinics of North America, 13*(4), 497-509.

Whicher, D. M., Miller, J. E., Dunham, K. M., & Joffe, S. (2015). Gatekeepers for pragmatic clinical trials. *Clinical Trials, 12*, 442-448.

Whittemore, R. & Grey, M. (2002). The systematic development of nursing interventions. *Journal of Nursing Scholarship, 34*, 115-120.

Williams, C. M., Skinner, E. H., James, A. M., Cook, J. L., McPhail, S. M., & Haines, T. P. (2016). Comparative effectiveness research for the clinician researcher: A framework for making a methodological design choice. *Trials, 17*, 406-411. https://doi.org/10.1186/s13063-016-1535-6

Woolf, S. H. (2008). The meaning of translational research and why it matters. *JAMA, 299*, 211-213.

Wyman, J. F. (2014). Council for the Advancement of Nursing Science: Council news. *Nursing Outlook, 62*, 299-300.

Zerhouni, E. (2003). The NIH roadmap. *Science, 302*(5642), 63-72.

Zoellner, J. M., & Porter, K. J. (2017). Translational research: Concepts and methods in dissemination and implementation research. In A. M. Coulston, C. J. Boushey, M. G. Ferruzzi, & L. M. Delahanty (Eds.), *Nutrition in the prevention and treatment of disease* [Digital Edition version] (4th ed., pp. 125-143). Elsevier. http://dx.doi.org/10.1016/B978-0-12-802928-2.00006-0

THEORIES, FRAMEWORKS, AND MODELS IN IMPLEMENTATION AND DECISION SCIENCE

Cynthia Peltier Coviak, PhD, RN, FNAP

CHAPTER OBJECTIVES

- Describe major theories, models, and frameworks that guide implementation science
- Outline dissemination frameworks and their implications for messaging and the spread of evidence-based practice uptake
- Identify instruments, checklists, and methods associated with dissemination and implementation frameworks

KEY WORDS

- Dissemination frameworks
- Implementation checklist
- Implementation measurement
- Implementation science frameworks
- Implementation science models

- Implementation science theories
- Implementation tools
- Knowledge translation
- Translational science

Roussel, L. A., & Thomas, P. L. (Eds.). *Implementation Science in Nursing: A Framework for Education and Practice* (pp. 39-53).
© 2022 Taylor & Francis Group.

Building on the concepts presented in Chapter 2, this chapter examines the theories, frameworks, and models in implementation and dissemination. Major theorists and scientists who have contributed to this work are highlighted in discussion about the study design. The adaptation of randomized controlled trials (RCTs), cluster RCTs, and comparative effectiveness research is offered; an evolving design known as *pragmatic clinical trials* (PCTs) is also explored.

THEORIES, FRAMEWORKS, AND MODELS IN IMPLEMENTATION AND DISSEMINATION SCIENCE

Major Theorists and Scientists

Previous discussions of the fields of implementation science (IS) and dissemination science (DS) have included their origins, unique concerns in research designs and methods, and the likely products of IS and DS. The focus now shifts to the reciprocal relationship between theory and research that creates the foundations of science. Benoliel (1977) portrayed practice as the usual first stimulus for research. She maintains that this is through an interaction that occurs with theory. It has been noted previously that Carper (1978) identified empirics as one "pattern of knowing." By this statement, the research foundation providing an element of nursing knowledge is recognized. However, the relationship among practice, research, and theory is more than that. Fawcett (1978) depicted a structure, the "double helix," as representing the relationship of nursing theory and research, pointing to theory as vital to establishing research as "non-trivial" (p. 49). This intimates that theory constitutes the means for interpreting research findings that otherwise would make little sense for the discipline's body of knowledge. Similar observations about theory and research are noted in the fields of IS and DS. IS and DS theory and research are intertwined, as Fawcett (1978) observed for nursing knowledge development.

It is acknowledged here that the terms *theories*, *frameworks*, and *models* for IS and DS are not synonymous, although in many cases in the current discussion they are used interchangeably. Theories are sets of abstract concepts and constructs that label phenomena and that are linked together by statements that describe or explain the relationships among them (Glanz et al., 2008; Kim, 2010; McEwan, 2014). They may also predict events or situations or prescribe actions that should be taken in a circumstance (Dickoff et al., 1968).

Frameworks are less formal but still are based on theories that underlie a field or sector of knowledge. They help a researcher to operationalize the concepts of the theories upon which scholarly work is based. "[T]he theoretical framework is a structure that summarizes concepts and theories, which you develop from previously tested and published knowledge which you synthesize to help you have a theoretical background, or basis for your data analysis and interpretation of the meaning contained in your research data" (Kivunja, 2018, p. 46).

Finally, models are depictions of phenomena in the real world. Models may be objects that can be manipulated, such as models of human organs, but if they are theoretical, they use language and symbols to represent the phenomenon in diagrams (McEwan, 2014). What is important about models is that they are concrete and assist a scientist to choose data collection techniques and measures, which facilitates the organization of data from an investigation (Rycroft-Malone & Bucknall, 2010). Several authors who have reviewed the IS and DS literature note that theories, frameworks, and models are terms that are often not differentiated (Damschroder et al., 2009; Nilsen, 2015; Tabak et al., 2012).

Currently, few formal theories exist in IS and DS. However, theories are developed over time, and some frameworks and models are now incorporating theoretical propositions that underlie their various components. For example, Promoting Action on Research Implementation in Health Services (PARIHS) was developed by Kitson et al. (1998) and later expanded with the collaboration of Rycroft-Malone (2004) and others. Propositional statements about the functions of evidence, context, and facilitation in fostering the use of evidence-based practice (EBP) by nurses in a health care setting have evolved (Rycroft-Malone, 2004). Other theories are developing through theory synthesis and often include propositions of the theories they have incorporated. For example, the normalization process theory (May, 2013) includes social cognitive and systems theories as foundations and accepts the premises of other authors, such as Bandura (1997), for the integrated theory. Still others, such as RE-AIM (Reach, Effectiveness, Adoption, Implementation, Maintenance; Glasgow et al., 1999), guide researchers to incorporate theories to support interventions and do not attempt to propose relationships among concepts.

However, frameworks and models for IS and DS are multiplying rapidly, especially considering the overall newness of translational science (TS). The value of a firm theoretical foundation for a DS or IS investigation is borne out by the observations of several authors; by 2018, there were more than 100 frameworks for IS and DS (Battaglia & Glasgow, 2018; Dintrans et al., 2019; Mitchell et al., 2010; Tabak et al., 2018). As noted earlier, theories may be arising from these frameworks.

Why are theoretical frameworks so needed in IS and DS? Drolet and Lorenzi (2011) provided rationale, noting that frameworks are needed (a) to find gaps in the translation process to be able to move research to practice and (b) to allow researchers and clinicians to fix the process by addressing the gaps. In practical language, they help us plan for research and evaluate the outcomes of our efforts. Some authors of IS and DS frameworks have been quite direct about these being their ambitions (Damschroder et al., 2009; Dzewaltowski et al., 2004; Glasgow et al., 1999). An eventual goal, as noted by Glasgow et al. (1999), is having the ability to ascertain the public health impact of an intervention, reaching that last step in intervention testing that had been identified by Whittemore and Grey (2002) as the aim.

With the many TS frameworks already in the literature, it was decided to limit the discussion in this chapter to six frameworks that have a history of use in nursing and community or public health. The frameworks developed in community and public health are important to nursing because of the discipline's ongoing involvement in and concern for population health initiatives and interventions. Other frameworks used in nursing have often been adapted from models that were originally used for the implementation of EBP. Rycroft-Malone (2004) noted that the research team developing PARIHS (Kitson et al., 1998) "accumulated experience and knowledge about implementation and changing practice from their involvement in a number of researches, practice development, and quality improvement projects" (p. 298). Thus, the development of the framework moved away from being primarily to foster EBP to the expansion of IS in nursing. It provides an example of the research–theory double helix relationship as its shift to IS stimulated more formal theoretical advancement.

The frameworks that are discussed in this chapter include two used in DS, two used in IS, and two used for either. Readers who wish to explore frameworks that are not discussed here are encouraged to consult reviews by Mitchell et al. (2010), Tabak et al. (2012), and Nilsen (2015), which provide information about the primary foci of the frameworks (IS, DS, or both). In addition, a very helpful website is hosted at http://dissemination-implementation.org where models and frameworks can be searched and compared by their foci and major concepts. The website also provides other information, such as links to measures for the concepts of many of the frameworks.

As the frameworks are reviewed, it should be noted that TS has been a global priority. Canada, the United Kingdom, and other countries use slightly different terminology in their efforts. *Knowledge translation* is the term used by the Canadian Institutes of Health Research (CIHR) for efforts that in the United States are called TS. The focus on translation is evident in CIHR's mandate, stating it "... facilitates the application of the results of research and their transformation into new policies, practices, procedures, products and services" (CIHR, 2013, section 2, bullet 3). The definition of knowledge translation is inclusive of the concept of dissemination but also includes statements that reflect the actions as part of a process. CIHR defines it as "A dynamic and iterative process that includes synthesis, dissemination, exchange and ethically-sound application of

TABLE 3-1
Selected Dissemination Frameworks of Translational Science

TITLE OF FRAMEWORK	MAJOR PUBLICATIONS ABOUT FRAMEWORK	DESCRIPTION OF PREMISES, NOTABLE FEATURES
Rogers' diffusion of innovations	Rogers (2003) Dearing & Cox (2018)	Diffusion (a) is a social process, (b) about an innovation, (c) communicated through "certain channels," (d) that are members of a social system Adoption of the innovation depends on (a) characteristics of the innovation, (b) motivations/needs of adopters, (c) the larger social context (Rogers, 2003; Dearing & Cox, 2018)
RAND model of persuasive communication and diffusion of medical innovation	Winkler et al. (1985)	Derived from persuasion theory and research "Medical technology assessment" communication features of importance: sources of information, message content, channels or medium used, audience characteristics, and settings in which communication is received (Winkler et al., 1985)

knowledge to improve the health of Canadians, provide more effective health services and products and strengthen the health care system" (CIHR, 2019, para. 1).

The term *knowledge translation* is also sometimes used by researchers in other countries. Several frameworks have been developed through CIHR grant funding; therefore, they may include the term *knowledge* or *knowledge translation* in their titles. The Knowledge to Action framework (Graham et al., 2006) is an example of one of these.

Dissemination Frameworks

As a group, the frameworks of TS that are solely devoted to dissemination are greatly outnumbered by the implementation and mixed DS-IS frameworks. However, among TS frameworks, two of the dissemination frameworks have the longest history and have had an impact across many disciplines (Table 3-1). Rogers' diffusion of innovations model (2003) was first formulated in 1962 and has undergone much revision in the nearly 60 years since he published his first edition. Rogers' fields were communication and sociology, and his work arose from reviewing research of these and other disciplines and subdisciplines, such as medical sociology. Factors that affect the adoption of innovations have undergone the most revision and maturation in the model over time. Some of the modifications have come about because of the expansion of diffusion research beyond individuals to organizations. Other changes have resulted from its use and adaptations for use in global communities, which made the model less culture bound (Rogers, 1983). With its long history and broad applicability for the introduction of various novel practices, the influence of Rogers' many iterations of diffusion theory can be readily seen by the entry of "diffusion of innovation and nursing" as search terms in library databases. It has been widely used in the initiation of EBPs in nursing, including those developed for use in nursing education. However, the long-standing influence of Rogers' work in nursing may also be its theoretical influence in other frameworks and models. For example, authors of the PARIHS framework have explicitly cited their reliance on Rogers' diffusion of innovations theory as a foundation to the framework as they have engaged in its revision to the integrated Promoting Action on Research Implementation in Health Services (i-PARIHS; Harvey & Kitson, 2016).

The RAND model of persuasive communication and diffusion of medical innovation (Winkler et al., 1985) was originally developed during the 1970s when Cochrane's call for the use of research in medicine was drawing much attention by physicians and other health care stakeholders. The use of the term *medical technology assessment* referred to the evaluation of characteristics such as safety, efficacy, and costs of new treatments or procedures (Winkler et al., 1985). The communications about the new practices were intended to encourage adoption. The communication in this context was more focused, tailored, and direct than that described by Rogers' diffusion model. The RAND persuasive communication model and diffusion of medical innovation continues to be important in the policy work and research for which the corporation is famous (RAND Health Care, 2019).

Implementation Frameworks

The Consolidated Framework for Implementation Research (CFIR), which was created by Damschroder et al. (2009), and PARIHS, which was developed by Kitson et al. (1998), Rycroft-Malone (2004), Laycock et al. (2018), and many others, grew from the field of health systems research and were established primarily through the efforts of nursing leaders (Table 3-2). As has been discussed previously, PARIHS originated as a framework for introducing EBPs to nurses in health organizations. CFIR was created to address both the constructs the authors deemed to be missing from the existing implementation frameworks and the inconsistencies and overlap perceived to typify them (Damschroder et al., 2009). These two models have undergone extensive testing and development since they were first published. The authors of each are also actively involved in their operationalization and modification, which have come about through critique, reports of research using the frameworks, and systematic reviews (Helfrich et al., 2010; Kirk et al., 2016).

PARIHS' original constructs of successful implementation, evidence, facilitation, and context were combined in a propositional statement. The growth in IS research that expanded notions of the important factors in supporting practice changes and consideration of the criticisms identified by IS researchers and authors of systematic reviews led to concerted efforts by the developers to update the framework. The i-PARIHS, which highlighted the importance of the facilitation construct for success in using the framework, was introduced in 2015 (Harvey & Kitson, 2015). This revision also proposed the addition of recipient as a new construct with the previous three (i.e., evidence, context, and facilitation) and the replacement of evidence by innovation in alignment with Rogers' diffusion of innovations theory (Harvey & Kitson, 2016). The original proposition was revised (see Table 3-2) and now suggests that "successful implementation (SI) is achieved by facilitation (Fac) of an innovation (I) with recipients (R) in their . . . context (C)" (Harvey & Kitson, 2016, p. 2). This new formulation of the major proposition of i-PARIHS is now in further testing.

With the introduction of i-PARIHS and the added emphasis that it places on facilitation in implementation processes, the development team has created materials designed to assist facilitators in their roles. Some are available as attachments to journal articles (Harvey & Kitson, 2016), whereas others are associated with an edited book (Harvey & Kitson, 2015). In addition, over the history of PARIHS use, various instruments have been developed for measuring its original constructs, such as context. Some of the websites that were developed for translational scientists include links to these concepts. Those websites are addressed later.

TABLE 3-2
Selected Implementation Frameworks of Translational Science

TITLE OF FRAMEWORK	MAJOR PUBLICATIONS ABOUT FRAMEWORK	DESCRIPTION OF PREMISES, NOTABLE FEATURES
Consolidated Framework for Implementation Research	Damschroder et al. (2009) Website: https://cfirguide.org/	Developed from a comprehensive review of health services research frameworks published through 2008 identified from two published reviews, *Implementation Science* journal, and snowball technique Identified five major domains and constructs associated with each: 1. Intervention characteristics (eight constructs) 2. Outer setting (four constructs) 3. Inner setting (12 constructs) 4. Characteristics of involved individuals (five constructs) 5. Process of implementation (eight constructs)
Promoting Action on Research Implementation in Health Services Integrated Promoting Action on Research Implementation in Health Services	Kitson et al. (1998) Harvey & Kitson (2015, 2016) Laycock et al. (2018)	Original Promoting Action on Research Implementation in Health Services: three main constructs in implementation of evidence-based practice in health systems 1. Evidence 2. Context 3. Facilitation Successful implementation (SI) is function (f) of evidence, context, and facilitation (E, C, F): $SI = f(E, C, F)$ Integrated Promoting Action on Research Implementation in Health Services reformulation of above proposition: $SI = Fac (I + R + C)$ Innovation (I) replaces evidence, and recipients (R) is a new construct ("Fac" is new abbreviation for facilitation)

The CFIR came about because of efforts in the U.S. Department of Veterans Affairs' Quality Enhancement Research Initiative (CFIR, 2019a). At a time when implementation research was in an upsurge, the framework was developed to organize the constructs that researchers were identifying. A list of five domains and their associated constructs was created through a review of 19 frameworks that were in use at the time. The authors were careful to note that they did not aim to create relational statements among the constructs—only to organize the information in logical categories (Damschroder et al., 2009). They consider the CFIR to be a metatheoretical framework.

The CFIR (2019b) has a detailed website that includes descriptions of the domains and associated constructs, suggested evaluation approaches and methods, links to selected measures, relevant publications, and a variety of other resources. It should be noted that because the CFIR was created to organize the numerous constructs in IS literature, measures that are included on the website (e.g., organizational assessment tools) could be used for multiple frameworks that include a construct and define it as observed in the CFIR. Having been developed as a descriptive rather than explanatory or predictive model, it is unsurprising that the authors of a systematic review published in 2016 (Kirk et al.) found that all but one of the researchers authoring manuscripts of the review used the framework only for planning of their studies and data analysis. Also, use of the CFIR to provide theoretical explanations for study findings was limited to only two studies. Linkages of constructs to the findings of the studies were also lacking.

Despite these concerns, the CFIR's use in the Quality Enhancement Research Initiative and operationalization of the constructs support its ongoing development. Care in the selection of constructs within a study and reflection about the relationships among them will be required for what some authors have called *meaningful use* of the framework (Kirk et al., 2016). With these actions as foundations, the many frameworks from which concepts of the CFIR are derived may, in turn, be further developed.

Frameworks for Either Dissemination or Implementation

The last two frameworks in our discussion are ones that can be used across the dissemination–implementation spectrum (Table 3-3). The PRECEDE-PROCEED (Green & Kreuter, 2005) and RE-AIM (Glasgow et al., 1999) frameworks were developed in the public health field, with the original intent of providing models for planning and evaluating programs and health promotion initiatives. Well before the many calls for quality, safety, and cost-effectiveness of health care interventions stimulated the launch of TS in the later part of the 1900s, public health departments were expected to provide evidence of the worth of their programming considering these issues. Thus, the PRECEDE-PROCEED model (PPM) had its origins in the early 1970s and was fully formulated in 1991 for the evaluation of health education programs (Nair, 2016). Glasgow et al. (1999), who were affiliated with major health research organizations involved with prevention research, had great concerns about the ongoing emphasis on interventions that were not practical for real-world community settings. They formulated RE-AIM as an evaluation model to move public health interventions from the efficacy paradigm prominent at that time to more realistic yet beneficial remedies for enhancing the well-being of populations. With the emphasis these models gave to evaluation, which often uses techniques like those of research, their adaptation for use in translation research was readily accomplished, and they have been very influential in the field.

In 1974, an article by Green proposing a model for cost-benefit analysis of health education programs was the foundation for the Precede portion of the PPM. In that publication, the predisposing, reinforcing, and enabling constructs of the model were first described. These are characteristics of an individual or community that are assessed for planning and guide evaluation. When the Proceed portion was added in 1991 (Nair, 2016) and thereafter, the model added focus on the assessment and evaluation of policy, regulation, and organization that were identified as adding an ecological frame to the model (Porter, 2016). This was significant because at the time there was much more focus on

TABLE 3-3
Selected Frameworks for Dissemination or Implementation Science

TITLE OF FRAMEWORK	MAJOR PUBLICATIONS ABOUT FRAMEWORK	DESCRIPTION OF PREMISES, NOTABLE FEATURES
PRECEDE-PROCEED Model	Green (1974) Green & Kreuter (2005) Porter (2016) Websites: http://www.lgreen.net/precede.htm	Eight-stage process for planning, designing, implementing, and evaluating health promotion programs PRECEDE: Predisposing Reinforcing & Enabling Constructs in Educational Diagnosis & Evaluation PROCEED: Policy Regulatory & Organizational Constructs in Educational & Environmental Development
Reach, Effectiveness (originally Efficacy), Adoption, Implementation, Maintenance	Glasgow et al. (1999) Glasgow et al. (2019) Website: http://www.re-aim.org/	Model originally designed for evaluation of programs and then for planning Considered to be "compatible" with systems science and social–ecological foundations of many interventions Early in development, authors encouraged greater reporting of external validity—change made in constructs from efficacy to effectiveness

individual responsibility for one's own health and less on social, political, and contextual influences on health behaviors. The expansion of emphasis to the contextual influences was believed to add an ethical dimension to the factors that come into play for health intervention success.

A unique and often confusing characteristic of PRECEDE-PROCEED is that the eight phases it describes begin at the desired outcome (the desired end point). The rationale is to focus on a higher quality of life for a population rather than behaviors or health conditions (Porter, 2016). There are four assessment and planning phases that comprise the Precede activities, and four implementation and evaluation phases that combine as the Proceed actions. The phases are: (a) social assessment, (b) epidemiological assessment, (c) educational and ecological assessment, (d) administrative and policy assessment and intervention adjustment, (e) implementation, (f) process evaluation, (g) impact evaluation, and (h) outcome evaluation (Green & Kreuter, 2005). Particularly because of the phases that examine social, ecological, policy, and process evaluation, the model presents many foci for implementation research. Also, the authors very deliberately direct users of the model to incorporate appropriate theories of individual, organizational, or population behavior when conducting the assessments (Green & Kreuter, 2005; "New Features," 2005). Therefore, instruments that have been developed for those theories can be used for operationalizing the constructs of the model for implementation research.

RE-AIM was developed in the 1990s to help researchers gauge the public health impact of an intervention. Each of the words associated with the acronym represent a dimension of an intervention that should be evaluated to make this determination of impact. The idea put forward by the developers was that each dimension would be rated on a 0 to 1 (or 0% to 100%) scale. The Reach and Effectiveness dimensions were to be rated at the individual level. Adoption and Implementation were to have organizational- or community-level ratings, and Maintenance could be evaluated by individual and/or organizational ratings (Glasgow et al., 1999).

Reach, as a dimension evaluated in individuals, is the percentage and risk level of participants in an intervention compared with those who are not. Effectiveness, also rated on the individual level, has two subdimensions, positive and negative outcomes, and outcomes chosen for measurement. For this dimension, outcomes that are appropriate for the theory underlying the intervention would be chosen. For instance, if the theory postulated that certain behaviors would be changed because of the intervention, those behaviors should be assessed. Adoption was to be assessed in relation to the proportion of settings and the representativeness of the settings adopting the intervention. Implementation is judging the degree to which an intended intervention is implemented (in other words, the fidelity of the implementation). Lastly, Maintenance at the individual level pertains to the long-term continuance of the changed behaviors. At the organization level, Maintenance is judged to be the degree to which a new intervention becomes routine in the setting or community (Glasgow et al., 1999). As TS became a priority in health research, the developers then created a website (http://www.re-aim.org) to host resources that would support and foster IS (Dzewaltowski et al., 2004).

The efforts of the RE-AIM developers have greatly impacted IS. Glasgow et al. (2019) recently completed a review of the work that has been published using the RE-AIM framework. They noted that more than 450 publications have reported its use, both in North America and globally. They reported that it has been used in clinical sites, which is an expansion of its originally intended settings. Its usefulness in assisting researchers to document changes in their methods during an investigation and in exploration of cost issues in programs were noted, whereas ongoing needs to document maintenance of practice changes or programs over time were recognized. They identified needs for additional exploration of contextual factors that impact programs and their participants. This would bring the use of RE-AIM to be more in alignment with other frameworks that have recognized context as important in the implementation of new interventions and programs.

IS and DS frameworks have been developed to assist researchers in choosing appropriate methods for exploring factors that promote or present barriers to the successful adoption and integration of evidence-based and novel interventions in health care. Nurses engaged in IS and DS can use the frameworks for guidance in the measurement of relevant concepts and as structures for interpreting and reporting the findings of their research. Damschroder et al. (2009) observed that there were common domains of constructs across frameworks, and this should be apparent among the six frameworks discussed here. Resources and methods of use of the frameworks are addressed in the next section.

INSTRUMENTS, CHECKLISTS, AND METHODS ASSOCIATED WITH DISSEMINATION AND IMPLEMENTATION FRAMEWORKS

As this chapter draws to conclusion, it is time to consider one of the many challenges of engagement in DS and IS. Because various DS and IS frameworks have been described, operationalizing and measuring concepts of the frameworks have become a critical undertaking and are receiving great attention. The nurse scientist who engages in translational research will have to address the difficulties that have been encountered in the measurement challenge and are yet to be resolved.

Because of its early applications in TS and designation as an evaluation framework, developers of the RE-AIM framework (Glasgow et al., 1999) were among the first authors to bring measurement concerns forward (Glasgow, 2009). Development of the CFIR by Damschroder et al. (2009) also drew attention to the need for uniform definitions of the many concepts that were multiplying in DS and IS frameworks. The variability among concept definitions was soon identified as creating obstacles for the development of reliable and valid instruments that would allow precision in measurement while being practical for use in real-world settings (Martinez et al., 2014; Rabin et al., 2012). Precision in measurement is necessary in any translation research in order to detect changes in participants, staff members delivering interventions, or organization or communities. It is needed to capture change in the unique concepts of DS and IS such as reach, adoption, and maintenance or sustainability. Also, because DS and IS research is often focused on various units of measurement (individuals, organizations, and groups), the task of measuring concepts has additional complexity (Glasgow, 2009; Lewis et al., 2018; Martinez et al., 2014; Rabin et al., 2012).

Martinez et al. (2014) provided guidance regarding measurement issues to those who may embark on DS or IS investigations. They identified the following six critical issues impacting the measurement of concepts in translational research:

1. A growing number of frameworks, theories, and models
2. A need to establish instrument psychometric properties
3. Use of "homegrown" and adapted instruments
4. Choosing the most appropriate evaluation method and approach
5. Practicality of the instrument for use in real-world settings
6. A need for decision-making tools (Martinez et al., 2014, pp. 2-6)

For each of the identified issues, a discussion of the problems created by the issue and recommendations for a resolution were provided. For example, issue number one, the growth in frameworks, theories, and models, creates the problems of homonymy and synonymy. Homonymy is a situation in which a concept's definition is represented by different items in different instruments, whereas synonymy is a circumstance in which measures for different concepts have overlapping or the same items representing them (Lewis et al., 2018; Martinez et al., 2014). To combat these problems, Martinez et al. (2014) recommended a process among translation scientists to develop consensus definitions of major concepts in the field so that psychometric testing on instruments representing the concepts could commence in a systematic manner.

The identification of measurement problems by Martinez et al. (2014) and others has been fruitful in stimulating action to address them. The Society for Implementation Research Collaboration (SIRC) created an instrument review project (IRP), and the National Institute for Mental Health at the National Institutes of Health has provided funding to members of the SIRC to review, synthesize, and rate the psychometric properties and practicality of instruments designed to measure DS and IS outcomes (Lewis et al., 2015; SIRC IRP, 2019; Zoellner & Porter, 2017). As a result of that work, a repository has been created wherein instruments for concepts from the CFIR are reviewed, and data summarizing their psychometric characteristics are available for a society membership fee (SIRC IRP, 2019).

These important efforts aside, there are recommendations available for measures representing some of the major DS and IS concepts. During the development of the RE-AIM model, Glasgow (2009) proposed using a journalist approach of who, what, where, why, how, and how long as a method of capturing program participation, implementation variables, and outcomes of a program. For some of the measures, a simple count obtained through tracking of participants, activities, or other aspects of the program followed by the use of a numerator-denominator calculation may suffice in creating percentages of the maximum possible occurrences for a variable. For example, the reach of a program could be estimated by dividing the number of actual participants in a program by the total number of eligible members of an organization or population. Other numerators and denominators could be selected for adoption and for concepts representing other possible outcomes.

In addition to author recommendations for concept measurement, nurse scientists involved in DS and IS work can access a variety of online resources that have been created by various research groups. The authors of RE-AIM (Glasgow et al., 1999), the CFIR (Damschroder et al., 2009), and several research initiatives have created and hosted websites that include information on the measurement of major concepts. Table 3-4 provides a list of several of the available websites that include

TABLE **3-4**

Resource Websites for Translational Science Concept Measurement

FRAMEWORK/ INITIATIVE NAME	WEB ADDRESS, AVAILABLE INFORMATION
Consolidated Framework for Implementation Research	https://cfirguide.org/ Interactive website including construct definitions, links to selected measures and the work of Society for Implementation Research Collaboration Instrument Review Project, and guidance for linking implementation strategies with contexts of use of the Consolidated Framework for Implementation Research
Dissemination & Implementation Models in Health Research & Practice	https://dissemination-implementation.org/index.aspx Interactive website to assist researchers to develop a logic model for choosing and applying dissemination and implementation science frameworks to a proposed project and selecting measures that will represent model concepts
National Cancer Institute's Grid-Enabled Measures	https://www.gem-measures.org/public/ Searchable database of measures for constructs in the behavioral, social, and other relevant sciences (e.g., implementation science) Links from Dissemination & Implementation Models measurement database land in the National Cancer Institute's Grid-Enabled Measures database
Pragmatic–explanatory continuum indicator summary	https://precis-2.org/ Website providing information on pragmatic-explanatory continuum indicator summary and pragmatic-explanatory continuum indicator summary-2 tools for planning pragmatic trials and gauging the degree to which each of the implementation dimensions are more controlled, or more pragmatic A tool kit document can be downloaded that provides instructions on use of the tool
Reach, Effectiveness, Adoption, Implementation, Maintenance	http://www.re-aim.org/ Website providing up-to-date information about the framework, how to apply it, tools for planning a project using RE-AIM, measures and checklists that can be used for concepts, and training modules
Society for Implementation Research Collaboration Instrument Review Project	https://societyforimplementationresearchcollaboration.org/sirc -instrument-project/ Describes the progress of the Society for Implementation Research Collaboration Instrument Review Project work and provides a link to the repository of measures with psychometric properties that is available through a membership fee

information about measuring concepts in DS and IS, as well as other guidance for planning research designs and methods appropriate for TS.

To contribute to progress in TS, the concept of measurement problems in the field must be addressed. Measures must be reliable and valid to enhance the internal validity of a study, allowing for confidence in interpreting study findings and reporting outcomes of a project. As important as measurement is to IS and DS, there are as many concerns for overall design and methodology of an investigation because the emphasis in these studies is the external validity (generalizability) of interventions and procedures to implement them in real-world settings. Procedures as well as measurements must be appropriate in order to generate confidence in the observed outcomes of research and their applicability to other contexts. Creating a balance of control and flexibility in the methods of an investigation is another challenge for TS.

In Chapter 2, we identified PCTs as designs appropriate for TS. To plan a rigorous PCT that accounts for the participants and contexts of real-world settings, many decisions about control balanced with flexibility in procedures must be made. An instrument has been developed that assists researchers to gauge how much a study's procedures adhere to the characteristics of a controlled experiment or allow flexibility, which is the intent of a PCT. The pragmatic–explanatory continuum indicator summary (PRECIS; Thorpe et al., 2009) and its revision, PRECIS-2 (Loudon et al., 2015), are measures in which 10 (PRECIS) or 9 (PRECIS-2) dimensions of a translation study are rated as similar to a RCT or are flexible as in a PCT.

PRECIS (Thorpe et al., 2009) was one of the outcomes of work completed to modify the Consolidated Standards of Reporting Trials statement (a standard list of elements of a research report for RCTs; see http://www.consort-statement.org/) to assess PCTs and a work group created by international researchers to develop web-based pragmatic trials in developing countries (Treweek et al., 2006; Zwarenstein et al., 2008). This work was performed with the acknowledgment that the degree to which any particular study adhered to standards for RCTs, or aimed to achieve a more realistic implementation, should be considered as falling along a continuum rather than being judged as representing opposite poles of design for efficacy or pragmatism. Rating scales for design elements such as sampling, intervention fidelity (or flexibility), expertise of interveners, intensity of monitoring of participant adherence to the protocol, and other procedures were developed. To use the tool, researchers make judgments about how procedures of each dimension follow the principles of control or were planned and implemented to be more flexible. The ratings for each set of procedures are then plotted on a wheel-like diagram in which each "spoke" represents a design dimension. The connection of the points at which the dimensions were rated gives an overall picture of the study as being more controlled or more pragmatic. It should be noted that each dimension is rated independently, and some dimensions could be designed to maintain a great deal of control, whereas others in the same study might be very flexible (Thorpe et al., 2009). Since the development of PRECIS, some work has been done to establish inter-rater reliability in ratings of specific trials (Gaglio et al., 2014; Glasgow et al., 2012), as well as criterion and construct validity. Table 3-4 includes information about the website created to assist researchers with the use of PRECIS-2 (Loudon et al., 2015), which was a modification of PRECIS to 9 rather than 10 dimensions and changes of the rating scale from 1 (*very controlled*) to 5 (*very pragmatic*). The available assistance includes a downloadable tool kit document.

CONCLUSION

Theories, frameworks, and models arising from nursing and other disciplines that can guide TS investigations were described in this chapter. Resources for further exploration of these frameworks were provided. Finally, challenges encountered in DS and IS investigations, including the identification of psychometrically sound measures and achieving appropriate balance between control and pragmatic procedures, were presented, and resources for addressing the challenges were reviewed.

REFLECTIVE QUESTIONS

1. Define models, frameworks, and theories related to TS.
2. Select at least one implementation model (framework) and apply the major concepts to your implementation plan of a project.
3. Identify at least one dissemination framework that you would include in your dissemination plan for your project.
4. Identify measurement concerns related to implementation and dissemination frameworks.

REFERENCES

Bandura, A. (1997). Sources of self-efficacy. In A. Bandura (Ed.), *Self-efficacy: The exercise of control* (pp. 79-115). W. H. Freeman.

Battaglia, C., & Glasgow, R. E. (2018). Pragmatic dissemination and implementation research models, methods and measures and their relevance for nursing research. *Nursing Outlook, 66*, 430-445.

Benoliel, J. Q. (1977). The interaction between theory and research. *Nursing Outlook, 25*(2), 108-113.

Canadian Institutes of Health Research. (2013). Our mandate. http://www.cihr-irsc.gc.ca/e/7263.html

Canadian Institutes of Health Research. (2018). About us—CIHR. http://www.cihr-irsc.gc.ca/e/37792.html

Canadian Institutes of Health Research. (2019). Knowledge translation. http://www.cihr-irsc.gc.ca/e/29529.html

Carper, B. (1978). Fundamental patterns of knowing in nursing. *Advances in Nursing Science, 1*(1), 13-23.

Consolidated Framework for Implementation Research. (2019a). CFIR technical assistance website. https://cfirguide.org/

Consolidated Framework for Implementation Research. (2019b). What is the CFIR? https://cfirguide.org/

Damschroder, L. J., Aron, D. C., Keith, R. E., Kirsh, S. R., Alexander, J. A., & Lowery, J. C. (2009). Fostering implementation of health services research findings into practice: A consolidated framework for advancing implementation science. *Implementation Science, 4*, 50. https://doi.org/10.1186/1748-5908-4-50

Dearing, J. W., & Cox, J. G. (2018). Diffusion of innovations theory, principles, and practice. *Health Affairs, 37*(2), 183-190.

Dickoff, J., James, P., & Weidenbach, E. (1968). Theory in a practice discipline part II: Practice oriented research. *Nursing Research, 17*(6), 545-554.

Dintrans, P. V., Bossert, T. J., Sherry, J., & Kruk, M. E. (2019). A synthesis of implementation science frameworks and application to global health gaps. *Global Health Research and Policy, 4*, 25. https://doi.org/10.1186/s41256-019-0115-1

Drolet, B. C., & Lorenzi, N. M. (2011). Translational research: Understanding the continuum from bench to bedside. *Translational Research, 157*, 1-5.

Dzewaltowski, D. A., Glasgow, R. E., Klesges, L. M., Estabrooks, P. A., & Brock, E. (2004). RE-AIM: Evidence-based standards and a web-resource to improve translation of research into practice. *Annals of Behavioral Medicine, 28*(2), 75-80.

Fawcett, J. (1978). The relationship between theory and research: A double helix. *Advances in Nursing Science, 1*(1), 49-62.

Gaglio, B., Phillips, S. M., Heurtin-Roberts, S., Sanchez, M. A., & Glasgow, R. E. (2014). How pragmatic is it? Lessons learned using PRECIS and RE-AIM for determining pragmatic characteristics of research. *Implementation Science, 9*, 1-11. https://doi.org/10.1186/s13012-014-0096-x

Glanz, K., Rimer, B. K., & Viswanath, K. (2008). Theory, research, and practice in health behavior and health education. In K. Glanz, B. K. Rimer, & K. Viswanath (Eds.), *Health behavior and health education: Theory, research, and practice* (4th ed., pp. 23-40). Jossey-Bass.

Glasgow, R. E. (2009). Critical measurement issues in translational research. *Research on Social Work Practice, 19*, 560-568. https://doi.org/10.1177/1049731509335497

Glasgow, R. E., Green, L. W., Taylor, M. V., & Stange, K. C. (2012). An evidence integration triangle for aligning science with policy and practice. *American Journal of Preventive Medicine, 42*(6), 646-654. https://doi.org/10.1016/j.amepre.2012.02.016

Glasgow, R. E., Harden, S. M., Gaglio, B., Rabin, B., Smith, M. L., Porter, G. C., Ory, M. G. & Estabrooks, P. A. (2019). RE-AIM planning and evaluation framework: Adapting to new science and practice with a 20-year review. *Frontiers in Public Health, 7*(64). https://doi.org/10.3389/fpubh.2019.00064

Glasgow, R. E., Vogt, T. M., & Boles, S. M. (1999). Evaluating the public health impact of health promotion interventions: The RE-AIM framework. *American Journal of Public Health, 89*, 1322-1327.

Graham, I. D., Logan, J., Harrison, M. B., Straus, S. E., Tetroe, J., Caswell, W., & Robinson, N. (2006). Lost in knowledge translation: Time for a map? *The Journal of Continuing Education in the Health Professions, 26*(1), 13-24. https://doi.org/10.1002/chp.47

Green, L. (1974). Toward cost-benefit evaluations of health education: Some concepts, methods, and examples. *Health Education & Behavior, 2*(1, Suppl.), 34-64.

Green, L., & Kreuter, M. K. (2005). *Health program planning: An educational and ecological approach.* McGraw-Hill.

Harvey, G., & Kitson, A. (2015). PARIHS re-visited: Introducing i-PARIHS. In G. Harvey, & A. Kitson (Eds.), *Implementing evidence-based practice in health care: A facilitation guide* (pp. 25-46). Routledge.

Harvey, G., & Kitson, A. (2016). PARIHS revisited: From heuristic to integrated framework for the successful implementation of knowledge into practice. *Implementation Science, 11*, 33, 1-13. https://doi.org/10.1186/s13012-016-0398-2

Helfrich, C. D., Damschroder, L. D., Hagedorn, H.J., Daggett, G. S., Sahay, A., Ritchie, M., Damush, T., Guihan, M., Ullrich, P. M., & Stetler, C. B. (2010). A critical synthesis of literature on the promoting action on research implementation in health services (PARIHS) framework. *Implementation Science, 5*(82). http://www.implementationscience.com/content/5/1/82

Kim, H. S. (2010). *The nature of theoretical thinking in nursing* (3rd ed.). Springer.

Kirk, M. A., Kelley, C., Yankey, N., Birken, S. A., Abadie, B., & Damschroder, L. (2016). A systematic review of the consolidated framework for implementation research. *Implementation Science, 11*, 72. https://doi.org/10.1186/s13012-016-0437-z

Kitson, A., Harvey, G., & McCormack, B. (1998). Enabling the implementation of evidence-based practice: A conceptual framework. *Quality in Health Care, 7*(3), 149-158.

Kivunja, C. (2018). Distinguishing between theory, theoretical framework, and conceptual framework: A systematic review of lessons from the field. *International Journal of Higher Education, 7*(6), 44-53. https://doi.org/10.5430/ijhe.v7n6p44

Laycock, A., Harvey, G., Percival, N., Cummingham, F., Bailie, J., Matthews, V., Copley, K., Patel, L., & Bailie, R. (2018). Application of the i-PARIHS framework for enhancing understanding of interactive dissemination to achieve wide-scale improvement in Indigenous primary healthcare. *Health Research Policy and Systems, 16*(117). https://doi.org/10.1186/s12961-018-0392-z

Lewis, C. C., Proctor, E. K., & Brownson, R. C. (2018). Measurement issues in dissemination and implementation research. In R. C. Brownson, G. A. Colditz, & E. K. Proctor (Eds.), *Dissemination and implementation research in health: Translating science to practice* (2nd ed., pp. 441-470). Oxford University Press.

Lewis, C. C., Weiner, B.J., Stanick, C., & Fischer, S. M. (2015). Advancing implementation science through measure development and evaluation: A study protocol. *Implementation Science, 10*, 102. https://doi.org/10.1186/s13012-015-0287-0

Loudon, K., Treweek, S., Sullivan, F., Donnan, P., Thorpe, K. E., & Zwarenstein, M. (2015). The PRECIS-2 tool: Designing trials that are fit for purpose. *British Medical Journal, 350*, h2147. https://doi.org/10.1136/bmj.h2147

Martinez, R. G., Lewis, C. C., & Weiner B. J. (2014). Instrumentation issues in implementation science. *Implementation Science, 9*, 118, 1-9. https://doi.org/10.1186/s13012-014-0118-8

May, C. (2013). Towards a general theory of implementation. *Implementation Science, 8*, 18. https://doi.org/10.1186/1748-5908-8-18

McEwan, M. (2014). Overview of theory in nursing. In M. McEwan, & E. M. Wills (Eds.), *Theoretical basis for nursing* (4th ed., pp. 23-48). Wolters Kluwer.

Mitchell, S. A., Fisher, C. A., Hastings, C. E., Silverman, L. B., & Wallen, G. R. (2010). A thematic analysis of theoretical models for translational science in nursing: Mapping the field. *Nursing Outlook, 58*(6), 287-300.

Nair, S. (2016). A resource for instructors, students, health practitioners, and researchers using the PRECEDE-PROCEED model for health program planning and evaluation. http://lgreen.net/index.html

New Features, Flow, and Updated References in 4th Edition, 2005. (2005). http://www.lgreen.net/hpp/Endnotes/Endnotes.htm

Nilsen, P. (2015). Making sense of implementation theories, models and frameworks. *Implementation Science, 10*, 53.

Porter, C. M. (2016). Revisiting Precede-Proceed: A leading model for ecological and ethical health promotion. *Health Education Journal, 75*(6), 753-764. https://doi.org.ezproxy.gvsu.edu/10.1177/0017896915619645

Rabin, B. A., Purcell, P., Naveed, S., Moser, R. P., Henton, M. D., Proctor, E. K., Brownson, R. C., & Glasgow, R. E. (2012). Advancing the application, quality and harmonization of implementation science measures. *Implementation Science, 7*, 119. https://doi.org/10.1186/1748-5908-7-119

RAND Health Care. (2019). What we do. https://www.rand.org/health-care.html

Rogers, E. M. (1983). *Diffusion of innovations* (3rd ed.). Free Press.

Rogers, E. M. (2003). *Diffusion of innovations* (5th ed.). Free Press.

Rycroft-Malone, J. (2004). The PARIHS framework—A framework for guiding the implementation of evidence-based practice. *Journal of Nursing Care Quality, 19*(4), 297-304.

Rycroft-Malone, J., & Bucknall, T. (2010). Theories, frameworks, and models: Laying down the groundwork. In J. Rycroft-Malone, & T. Bucknall (Eds.), *Models and frameworks for implementing evidence-based practice: Linking evidence to action* (pp. 35-53). Wiley-Blackwell.

Society for Implementation Research Instrument Review Project. (2019). The SIRC Instrument Review Project (IRP): A systematic review and synthesis of implementation science instruments. https://societyforimplementationresearchcol laboration.org/sirc-instrument-project/

Tabak, R. G., Chambers, D. A., Hook, M., & Brownson, R. C. (2018). The conceptual basis for dissemination and imple-mentation research: Lessons from existing models and frameworks. In R. C. Brownson, G. A. Colditz, & E. K. Proctor (Eds.), *Dissemination and implementation research in health: Translating science to practice* (2nd ed., pp. 164-191). Oxford University Press.

Tabak, R. G., Khoong, E. C., Chambers, D. A, & Brownson, R. C. (2012). Bridging research and practice: Models for dis-semination and implementation research. *American Journal of Preventive Medicine, 43*(3), 337-350.

Thorpe, K. E., Zwarenstein, M., Oxman, A. D., Treweek, S., Furberg, C. D., Altman, D. G., Tunis, S., Bergel, E., Harvey, I., Magid, D. J., & Chalkidou, K. (2009). A pragmatic–explanatory continuum indicator summary (PRECIS): A tool to help trial designers. *CMAJ: Canadian Medical Association Journal, 180*(10), E47-E57.

Treweek, S., McCormack, K., Abalos, E., Campbell, M., Ramsay, C., Zwarenstein, M. (2006). The Trial Protocol Tool: The PRACTIHC software tool that supported the writing of protocols for pragmatic randomized controlled trials. *Journal of Clinical Epidemiology, 59*(11), 1127-1133. https://doi.org/10.1016/j.jclinepi.2005.12.019

Whittemore, R., & Grey, M. (2002). The systematic development of nursing interventions. *Journal of Nursing Scholarship, 34*, 115-120.

Winkler, J. D., Lohr, K. N., & Brook, R. H. (1985). Persuasive communication and medical technology assessment. *Archives of Internal Medicine, 145*(2), 314-317.

Zoellner, J. M., & Porter, K. J. (2017). Translational research: Concepts and methods in dissemination and implementation research. In A.M. Coulston, C. J. Boushey, M. G. Ferruzzi, & L. M. Delahanty (Eds.), *Nutrition in the prevention and treatment of disease* (4th ed., pp. 125-143). Elsevier. https://dx.doi.org/10.1016/B978-0-12-802928-2.00006-0

Zwarenstein, M., Treweek, S., Gagnier, J. J., Altman, D. G., Tunis, S., Haynes, B., Oxman, A. D., Moher, D., CONSORT Group., & Pragmatic Trials in Healthcare Group. (2008). Improving the reporting of pragmatic trials: An extension of the CONSORT statement. *British Medical Journal, 337*, a2390. https://doi.org/10.1136/bmj.a2390

SCHOLARSHIP FOR ACADEMIC NURSING
Alignment With Implementation and Dissemination Sciences?

Cynthia Peltier Coviak, PhD, RN, FNAP

CHAPTER OBJECTIVES

- Define scholarship for academic nursing inclusive of discovery, integration, application, and teaching
- Explore scientific inquiry and the scholarship of practice and teaching in the context of implementation frameworks
- Examine Carper's ways of knowing and how this theoretical framework intersects with nursing's knowledge, scholarship, and practice as a value proposition for nursing
- Consider implementation and dissemination science applications of population health in scholarship, education, and practice

---

Roussel, L. A., & Thomas, P. L. (Eds.). *Implementation Science in Nursing: A Framework for Education and Practice* (pp. 55-71).

KEY WORDS

- Application
- Collaboration
- Discovery
- Dissemination science
- Implementation science
- Inquiry
- Integration
- Interprofessional

- Nurse scientist
- Patterns of knowing
- Programs of scholarship
- Scholarship
- Scholarship of practice
- Scholarship of teaching
- Translational science

In this chapter, scholarship for academic nursing (American Association of Colleges of Nursing [AACN], 2018) and its foundations in the work of Boyer (1990, 1996) are described. The enactment of the scholarship of discovery, integration, application, teaching, and engagement is illustrated for the pursuit of implementation science (IS) and dissemination science (DS) through the discussion of case examples of nurse scientist involvement in health informatics and community evidence-based health promotion programs. The intersection of the types of nursing scholarship, partnerships with clinical entities, and a commitment to the use of Carper's ways of knowing (1978) in translational science (TS) activities is recognized as a position from which collaboration, advocacy, and quality improvement can occur.

SCHOLARSHIP FOR ACADEMIC NURSING: HOW IS IT ALIGNED WITH IMPLEMENTATION AND DISSEMINATION SCIENCES?

To meet the goals of the remaining consequential contributors in global health systems, nursing, medicine, and the other health professions are at an important point in their ongoing evolution. As discussed in previous chapters, health professionals in every field have been called to address the needs for reform in the health care enterprise (Institute for Healthcare Improvement [IHI], 2019; Institute of Medicine [IOM], 2000, 2001). Increasing the prevalence of evidence-based practice (EBP) is recognized as one way of impacting quality and safety in the health system (IOM, 2001, 2007). Emphasis on this strategy for improvement requires concerted efforts to bring appropriate, timely, and effective interventions to health professionals' contacts with clients. Accelerating the transfer of knowledge to care providers about effective interventions and monitoring the ways in which these are incorporated in routine practice are paramount to the goal of having clinical decisions "supported by accurate, timely, and up-to-date clinical information" reflecting "the best available evidence" (IOM, 2007, p. ix). TS in general and DS and IS specifically are forms of scientific inquiry that provide health professionals with data that can inform and substantiate the approaches taken to facilitate knowledge transfer, document the processes and outcomes of the knowledge transfer, and ensure ongoing use of the EBPs that are introduced. By engaging in DS and IS, nursing faculty can address many of the needs of the health care system while fulfilling the roles of academic professionals and scholars.

SCIENTIFIC INQUIRY, SCHOLARSHIP FOR PRACTICE AND TEACHING, AND TRANSLATIONAL SCIENCE

In successive position statements by the AACN, visions of the future of academic nursing (AACN, 2016) and the qualifications and skills of nursing faculty (AACN, 2017) created the foundations for a revised definition of scholarship for nursing (AACN, 2018), encompassing all four of the domains of scholarship identified in Boyer's (1990) famous report to the Carnegie Foundation titled *Scholarship Reconsidered: Priorities of the Professoriate*. The consensus position statement *Defining Scholarship for Academic Nursing* (AACN, 2018) and a document contributing to the statement titled *Advancing Healthcare Transformation: A New Era for Academic Nursing* (AACN, 2016) presented expectations that nursing faculty would "demonstrate a commitment to inquiry, generate new knowledge for the discipline, connect practice with education, and lead scholarly pursuits that improve health and health care" (AACN, 2016, as cited in AACN, 2018, p. 1).

AACN noted the nature of research, practice, and education in nursing as interprofessional as well as being multidisciplinary, interdisciplinary, and transdisciplinary (AACN, 2018, p. 2). Intersections among the interests of health system improvement, interprofessional and multidisciplinary scholarship, knowledge transfer, and connections to practice engender logical connections to the major concerns that DS and IS address and that are appropriate emphases for the practice and scientific bases of nursing. AACN's (2018) statement on scholarship "calls out" Boyer's (1990) views, including the scholarship of integration, application, and teaching, as well as discovery. Because the scholarship of application can be thought of as associated with practice, and integration is an activity that can occur in concert with practice and teaching as well as empirics, the major roles and responsibilities of nursing faculty fit Boyer's observations well. Practice and teaching are pursuits complementary to the ethical, esthetic, and personal patterns of knowing described by Carper (1978). Their inclusion in the academic scholarship of nursing augment and harmonize with the scholarship of discovery, which has been the traditional scholarly emphasis of the nursing professoriat. In addition, AACN (2018) advocates for scholarship expectations that place value on "all scholarly contributions" that are "inclusive and supports multiple ways of knowing" (p. 2). The position statement thereby promotes Carper's (1978) view of knowing in nursing united with Boyer's views.

Engagement in scholarship that aligns with Boyer's report has an additional relevance to the advancement of IS and DS because these new sciences gained prominence at a time when calls for cost containment and quality improvement and pressures to demonstrate how professional work was of benefit to society were intensifying. In higher education, the primary tensions arose around rededication of institutions to a well-rounded, recognizable involvement in the teaching and community service missions of academe, whereas in health care the challenge to incorporate the large amounts of evidence already available to professionals was the more crucial issue. With a prominent feature of IS and DS being the need for interdisciplinary and interprofessional collaboration, Boyer's scholarship of integration was relevant to collaboration among academic implementation scientists, including nurses. Boyer's call for the scholarship of application was certainly appropriate for academic disciplines like nursing that are devoted to the preparation of professionals who must bring the evidence generated through the scholarship of discovery to the practice environment. Also, the scholarship of teaching could not only address the best methods for educating health care professionals while in their preparatory programs but also could spawn new methods of disseminating evidence to professionals already in practice. This form of scholarship could prompt examination of the processes that best prepare health professionals to engage in team-based health care and scientific teams needed for IS and DS. The AACN (2018) statement on scholarship not only embraced all of the types of scholarship advocated by Boyer but also articulated the validity of IS as an area of discovery.

In accepting Boyer's (1990) work to frame the scholarship of nursing faculty, the underlying value of an academic institution to its community must be understood, as well as the concrete ways the faculty members contribute to the discovery, integration, and application of knowledge. In addition, a stance advanced by Boyer in later writings that is applicable but has received much less attention is the need for a scholarship of engagement among faculty and students in the communities in which their institutions are embedded (Boyer, 1996). Noting a parallel to the historical involvement of the land-grant institutions in addressing demands of life in rural America, Boyer (1996) called on academia to become engaged with communities to address the many challenges that are currently faced by their citizens. Specifically adding cities, schools, and their inhabitants as potential milieus for academic engagement, Boyer's ongoing call for relevance of those who fulfill academic roles provided another dimension of appropriate scholarship for nurses and for furthering TS. The advent of community-based participatory research as a method of investigation also supports this scholarly dimension as appropriate for nursing (Burrell et al., 2005).

To be of value to a community and its residents, interventions tested in discovery scholarship must be translated for widespread use. The translation of new interventions to practice environments in response to community needs can be facilitated through approaches interpreted and actualized by academic nurses using IS and DS frameworks that guide the adoption and evaluation of the intervention. As engaged partners in the processes of change, nursing faculty and their academic institutions become a community asset. In this way, engaged nursing faculty can refashion relationships with health care communities in the traditions of the land-grant institutions and agrarian communities.

Bringing the Scholarship of Practice and Teaching to Life: How Do We Do It?

To foster the adoption of its vision for scholarship in nursing, the AACN professed commitment to a premise that academia required diversity among the faculty. Diversity was needed to best address the varying missions of nursing programs in their larger institutions. Various levels and types of educational preparation, areas of expertise, preparation for roles, and potential contributions to the educational enterprise assist the professoriat to fulfill its responsibilities to society (AACN, 2017). In the enactment of these ideas, institutions have faculty bearing leadership and teaching roles who hold both research-intensive degrees and practice doctorates. Traditional research-focused degrees include the doctor of philosophy (PhD), doctor of nursing science (DNS), and doctor of the science of nursing (DSN). In contemporary nursing education, most faculty holding practice doctorates earned the doctor of nursing practice (DNP).

To accomplish the educational mission, the doctorally prepared nursing faculty partner with nurses within and outside their academic institutions who hold master's degrees and who have relevant clinical expertise. The areas of expertise represented among faculty include nursing science but also the science of related disciplines, such as psychology, business, educational leadership, health informatics and data science, health policy, and others. Because of the diversity of these faculty backgrounds, there is great potential for long-lasting and impactful engagement in IS and DS that is embedded in the scholarship dimensions espoused by Boyer (1990, 1996).

The scientific backgrounds of nurses who have research-intensive degrees provide knowledge and skills enabling the design of IS and DS research, the development of new or the expansion and testing of existing IS and DS frameworks, and contributions to TS knowledge through a scholarship program focused on discovery. Having completed coursework and projects that encompass theory critique and development, research methodologies, qualitative or quantitative analysis, and areas of science that augment their chosen research areas (Buchholz et al., 2015; Cygan & Reed, 2019; Trautman et al., 2018), they are prepared to answer many of the questions IS and DS pose.

Alternately, these faculty members can develop expertise in the evaluation of IS and DS efforts or in using the products of TS to develop and foster the adoption of health policy or innovative organizational practices. These efforts combine discovery, integration, and application dimensions of scholarship in succession or simultaneously.

To build a program of scholarship based on discovery, research-focused faculty may begin to inform IS and DS through descriptive studies of outcomes from practice or organizational changes and of the actions that contributed to the outcomes. Experimental designs may be used to test various interventions by using methods suggested by an IS or DS framework. To enhance the ability to generalize findings through increases in statistical power made possible by larger sample sizes, multiple settings may be included for IS and DS. Nurses who hold research-intensive doctorates have expertise for managing these complex data and facilitating analyses that they can bring to IS and DS investigations.

The completion and publication of an IS or DS study provide opportunities for expansion of the endeavor. Frameworks that were used for the study can be examined in light of the findings. The areas of the framework that were supported or would benefit from modification or expansion could be identified. The theories of IS and DS are drawn from many diverse disciplines. Through collaboration with scientists from other disciplines whose foci address the advantages or gaps of the tested framework, the scholarship of integration may be achieved. During the advancing careers of IS and DS scientists, their ongoing activities within the settings where TS is carried out provide rich opportunities for the scholarship of engagement. Rather than moving from setting to setting to conduct research, these nurse translational scientists can build their scholarship on various implementation needs of settings over time and become resources and advocates for the clinical enterprise.

Faculty members who come to academia with practice degrees such as the DNP are usually quite focused on the scholarship of application (Buchholz et al., 2015; Cygan & Reed, 2019; Moore, 2014; Trautman et al., 2018). The use of evidence in direct or indirect care of clients and for improvement in population health outcomes is a hallmark of the curriculum for the DNP-prepared nurse (AACN, 2006; Melnyk, 2013). The DNP graduate's focus on practice and quality improvement provides real-world experiences in using frameworks while assessing systems, facilitating and enacting changes in care settings, and evaluating the outcomes from these actions. While carrying out these activities, place-based knowledge may be generated (i.e., knowledge gained from experiencing, reflecting upon, and collecting evidence that addresses improvement in the patient experience and population health). Ultimately, as suggested by the IHI's Triple Aim (IHI, 2020), these activities may contribute to the reduction of per capita health care costs, but the knowledge is not generalizable to other contexts. For the faculty member holding a DNP degree, an intentional focus on the use of Carper's (1978) patterns of knowing can greatly enhance the scholarship of application while incorporating the scholarship of integration and engagement to ensure the fit of an implementation approach for the people, place, processes, and desired products of a practice change.

Several authors have examined frameworks for and examples of collaboration among PhD- and DNP-prepared faculty and students (Buchholz et al., 2015; Cygan & Reed, 2019; Murphy et al., 2015; Trautman et al., 2018). Some accounts have focused on the distribution of the responsibilities assumed by the different members of this type of intraprofessional team to bring a project to its successful conclusion. However, TS, like other sciences, is more than isolated scholarly projects. Completing a particular project is important, but to build TS, the optimal approach is to leverage each faculty member's unique preparation and expertise. Highly productive and beneficial scholarship programs can be achieved through collaborative research-focused and practice-focused faculty teams. As Carper (1978) suggested, empirical knowledge is only one of the patterns of knowing for nursing, and disciplinary and professional knowledge is gained from ethical, esthetic, and personal knowledge as well. A faculty team composed of practice-focused as well as research-focused nurses can more fully address all of the patterns of knowledge described by Carper (1978). In addition to actualizing the various types of scholarship and the patterns of knowing outlined for nursing, the faculty team engaged in IS or DS research can deliver products that fulfill the value proposition

TABLE 4-1

Possible Research-Focused and Practice-Focused Questions for a Translational Science Project

PROJECT STAGE	PRACTICE-FOCUSED QUESTIONS	RESEARCH-FOCUSED QUESTIONS
Preparation/ exploration	• What is the best evidence associated with this phenomenon/practice problem? • What is a realistic approach for addressing the problem or examining the phenomenon? • How effective are the current approaches to the phenomenon/problem?	• What is the phenomenon/ problem? • What gaps in disciplinary knowledge exist around this phenomenon/problem? • How do relevant frameworks and theories direct actions for the phenomenon/problem? • What is the efficacy and/ or effectiveness of the current approaches to the phenomenon?
Design	• What are the characteristics of the setting? • What method best suits the context (people, place, processes, etc.)? • What resources are available to intervene and sustain interventions after the project? • What adaptations may be necessary for broad application of the approach? Will they still have fidelity to the intervention's theoretical premises? • What measures can realistically be used now and in the future? • What resources for data collection and/or management will be available? • What resources are available to intervene and sustain interventions after the project?	• Where and when could intervention be tested? Who is best suited or trained to do this? • What method best suits the question (qualitative, quantitative; experimental, quasi-experimental)? • What is the conceptual validity of the intervention (fidelity to theory in planning and enactment)? • What best measures the concepts of the theory or framework? • How and in what format can data be collected and managed?

(continued)

TABLE **4-1** (CONTINUED)
Possible Research-Focused and Practice-Focused Questions for a Translational Science Project

PROJECT STAGE	PRACTICE-FOCUSED QUESTIONS	RESEARCH-FOCUSED QUESTIONS
Analysis	• What analysis is most needed for judging the effects of the implementation (or dissemination)? • Were the measures realistic for ongoing use and monitoring of the processes and outcomes? • What is missing from the analyses that would be needed for ongoing implementation?	• What analyses answer the research questions in a manner that can be generalized? • Were the measures reliable and valid within the chosen sample? • Can one have confidence in the results of the analyses through their degrees of power or the procedures done to enhance trustworthiness of qualitative data?
Interpretation and judging implications of project	• Was the approach appropriate for the context? • What areas of the project did the chosen theory/framework guide well or not well?	• Do the results support a conclusion of implementation efficacy or effectiveness? • Is the theory/framework supported by the results? Complete? Or needing modification/revisions?

for nursing, which includes innovation, health improvement among consumers, and discovery (Miyamoto, as cited by Cashion et al., 2019).

To achieve the goals of a collaborative scholarship team, its members' unique strengths and views of the phenomena studied should be recognized. With some members more focused on application and others more concerned with discovery, the questions arising from each team member's interests may reflect the differing emphases. Table 4-1 provides examples of the contrasting but complementary questions that scholarship team members may bring to an IS or DS project. As a team is formed, members may wish to use these or similar questions to discern the thoughts and foci of each collaborator.

Thus far, our discussion has addressed the ways that IS and DS can represent the enactment of the scholarship of discovery, application, integration, and engagement. The scholarship of teaching is also an important focus for the nursing professoriat, and leaders in IS and DS have documented the need to expand the numbers of students prepared specifically for the TS field (Baldwin et al., 2017; Meissner et al., 2013; Padek et al., 2015; Proctor et al., 2013, 2015). Nursing professors, with their ongoing focus on teaching the next generation of nursing professionals and scientists, have already been called to prepare students to function effectively in interprofessional teams (AACN, 2006, 2008, 2011; Interprofessional Education Collaborative, 2016; Interprofessional Education Collaborative Expert Panel, 2011; IOM, 2003). Methods that have been used in the study of interprofessional education may include designs and activities adaptable to the preparation of intra- and interdisciplinary TS teams.

A nursing professor seeking to pursue the scholarship of teaching could compare the knowledge, skills, or attitude outcomes between students receiving mentoring in TS from faculty teams that are interdisciplinary and those who were not in such teams. Alternately, student outcomes after participation in teams with both research-focused and practice-focused faculty mentors could be evaluated. The examination of faculty ratings of student performance within teams, student knowledge of IS and DS frameworks, and student perceptions of their abilities to use frameworks for advocacy efforts could be pursued. There are many desired TS competencies that could be explored (Padek et al., 2015; Strauss et al., 2011).

Other emphases for the scholarship of teaching could include the processes occurring during students' participation in IS or DS teams. For instance, studies describing the types of activities undertaken by students in practice-focused, contrasted with research-focused, degree programs could be completed during their involvement in faculty-led TS projects. This type of information may not only be of importance to educators but also to those who develop and direct TS training programs. The value of these projects is in their capacity to inform the creation of curricula for IS and DS research team members of the future.

Establishing, Nurturing, and Sustaining Translational Science Scholarship

To this point, many of the published accounts of TS undertaken by nurses have occurred in the contexts of large academic health centers and research-intensive academic institutions. However, the intent of the AACN statements on scholarship were to provide guidance for nursing faculty across the spectrum of constituent institutions (i.e., small liberal arts colleges to large research universities). The statements were designed to assist faculty with many variations in responsibilities, from highly weighted to practice, teaching, research, or a combination of the three. The majority of nursing programs in the United States are not housed within research-intensive universities that have the greatest resources to enable the scholarship of discovery. Even in the research institutions, there are likely to be many nursing faculty whose responsibilities are weighted toward practice and teaching who must still provide evidence of scholarship to advance in their academic careers (AACN, 2019; Shieh & Cullen, 2019).

Across these settings, no matter the composition or work responsibilities of their faculty, the schools are likely to be affiliated with clinical sites that would benefit from assistance of the faculty advancing the use of EBPs in their care activities or general operations. Many of the clinical sites would welcome the expertise of nursing faculty who have skill in applying frameworks for change and evaluating outcomes. Thus, nearly every nursing faculty member with interest in TS could devise plans to engage with their clinical affiliates or with TS teams to initiate and build programs of scholarship based in IS or DS.

To provide illustrations of some ways that scholarship based in IS or DS can be central to scholarship in academic nursing, two cases are presented. For each, characteristics of the projects, including people, places, processes, and products, are described, and the engagement of faculty in providing assistance to organizations and building the science are explained. One of the cases is a project that originated in the field of health and nursing informatics. The other describes a community-based project in which an evidence-based chronic disease self-management program was implemented.

Case Example 1

Case example 1 presents an illustration of a typical work team in the contemporary health informatics field. Because this team was led by a nursing faculty member whose scholarly focus was research, the student members could have perceived the project as irrelevant because they were preparing for professional practice roles. However, the nursing faculty member kept the team's focus on the requests of the clinical partner while highlighting the information that was discovered about the nursing practice on the unit. This being the case, the project represented the scholarship of engagement, application, and integration as well as of discovery.

The project described in the case example was not concentrated on IS, but as an initial step toward practice change in the health system, it could readily shift to an IS focus through discovery, engagement, and integration scholarship. For this, the implementation of a joint academic–community initiative would become the phenomenon of scrutiny. The process aspects of the implementation that might be considered could include how the academic team negotiated its role in the initiative and perceptions of each of the project team members regarding the way that implementation was enhanced or impediments arose because of the team's composition. The interactions of the student team members with health system representatives could be examined.

To further inform the implementation, a framework could be adopted that could guide actions, measures, and products of the team. In the informatics field, a number of implementation models have been used for the initiation and ongoing sustainability of technology interventions (Taherdoost, 2018). One of these could be used or one of the more general IS or DS frameworks might be more helpful. The Promoting Action on Research Implementation in Health Services framework (Harvey & Kitson, 2016; Kitson et al., 1998), which uses ideas such as a supportive context and beneficial facilitation as factors fostering organizational change, might be an appropriate model to use for the setting and personnel who were involved. Measures for many relevant concepts from these frameworks are available and could be used to contribute to TS. Members of the project team who had research-focused degrees could fashion their scholarship to test and evaluate the premises of theories used in the implementation. These questions would emphasize the use of the empirical pattern of knowing. Practice-focused members of the team could pursue application-based scholarship, focusing on processes, team member activities, and clinical and systems knowledge gained from their efforts. For them, the ethical, esthetic, and personal ways of knowing would be indispensable.

The health system's request and the involvement of the students in the implementation could have also been the basis for a project rooted in the scholarship of teaching. The unique combination of student and faculty expertise, backgrounds, knowledge, and skills would provide a distinctive portrayal of an interprofessional group educational exercise. Descriptions of the competencies addressed in the students' specific fields of study as well as in the domains of leadership and interprofessional team functioning could be developed. Comparisons of communication patterns that were exhibited by the team members, student and faculty opinions about insights they gained regarding unique and shared roles among the students of various disciplines, and the measurement of actual discipline-specific knowledge and skills that were transferred from team members of one field to another would have all been distinctive topics for a project directed toward teaching and learning. The curricular implications for the graduate programs whose students were members of the team could be inferred from what was discovered.

Overall, this case provides an example of how a typical student clinical or internship experience is adaptable to IS projects. By attending to the ways that faculty and students are engaged with clinical settings, nursing faculty can identify multiple opportunities for IS or DS projects representing forms of scholarship promoted by AACN (2018). In the next case, a faculty member's involvement in a community-based program implementation incorporates many of the scholarship dimensions we are discussing.

Case Example 2

Case example 2 is unique in that it involved one of the earliest efforts to translate evidence-based interventions to the community and had federal funding to back it up. Being an early effort, the intended activities of research partners were not clear; there were no previous projects on which to model the researchers' roles. Furthermore, TS in the community was not yet defined. In fact, the grants made by the Administration on Aging (AoA) coincided with the development of the National Institutes of Health's Roadmap (Zerhouni, 2003) and predated the 2006 funding of the Clinical and Translational Science Awards from the National Institutes of Health. Therefore, undertaking these projects and establishing the activities as distinct areas of scholarship could have been a perilous endeavor for an inexperienced faculty member who was not yet tenured. Fortunately, neither of these circumstances were the case for the nurse scientist engaged with community A.

Several of the concerns of IS and DS were enmeshed with the overriding goals of the evidence-based health promotion projects funded by the AoA. First, although the AoA was certainly interested in the population effects and client outcomes from the projects that were funded, the agency was just as invested in uncovering and publicizing effective and ineffective approaches for the initiation and ongoing success of the programs in communities. These process topics are major emphases of IS and DS. To address these issues, the nurse scientist and the Area Agency on Aging (AAoA) team maintained detailed records of the success of recruitment efforts; participant numbers and characteristics; attendance and dropout from program sessions; recruitment and involvement of volunteer program leaders; and participant perceptions of the program sessions' content, atmosphere, and helpfulness. As time went on, the perceptions of the community partners about involvement in the project were also obtained. The scholarly products that were the culmination of these efforts were several national presentations to the National Council on Aging constituency. Population needs, as well as implementation insights, were shared.

A second focus of the nurse scientist was in guiding the community partners in delivering the Chronic Disease Self-Management Program (CDSMP) accurately and reliably in accord with the guidelines available for the sessions. To obtain licenses to offer the program, the AAoA was required to have a number of master trainers educated by the Stanford Patient Education Center, but ongoing assessment of the trainers' fidelity to the program and their commitments to monitor the delivery of the program by their trainees were still important aspects of the nurse scientist's efforts. Because of her extensive knowledge of the ways that fidelity to a tested intervention could affect the expected outcomes of the intervention (Hanafin & O'Reilly, 2015), the nurse scientist knew that fidelity measurement was an important implementation metric. Special checklists that were adaptable for both the project staff and master trainers' uses were created by the nurse scientist for the assessment of the group leaders' performance in guiding the sessions and for consideration in relation to the eventual evaluation of the project outcomes. The statistical analyses published in the original descriptions of the CDSMP's testing were also used to benchmark the outcomes expected in the community research translation project. At each report period, the available data were analyzed, and changes in self-reported measures of overall health, self-efficacy for disease management, experiences of symptoms (e.g., fatigue, shortness of breath, pain), communication with health providers, and health system utilization were reported in relation to the data in published accounts. The project team could judge their success in facilitating disease management by comparing their clients' measures to the original CDSMP results.

Because the AoA community health promotion projects predated the publication of most implementation frameworks and the endorsement of the DNP as a terminal practice degree by the AACN, at the outset the nurse scientist approached the project in community A using general principles of community-based participatory research. This was a situation when using ethical, esthetic, and personal patterns of knowing served the nursing faculty member well. There were instances when the nurse scientist's prior experiences as a clinical nurse specialist were the practice foundations drawn on to negotiate the roles and responsibilities among the project leaders and to resolve disagreements and interpersonal tensions. For example, community partners were not always aware of the ethical responsibilities they had in collecting client data for research. They questioned the need for informed consent, and at first the nurse scientist's insistence on the consent procedures was perceived as inflexible. Having no process framework to guide her actions, her personal pattern of knowing was counted on to direct the steps to resolve the disagreement. This situation illustrated how the challenges of IS are not always described or predicted by the existing frameworks and standard procedures of scholarship. In this instance, the complementary guidance of multiple patterns of knowing was an asset for the advancement of IS.

Although an implementation framework was not initially applied to the project by the nurse scientist, the national resource center facilitated the consideration of several emerging models of health promotion and prevention that might be applicable across the multiple AoA funded projects. The RE-AIM (Reach, Effectiveness, Adoption, Implementation, Maintenance) framework (Glasgow et al., 1999) was being described in the public health literature and has since become one of the most widely used IS frameworks. Combining the evaluation and science-building aims of the AoA projects, RE-AIM was adopted to guide the consideration of project implementation and outcomes. Using each of the main concepts of the framework, the nurse scientist and several of the other research partners for the funded projects published an article in which they described aspects of project execution important for future evidence-based implementation endeavors. The article placed major weight on the ways that fidelity to the original health promotion programs was maintained, an important focus of IS.

In this case, a nurse scientist was invited to assist a community in the implementation of a health promotion program for older adults. Although this project was significantly removed from her usual areas of research, it represented a unique opportunity to engage with a diverse collective of service providers in program implementation. The nursing faculty member was given the chance to demonstrate the scholarship of application, integration, engagement, and discovery while experiencing the early emergence of IS science in the community.

CONCLUSION

The nursing professoriat has been challenged to contribute to nursing's value proposition by engaging in multiple forms of scholarship. As members of the academy, nursing faculty members can use Boyer's categorizations to advance TS while using unique backgrounds and expertise to improve the patient experience and population health while reducing health care costs—challenges posed by the IHI (2020). This chapter described a variety of approaches that can be used by faculty with diverse backgrounds and expertise to accomplish these goals. Two case examples were presented to illustrate the pursuit of IS and DS from the perspectives of these several forms of scholarship.

REFLECTIVE QUESTIONS

1. Case example 1 provides an illustration of Boyer's model of scholarship, specifically engagement, application, and integration as well as discovery. This can readily shift to an IS focus through discovery, engagement, and integration scholarship. Select at least two areas of focus (discover, engagement, or integration) and provide examples of IS using the Promoting Action on Research Implementation in Health Services framework.

2. Case example 2 integrates RE-AIM as a framework for this community health initiative. Using this framework provide another example of how a community health promotion project can be informed by scholarship of integration and improvement science.

REFERENCES

American Association of Colleges of Nursing. (2006). *The essentials of doctoral education for advanced nursing practice.* Author. https://www.aacnnursing.org/Portals/42/Publications/DNPEssentials.pdf

American Association of Colleges of Nursing. (2008). *The essentials of baccalaureate education for professional nursing practice.* Author. https://www.aacnnursing.org/Portals/42/Publications/BaccEssentials08.pdf

American Association of Colleges of Nursing. (2011). *The essentials of master's education in nursing.* Author. https://www.aacnnursing.org/Portals/42/Publications/MastersEssentials11.pdf

American Association of Colleges of Nursing. (2016). *Advancing healthcare transformation: A new era for academic nursing.* Author. https://www.aacnnursing.org/Portals/42/Publications/AACN-New-Era-Report.pdf

American Association of Colleges of Nursing. (2017). *Preferred vision of the professoriate in baccalaureate & graduate nursing programs.* Author. https://www.aacnnursing.org/News-Information/Position-Statements-White-Papers/Professoriate

American Association of Colleges of Nursing. (2018). *Defining scholarship for academic nursing.* Task Force Consensus Position Statement. Author. https://www.aacnnursing.org/News-Information/Position-Statements-White-Papers/Defining-Scholarship-Nursing

American Association of Colleges of Nursing. (2019). *FactSheet: AACN in brief.* https://www.aacnnursing.org/Portals/42/News/Factsheets/AACN-Fact-Sheet.pdf

Baldwin, J. A., Williamson, H. J., Eaves, E. R., Levin, B. L., Burton, D. L., & Massey, O. T. (2017). Broadening measures of success: Results of a behavioral health translational research training program. *Implementation Science, 12*(92), 1-11.

Boyer, E. L. (1990). *Scholarship reconsidered: Priorities of the professoriate.* The Carnegie Foundation for the Advancement of Teaching.

Boyer, E. L. (1996). The scholarship of engagement. *Journal of Public Service & Outreach, 1*(1), 11-20.

Buchholz, S. W., Yingling, C., Jones, K., & Tenfelde, S. (2015). DNP and PhD collaboration: Bringing together practice and research expertise as predegree and postdegree scholars. *Nurse Educator, 40*(4), 201-206. https://doi.org/10.1097/NNE.0000000000000141

Burrell, J., Shattell, M., & Habermann, B. (2005). The scholarship of engagement in nursing. *Nursing Outlook, 53,* 220-223. https://doi.org/10.1016/j.outlook.2005.02.003

Carper, B. (1978). Fundamental patterns of knowing in nursing. *Advances in Nursing Science, 1*(1), 13-23.

Cashion, A. K., Dickson, V. V., & Gough, L. L. (2019). The value and importance of PhD nurse scientists [Editorial]. *Journal of Nursing Scholarship, 51*(5), 611-613.

Cygan, H. R., & Reed, M. (2019). DNP and PhD scholarship: Making the case for collaboration. *Journal of Professional Nursing, 35,* 353-357. https://doi.org/10.1016/j.profnurs.2019.03.002

Glasgow, R. E., Vogt, T. M., & Boles, S. M. (1999). Evaluating the public health impact of health promotion interventions: The RE-AIM framework. *American Journal of Public Health, 89,* 1322-1327.

Hanafin, S., & O'Reilly, E. D. (2015). Implementation science: Issues of fidelity to consider in community nursing. *British Journal of Community Nursing, 20,* 437-443.

Harvey, G., & Kitson, A. (2016). PARIHS revisited: From heuristic to integrated framework for the successful implementation of knowledge into practice. *Implementation Science, 11,* 33. https://doi.org/10.1186/s13012-016-0398-2

Institute for Healthcare Improvement. (2019). Science of improvement. http://www.ihi.org/about/Pages/ScienceofImprovement.aspx

Institute for Healthcare Improvement. (2020). What is the Triple Aim? http://www.ihi.org/Topics/TripleAim/Pages/Overview.aspx

Institute of Medicine. (2000). *To err is human: Building a safer health system.* National Academies Press. https://doi.org/10.17226/9728

Institute of Medicine. (2001). *Crossing the quality chasm: A new health system for the 21st century.* National Academies Press. https://doi.org/10.17226/10027

Institute of Medicine. (2003). *Health professions education: A bridge to quality.* National Academies Press. https://doi.org/10.17226/10681

Institute of Medicine. (2007). *The learning healthcare system: Workshop summary.* National Academies Press. https://doi.org/10.17226/11903

Interprofessional Education Collaborative Expert Panel. (2011). *Core competencies for interprofessional collaborative practice: Report of an expert panel.* https://ipec.memberclicks.net/assets/2011-Original.pdf

Interprofessional Education Collaborative. (2016). *Core competencies for interprofessional collaborative practice: 2016 update.* Interprofessional Education Collaborative. https://ipec.memberclicks.net/assets/2016-Update.pdf

Kitson, A., Harvey, G., & McCormack, B. (1998). Enabling the implementation of evidence based practice: A conceptual framework. *Quality in Health Care, 7*(3), 149-158.

Meissner, H. I., Glasgow, R. E., Vinson, C. A., Chambers, D., Brownson, R. C., Green, L. W., Ammerman, A. S., Weiner, B. J., & Mittman, B. (2013). The U.S. training institute for dissemination and implementation research in health. *Implementation Science, 8*, 12. https://doi.org/10.1186/1748-5908-8-12

Melnyk, B. (2013). Distinguishing the preparation and roles of doctor of philosophy and doctor of nursing practice graduates: National implications for academic curricula and health care systems. *Journal of Nursing Education, 52*(8), 442-448.

Moore, K. (2014). How DNP and PhD nurses can collaborate to maximize patient care. *American Nurse Today, 9*(1), 48-49.

Murphy, M. P., Staffileno, B. A., & Carlson, E. (2015). Collaboration among DNP- and PhD-prepared nurses: Opportunity to drive positive change. *Journal of Professional Nursing, 31*(5), 388-394.

Padek, M., Brownson, R., Proctor, E., Colditz, G., Kreuter, M., Dobbins, M., Sales, A., & Pfund, C. (2015). Developing dissemination and implementation competencies for training programs. *Implementation Science, 10*(Suppl. 1), A39. https://doi.org/10.1186/1748-5908-10-S1-A39

Proctor, E., Carpenter, C., Brown, C. H., Neta, G., Glasgow, R., Grimshaw, J., Rabin, B., Fernandez, M., Brownson, R., Curran, G., Mittman, B., Collins, L., Palinkas, L., Duan, N., Wallace, A., Wells, K., Tabak, R., & Aarons, G. (2015). Advancing the science of dissemination and implementation: Three "6th NIH Meetings" on training, measures, and methods. *Implementation Science, 10*(Suppl. 1), A13. https://doi.org/10.1186/1748-5908-10-S1-A13

Proctor, E. K., Landsverk, J., Baumann, A. A., Mittman, B., Aarons, G. A., Brownson, R. C., Glisson, C., & Chambers, D. (2013). The implementation research institute: Training mental health implementation researchers in the United States. *Implementation Science, 8*, 105. https://doi.org/10.1186/1748-5908-8-105

Shieh, C., & Cullen, D. L. (2019). Mentoring nurse faculty: Outcomes of a three-year clinical track faculty initiative. *Journal of Professional Nursing, 35*, 162-169.

Strauss, S. E., Brouwers, M., Johnson, D., Lavis, J. N., Légare, F., Majumdar, S. R., McKibbon, K. A., Sales, A. E., Stacey, D., Klein, G., Grimshaw, J., & KT Canada Strategic Training Initiative in Health Research. (2011). Core competencies in the science and practice of knowledge translation: Description of a Canadian strategic training initiative. *Implementation Science, 6*, 127. https://doi.org/10.1186/1748-5908-6-127

Taherdoost, H. (2018). A review of technology acceptance and adoption models and theories. *Procedia Manufacturing, 22*, 960-967.

Trautman, D. E., Idzik, S., Hammersla, M., & Rossiter, R. (2018). Advancing scholarship through translational research: The role of PhD and DNP prepared nurses. *Online Journal of Issues in Nursing, 23*(2), 1-8. https://doi.org/10.3912/OJIN.Vol23No02Man02

Zerhouni, E. (2003). The NIH roadmap. *Science, 302*(5642), 63-72.

Exemplar 4-1

Knowledge Discovery From Electronic Data

Cynthia Peltier Coviak, PhD, RN, FNAP

For nearly 4 decades, nurse researchers who study health and nursing informatics have been attempting to describe the care provided to patients by examining nursing documentation in electronic health records (EHRs). A wide range of research interests underlie researcher efforts, from creating descriptions of the dimensions of nursing practice with particular populations to the development of statistical prediction models that weight various nursing interventions in their contributions to specific health care outcomes. From the efforts of these researchers, it has become evident that to obtain the relevant data from EHRs and to interpret the data appropriately, a multidisciplinary and interprofessional team is needed. Successful health and nursing informatics research requires the clinical expertise of nurses and other health care providers, the technical expertise of computer and data scientists, and nursing informaticists.

In a project initiated by a PhD-prepared nursing professor in a Midwestern university, a multidisciplinary and interprofessional research team was constituted that included graduate students in the nursing PhD and DNP programs, health informatics, data science, and computer science fields, as well as a visiting postdoctoral (PhD) nurse scholar. The project originated from a request of a local community health care system that included primary, acute, and tertiary care settings and that had used a particular EHR for many years. During those years, many of which preceded the 2019 passage of the Health Information Technology for Economic and Clinical Health Act, the EHR had been modified by the health system's information technology department to meet the health system's unique needs. The project purpose was an exploration of the nursing documentation system to map nursing diagnoses to appropriate interventions. The eventual goal was to use the mapping to later reveal the patient outcomes resulting from the interventions. Thus, the project was the first step in an ongoing quality improvement initiative in which the health system's own evidence was to later be used to drive a practice change.

As the faculty member leading the research team, the nursing professor's interests were the discovery aspects of the project. She wished to explore the phenomenon of nursing practice as documented in the EHR to better describe the contributions of the nurses to patient care. The postdoctoral nurse scholar was interested in the discovery of practice information in the record but also in the actual structure of the data within the EHR and how it facilitated nursing work. She was working with the team to build her own knowledge of the informatics field but also was a clinical expert for the data that were going to be examined. The data were to be extracted from a neonatal intensive care unit, and this researcher had practiced and taught pediatric nursing for 30 years.

The DNP students were pursuing a nursing informatics specialty. They were immersing themselves in the application of informatics and systems frameworks to the health system's uses of the EHR. They were concerned with the ways the EHR facilitated or interfered with nursing workflow in the health system, the interoperability within the system, the system structure, and various features of the information housed and used in the system. One of the DNP students was both a content expert and a resource for workflow assessment because she had been a staff nurse in the neonatal intensive care unit and was familiar with the way the floor nurses used the EHR. The team was completed with the health informatics, data science, and computer science students, who were preparing for professional roles that would entail programming, data and database management, information systems assessment, and working with clinical staff to optimize the utility of the electronic systems.

During the project, team members assumed responsibilities that were appropriate for their expertise, interests, and goals. Workflow assessments, summaries of the recorded data from the EHR, and a gap analysis describing ways the documentation system could be improved to yield more complete information about the required and provided care were prepared and delivered to the health system. At the end of the academic semester, the team reached its initial goals of mapping the nursing diagnoses to interventions, and this mapping would become the foundation of the health system's next steps in quality improvement.

REFERENCE

Office of the National Coordinator for Health Information Technology. (2019). Laws, regulation, and policy. Health IT legislation. https://www.healthit.gov/topic/laws-regulation-and-policy

/⎺⎺⎺⎺⎺⎺⎺⎺⎺⎺⎺⎺⎺⎺\
Exemplar 4-2
\⎽⎽⎽⎽⎽⎽⎽⎽⎽⎽⎽⎽⎽⎽/

COMMUNITY HEALTH PROMOTION PROJECT IMPLEMENTATION

Cynthia Peltier Coviak, PhD, RN, FNAP

In the early 2000s, the U.S. AoA began a program for enhancing the health of older adults through community translation of evidence-based projects. A number of grants were made to communities, and a national research center was funded to offer and evaluate programs designed to address mental health, chronic disease self-management, fall prevention, physical activity, and nutrition of older adults (National Council on Aging Center for Healthy Aging, 2006). Grantee organizations were required to not only offer the programs but also to have a researcher contracted to assist them in designing the program so that project implementation and outcomes could be monitored and evaluated throughout the grant period and at its conclusion. The organizations could create these contracts with any qualified individual, but in most cases the researchers were affiliated with academic institutions.

In community A, the grantee organization was an AAoA, and the contracted researcher was an experienced nursing professor. A professor at the researcher's university who was a gerontology specialist and the AAoA had collaborated to apply for the grant. This specialist recruited the nursing professor to join the implementation team because the chosen program was the CDSMP previously developed by Dr. Kate Lorig and her colleagues at Stanford University (Lorig et al., 1999, 2001). It was believed that with the disease management focus of the program, the expertise of a nurse scientist was needed for the project's evaluation.

The project's goal was to disseminate the CDSMP throughout the community through collaboration with the various organizations serving older adults. Particular emphasis was on engaging organizations that served the community's Black and Spanish-speaking populations. Because of the desire to provide the program for this broad audience, the community team included social workers, staff case management nurses in a local health management organization and at the AAoA, psychologists, career and rehabilitation counselors, case workers, and health care interpreters. The volunteers already associated with many of the organizations were also members of the team. As the project progressed, more volunteers were recruited to be the lay group leaders, who were the core of the program delivery efforts; these included teachers and retired professionals, such as financial industry specialists, clergy, and others.

The relationship of the community grantee organization to the national research center provided opportunities for and consultation with national experts in exercise science, public health professionals, physical therapists, well-known gerontologists, nurse scientists who specialized in research on programs for older adults, methodologists, statisticians, and experts of other disciplines. The national goals for these associations included developing knowledge of how community aging service provider organizations could become resources for the health promotion of older adults but also to facilitate national information sharing on the ways to build and sustain the programs while documenting the health outcomes among program participants.

The grants to the organizations were originally provided for 3 years. During each year, the grantee organizations were convened in national meetings where progress of individual projects was shared, brainstorming and problem solving among the grantees and their researchers were facilitated, and consultation with the national resource center staff was provided. The contracted project researchers initiated various presentations that were delivered at national meetings and coauthored publications that were completed via the Internet in the following months. As the final funding years approached, additional funding was awarded for dissemination efforts. Online "tool kits" were created that provided concrete advice concerning resources and personnel needed for program success, preparatory and ongoing activities for establishing and sustaining a health promotion program, examples of publicity and messaging for recruitment and community partner engagement, examples of surveys and measurements that could be used to evaluate projects, and other materials for widespread distribution to other communities desiring to initiate their own health promotion programs.

REFERENCES

Lorig, K., Ritter, P., Stewart, A., Sobel, D., Brown, B. W., Bandura, A., González, V. M., Laurent, D. D., & Holman, H. (2001). Chronic disease self-management program: 2-year health status and health care utilization outcomes. *Medical Care, 39*(11), 1217-1223.

Lorig, K., Sobel, D. S., Stewart, A., Brown, B. W., Bandura, A., Ritter, P., González, V. M., Laurent, D. D., & Holman, H. (1999). Evidence suggesting that a chronic disease self-management program can improve health status while reducing hospitalization: A randomized trial. *Medical Care, 37*(1), 5-14.

National Council on Aging Center for Healthy Aging. (2006). *Using the evidence base to promote healthy aging: The Administration on Aging's evidence-based prevention programs for the elderly initiative.* Issue Brief: Evidence-Based Health Promotion Series, No. 3. Author. www.ncoa.org.

IMPLEMENTATION SCIENCE AND PRACTICE

Implications for Nursing Education Through Content, Context, and Projects

Linda A. Roussel, PhD, RN, NEA-BC, CNL, FAAN
Patricia L. Thomas, PhD, RN, FAAN, FACHE, FNAP, NEA-BC, ACNS-BC, CNL

CHAPTER OBJECTIVES

- Describe implementation sciences and practices with implications for entry-level nursing education
- Outline how implementation and dissemination sciences and practices impact graduate nursing education and advanced nursing practice roles
- Outline assignments for didactic and experiential learning that can be incorporated into selected coursework for entry and graduate level students

KEY WORDS

- Advanced nursing practice roles
- Didactic learning
- Experiential learning
- Graduate nursing education
- Implementation practice
- Implementation science
- Practice immersion

Roussel, L. A., & Thomas, P. L. (Eds.). *Implementation Science in Nursing: A Framework for Education and Practice* (pp. 73-87).
© 2022 Taylor & Francis Group.

This chapter integrates basic principles and concepts from implementation and dissemination sciences and practice centered on translational nursing. Specifically, this chapter serves as an overview to the chapters that follow with a focus on nursing education and systems. The authors describe implementation and dissemination sciences at the various levels in nursing education, including entry-level, graduate nursing, and advanced nursing practice. Content related to evidence-based implementation from the teaching–learning perspective is included. Selected implementation science (IS) content is introduced, and context is offered related to planning, development, and implementation of relevant assignments that culminate in scholarly projects.

EVOLUTION OF IMPLEMENTATION SCIENCE AND NURSING

Van Achterberg et al. (2008) underscored the importance of evidence-based nursing being supported by evidence-based implementation. The authors described nursing evidence-based frameworks that include implementation as a major step in the uptake of rigorous, well-designed research evidence. Evidence-based practice (EBP) and nursing implementation models are described as being important to understanding the role of implementation of quality nursing care and innovation. For example, the Promoting Action on Research Implementation in Health Care Services model developed by Kitson et al. (1998) described the critical step in making connections between innovation and evidence, emphasizing the importance of context in any change (Rycroft-Malone et al., 2004). After the culmination of information and critical appraisal, implementation is a key step in the Promoting Action on Research Implementation in Health Care Services model. Barriers to implementation are highlighted, and change strategies such as unfreezing–moving–freezing are important phases in evaluating improvement in practice. Van Achterberg et al. (2008) also referenced the Iowa Model of Evidence-Based Practice to promote quality care proposed by Titler et al. (2001), which delineates steps and decision points facilitating processes that nurses can take beginning with identifying problems or knowledge-focused triggers to completing a real change in practice. Implementation is key to improvement and innovation underpinned by Rogers' theory for diffusion of innovations (Rogers, 1983, 2003). According to Titler and Everett (2001), before implementation is accomplished, the developers take into account such elements as the characteristics of the change, messaging and communication about the change, implementers of the change, and the context (social system) in which the change takes place and is eventually embedded into practice patterns. There is further discussion of this model in this chapter as well as in Chapters 2 and 3.

Van Achterberg et al. (2008) provided the case of handwashing as an example of the challenges of implementation. In their work of drilling down the successes and failures of carrying out handwashing consistently, the authors identified patterns or common determinants including knowledge, cognitions, attitudes, routines, social influence, organization, and resources. The authors went on to describe unique determinants related to specific innovations, context, and target groups. Furthermore, individual professionals and voluntary approaches appear to be the overwhelming strategies identified in implementation research. In their article, van Achterberg et al. (2008) described implementation strategies such as decision support, information and communication technology, reminders, rewards, and multifaceted strategies that appear promising in moving research into EBP and innovation. The authors concluded that connecting determinants to theory-based strategies may optimize implementation plans and promote fidelity and consistent follow-through.

FRAMEWORKS FOR NURSING EDUCATION: IMPLICATIONS FOR IMPLEMENTATION MODELS

University of Iowa Hospitals and Clinics

An excellent framework for providing context for this chapter is the Implementation Strategies for Evidence-Based Practice developed by Lauren Cullen and the University of Iowa Hospitals and Clinics. This framework is an excellent evolution of EBP uptake focused on nursing practice, specifically on the phases of implementation, which are critical to success and sustained practice change. Before implementation occurs, the steps in determining the need and the strategies necessary to arrive at the implementation phase are considered. The revised Iowa EBP model provides a blueprint for beginning the journey to improvement (Figure 5-1), starting with identifying triggering issues and opportunities (Cullen et al., 2018). These triggers can come from several directions including failing clinical processes, new evidence to support a need for timely updates, accreditation/legislative issues, and organizational systems' identified improvements. Internal and external data drive the need, issue, or gap and provide important information guiding the question and purpose for the change in practice. Once the need or gap is determined, a team is formed using tools such as a project charter and best interdisciplinary team practices. External evidence in the form of rigorous performed research studies is assembled, appraised, and synthesized as the body of evidence supporting the improvement. The team works together to design and pilot a practice change and includes several strategies, such as engaging patients and providers, developing algorithms and protocols, creating an evaluation plan, collecting baseline data, designing an implementation and evaluation plan, and piloting the work. If the change is successful and adopted, the team integrates and implements strategies to sustain the practice change. The results are disseminated, and successes are celebrated. Building on this evidence-based model, the Implementation Strategies for Evidence-Based Practice developed by Cullen et al. (2018) provides the following implementation phases: create awareness, build knowledge and commitment, promote action and adoption, and pursue integration and sustained use (Figure 5-2). Each of the phases outlines individual implementation strategies. Moving along the phase continuum, two specific targeted areas are identified: connecting with clinicians, organizational leaders, and key stakeholders and building organizational system support (i.e., the phases begin with creating awareness through sustained change). For example, in the phase of create awareness and interest in the targeted area of connecting with clinicians, organizational leaders, and key stakeholders, implementation strategies, such as posters and postings/flyers, announcements and broadcasts, sound bites, slogans and logs, unit newsletter, unit in-services, and distributing key evidence, are a myriad of actions that can be used. Moving to the build knowledge and commitment phase, the implementation team considers change agents (e.g., change champions, core group, opinion leaders), clinician input, matching the practice change with resources and equipment, and case studies. Promote action and adoption moves the team into the third phase and involves implementation strategies to that end. This may include role modeling, skill competence, piloting the practice change, demonstration of a workflow or decision algorithm, resource materials, and quick reference guides, to name a few. Phase 4, pursue integration and sustained use, involves public recognition, personalized messaging to staff (reduced work, reduce infection exposure, etc.), peer influence, and updating practice reminders. The targeted area of building organizational systems supports advances the implementation strategies and includes actions and activities that encompass the larger perspective, such as audit and feedback, reporting to senior leaders, trending results, standing orders, checklists, and actionable and timely data feedback.

This framework, Implementation Strategies for Evidence-Based Practice, offers a systematic approach to building consensus on tailoring the best implementation actions and activities. Having a taxonomy of evidence-based implementation strategies provides a language that individuals

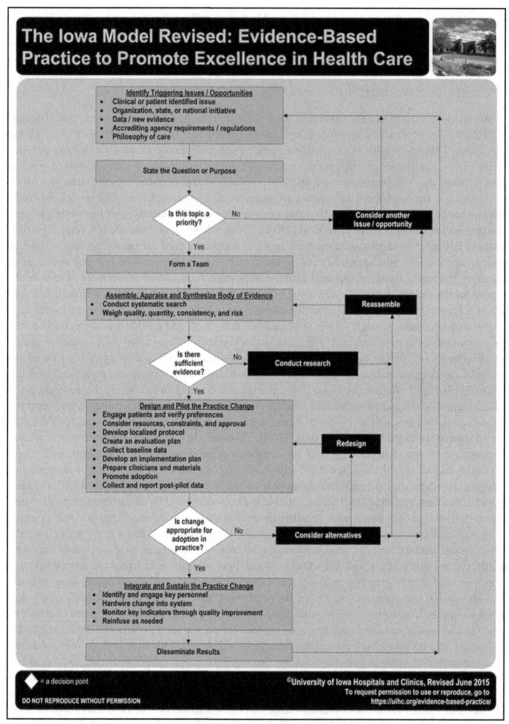

Figure 5-1. Used/reprinted with permission from the University of Iowa Hospitals and Clinics, Copyright 2015. For permission to use or reproduce the model, please contact the University of Iowa Hospitals and Clinics at 319-384-9098 or uihcnursingresearchandebp@uiowa.edu.

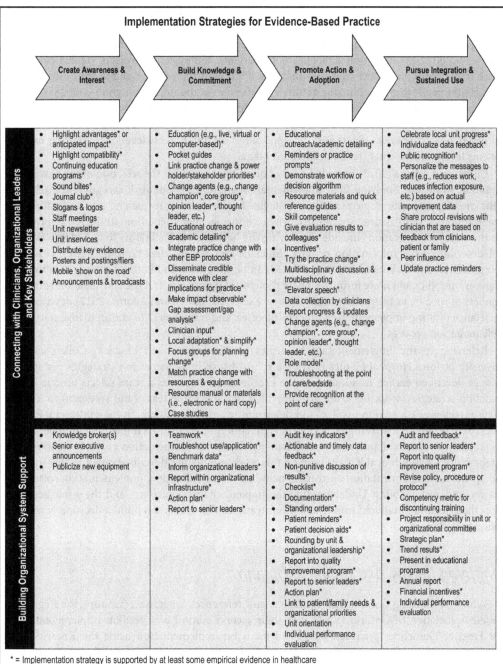

Implementation Strategies for Evidence-Based Practice

Create Awareness & Interest → **Build Knowledge & Commitment** → **Promote Action & Adoption** → **Pursue Integration & Sustained Use**

Connecting with Clinicians, Organizational Leaders and Key Stakeholders

Create Awareness & Interest
- Highlight advantages* or anticipated impact*
- Highlight compatibility*
- Continuing education programs*
- Sound bites*
- Journal club*
- Slogans & logos
- Staff meetings
- Unit newsletter
- Unit inservices
- Distribute key evidence
- Posters and postings/fliers
- Mobile 'show on the road'
- Announcements & broadcasts

Build Knowledge & Commitment
- Education (e.g., live, virtual or computer-based)*
- Pocket guides
- Link practice change & power holder/stakeholder priorities*
- Change agents (e.g., change champion*, core group*, opinion leader*, thought leader, etc.)
- Educational outreach or academic detailing*
- Integrate practice change with other EBP protocols*
- Disseminate credible evidence with clear implications for practice*
- Make impact observable*
- Gap assessment/gap analysis*
- Clinician input*
- Local adaptation* & simplify*
- Focus groups for planning change*
- Match practice change with resources & equipment
- Resource manual or materials (i.e., electronic or hard copy)
- Case studies

Promote Action & Adoption
- Educational outreach/academic detailing*
- Reminders or practice prompts*
- Demonstrate workflow or decision algorithm
- Resource materials and quick reference guides
- Skill competence*
- Give evaluation results to colleagues*
- Incentives*
- Try the practice change*
- Multidisciplinary discussion & troubleshooting
- "Elevator speech"
- Data collection by clinicians
- Report progress & updates
- Change agents (e.g., change champion*, core group*, opinion leader*, thought leader, etc.)
- Role model*
- Troubleshooting at the point of care/bedside
- Provide recognition at the point of care *

Pursue Integration & Sustained Use
- Celebrate local unit progress*
- Individualize data feedback*
- Public recognition*
- Personalize the messages to staff (e.g., reduces work, reduces infection exposure, etc.) based on actual improvement data
- Share protocol revisions with clinician that are based on feedback from clinicians, patient or family
- Peer influence
- Update practice reminders

Building Organizational System Support

Create Awareness & Interest
- Knowledge broker(s)
- Senior executive announcements
- Publicize new equipment

Build Knowledge & Commitment
- Teamwork*
- Troubleshoot use/application*
- Benchmark data*
- Inform organizational leaders*
- Report within organizational infrastructure*
- Action plan*
- Report to senior leaders*

Promote Action & Adoption
- Audit key indicators*
- Actionable and timely data feedback*
- Non-punitive discussion of results*
- Checklist*
- Documentation*
- Standing orders*
- Patient reminders*
- Patient decision aids*
- Rounding by unit & organizational leadership*
- Report into quality improvement program*
- Report to senior leaders*
- Action plan*
- Link to patient/family needs & organizational priorities
- Unit orientation
- Individual performance evaluation

Pursue Integration & Sustained Use
- Audit and feedback*
- Report to senior leaders*
- Report into quality improvement program*
- Revise policy, procedure or protocol*
- Competency metric for discontinuing training
- Project responsibility in unit or organizational committee
- Strategic plan*
- Trend results*
- Present in educational programs
- Annual report
- Financial incentives*
- Individual performance evaluation

* = Implementation strategy is supported by at least some empirical evidence in healthcare

Figure 5-2. Used/reprinted with permission from Laura Cullen, DNP, RN, FAAN. University of Iowa Hospitals and Clinics, Copyright 2011. For permission to use or reproduce the model, please contact the University of Iowa Hospitals and Clinics at 319-384-9098 or uihcnursingresearchandebp@uiowa.edu.

and organizational team members can come to an agreement on as interdisciplinary teams work together to solve problems and lead change.

Introducing nursing students to implementation language begins their capacity to apply evidence-based implementation strategies with patients and systems' projects. Teams can readily use frameworks and select strategies that best align with the changes and innovations that the organization needs to make. Nursing faculty can also access the implementation strategies as they design course content and tailor assignments for undergraduate and graduate nursing students. This is particularly critical as students apply evidence-based implementation strategies in their clinical and practicum experiences. Synthesis and application are the highest level of translating internal (systems level) and external (research literature) data.

Cullen and Adams (2012) provided a list of questions that guide the selection of the best implementation strategies. Applying their implementation strategies framework can guide the selection of the most appropriate implementation strategies for intervening in patient care and addressing organizational system issues. Specifically, when choosing implementation strategies, appropriate questions and considerations include identifying the barriers and facilitators to the adoption of the EBP, describing what information or data clinicians and stakeholders typically have access to in their practices, and discussing how the process can be simplified and built into the system to make adoption smoother and more intuitive. These thoughtful points can start the conversation with team members as specific implementation strategies are selected. Cullen and Adams (2012) described the importance of using implementation models, theories, and frameworks to conceptualize the overall implementation process.

Referring to the Implementation Strategies for Evidence-Based Practice, Cullen and the University of Iowa Hospital Clinics provide a robust list of implementation strategies per specific phase as described earlier. In addition to the excellent references, as a team selects unique implementation strategies, worksheets are also provided that guide the team (and students) to identify the resources needed, who to involve, and determining a date to initiate. In the same vein, Proctor et al. (2011) proposed a working taxonomy of eight conceptually distinct implementation outcomes: acceptability, adoption, appropriateness, feasibility, fidelity, implementation cost, penetration, and sustainability. Chaudoir et al. (2013) built on this work and further described qualities that increase EBP uptake and implementation outcomes, including fidelity, adoption, implementation costs, penetration, and sustainability. Understanding the implementation outcomes and the strategies reinforces the selection of tailored implementation strategies that teams can build a decision consensus around best choices.

Registered Nurses' Association of Ontario

When considering frameworks, resources, and references for nurse educators, the Registered Nurses' Association of Ontario (RNAO) in their second edition of a Toolkit: Implementation of Best Practice Guidelines provided a targeted focus on implementation using the Knowledge to Translation model to frame this revision. Using the Knowledge to Action framework (Straus et al., 2010) as adapted for the implementation of best practice guidelines, the model depicts the following seven essential components of knowledge translation necessary for the successful implementation of best practice guidelines:

1. Identify the problem: identify, review, and select knowledge tools/resources
2. Adapt knowledge tools/resources to local context
3. Assess barriers and facilitators to knowledge use
4. Select, tailor, and implement interventions
5. Monitor knowledge use
6. Evaluate outcomes
7. Sustain knowledge use (RNAO, 2012, p. 11)

The steps outline a process that is dynamic and iterative. The tool kit is grounded in theory, research, and experience of clinicians and is comprehensively written to provide practical information and strategies that support the implementation of best practice guidelines developed by RNAO to date. It brings useful tools and techniques to clinicians and stakeholders engaged in practice change for sustainable outcomes. The Knowledge to Translation framework is integrated throughout the tool kit and further reinforces how implementation models add value to the multifaceted interactions of the concepts. Nursing faculty can use the tool kit and the framework to provide resources for their students as they apply steps in the knowledge translation process.

Implementation Frameworks

When considering best teaching strategies when introducing IS and practices, it is important to return to some of the original work on theories, models, and frameworks. This was well covered in Chapter 3. Moving from conceptualization, it is in choosing which implementation framework is best suited to the interventions that provides the important grounding of the science. Specifically, identifying what are the ultimate aims of the intervention and deciding if it is acceptable to use more than one framework to progress implementation evidence into practice are important considerations. There are many implementation frameworks that are published in the literature with overlapping theories. Having a good solid knowledge base or a useful intervention is insufficient for practice and behavioral change, which prompted the discovery of the field of IS. Rogers (2003) provided a theory for successful change, identifying five qualities for successful innovation. These qualities include relative advantage to the users, compatibility with existing values and practices, simplicity and ease of use, "trialability," and the ease of observable results. Understanding this theory and how it relates to the successful implementation of useful interventions is the key to understanding IS. This is useful for nursing students at all levels of their nursing education. Furthermore, appreciating the context of the place or health care services where the intervention is to take place is essential for the successful adoption of any new interventions. Additionally, the requisite qualities to ultimate successful implementation include competency, leadership, organizational input, and performance assessment (Jordan et al., 2019).

Greenhalgh et al. (2004) provided a framework that outlines concepts that give greater context of implementation models and frameworks. According to the authors, implementation is considered in comparison to other ways that innovations spread in organizations, specifically diffusion, dissemination, and implementation. It is helpful for students to understand the differences between the concepts and phases. This can help nursing students frame their application and gain a better understanding of the importance of EBP.

Diffusion is described as the passive, unplanned, and untargeted spread of information or interventions. It is difficult to determine the effectiveness of an intervention if we are not able to plan and target our actions. Dissemination focuses on the targeted distribution of information and intervention materials to a specific audience. It is the messaging and the medium that are taken into account with EBP. Dissemination activities do propose to improve a practice or policy target audience's knowledge and awareness. We know that distributing or disseminating the material (e.g., through flyers or a tool kit) is not enough to make true behavioral change. Comparing diffusion and dissemination, implementation includes using deliberate strategies in specific settings to adopt new interventions, integrate them effectively, and change practice patterns. Specifically, implementation strategies are designed to improve implementation and service outcomes. Implementation outcomes refer to the effects of an implementation strategy on the new intervention, practice, or service. Examples of implementation outcomes also include adoption, fidelity, penetration, and reach.

Teaching–Learning Strategies

Using evidence-based implementation teaching strategies is a good place to start when describing best practices for teaching–learning at the entry and graduate advanced nursing practice levels. A basic understanding of implementation models, specifically evidence-based nursing implementation models, provides a foundational understanding to educate students about this phase of EBP update. Dolansky et al. (2017) provided an excellent review of using IS to better integrate Quality and Safety Education for Nurses (QSEN) competencies in nursing education. The authors give a historical perspective of IS and describe the Expert Recommendations for Implementation Change project's consensus document, which outlines terms and definitions for 73 discrete implementation strategies. The reader can refer to the work of Powell et al. (2015) for more information on how the team arrived at these implementation strategies. Waltz et al. (2015) further evaluated and refined the strategies based on the critical nature of intervention and the feasibility of the implementation. Seven categories were identified: (a) evaluative strategies such as audit and feedback, (b) interactive assistance strategies such as facilitation, (c) strategies for adapting and tailoring implementation to the local context such as with tailored strategy selection, (d) strategies for developing stakeholder inter-relationships such as with the use of champions and coalition building, (e) training and education strategies, (f) strategies for supporting clinicians/educators, and (g) engagement strategies for consumers/students. Building on this work, Dolansky et al. (2017) provided an excellent table that gives nurse educators robust implementation strategies with detailed action plans that can be readily adopted. Dolansky et al. (2017) describe the table as follows:

> The table uses the categories identified by the Expert Recommendations for Implementation Change project and provides specific action steps at both program (organizational) and course (individual) levels. The information in the table provides specific action steps to facilitate the implementation of the QSEN competencies into nursing education. (p. S16)

Horntvedt et al. (2018) completed a thematic literature review to identify strategies for teaching EBP in nursing education. In completing their review, four teaching strategy themes were identified, including subthemes within each theme (i.e., interactive teaching strategies, interactive and clinical integrated teaching strategies, learning outcomes, and barriers). The authors shared that the four studies they reviewed included a limited focus on teaching EBP principles; all studies reviewed included research utilization and interactive teaching strategies. The authors outlined learning outcomes in their review that supported enhanced analytical and critical skills and used research to ensure patient safety. Barriers to their review were challenging collaborations, limited awareness of EBP principles, and poor information literacy skills. Although the thematic review critically appraised a relatively small sample of evidence and included a relatively small sample of literature, their overall findings identified a need for more qualitative research. Furthermore, the authors emphasized the importance of reviewing research evidence to investigate interactive and clinically integrated teaching strategies toward further enhancing EBP undergraduate nursing students' knowledge and skills.

Khan and Coomarasamy (2006) outlined a three-level hierarchy of evidence-based medicine teaching and learning methods. The first level denotes the use of interactive clinical activities. Classroom didactics, the second level, uses both clinical and interactive activities. The third level, although less preferred for teaching evidence-based medicine, involves classroom didactic or stand-alone teaching. From teaching–learning theories, we know that engaging students from all perspectives of content introduction to return demonstration increases the retention of information (Knowles, 1980). The retention of information and changing attitudes toward research and EBP are enhanced by innovative teaching and blended approaches (Khan & Coomarasamy, 2006). Direct application in clinical settings has been shown to be an effective strategy for retaining information and learning hands-on skills. Teaching strategies such as online content, gaming, and simulation strategies are examples of direct application (Crookes et al., 2013). Although lecture continues to be a teaching–learning strategy, these authors suggest more active lectures with open-ended questions and reflection assignments that connect content and clinical skills.

Teaching EBP principles is considered foundational to other implementation strategies in nursing education. Specifically, research has described the importance of exposure to EBP frameworks and steps in the process (André et al., 2016; Cader et al., 2006; Malik et al., 2017). Active lectures, as well as teamwork and experiential learning, are reported as improving knowledge retention and application of the principles.

Irvine et al. (2008) described experiential learning as a strategy supplemented by collaborative group learning, including partnerships for learning course content. The authors presented experiential teaching approaches as a motivational tool for improving research learning. Specifically, the students used student-centered approaches and completed small group research studies. Group work or experiential learning teams were encouraged with assignments including activities such as performing a literature review, developing an evidence-based proposal, facing a mock ethics committee, and collecting and analyzing data. Student learning was enhanced using implementation strategies such as relevant lectures often presented through a virtual learning platform. The authors posited that student learning can be enhanced as they present their methodological and analytical approaches on virtual platforms, illustrating several implementation strategies supported in the literature.

A cornerstone to any evidence-based teaching strategy from an IS perspective includes the importance of partnering with a biomedical librarian who is engaged in teaching information literacy. Specifically, information literacy involves searching for relevant research in databases, critiquing, and using information to meet course requirements and assignments. We know there are barriers to the adoption of EBP that include difficulties with searching databases, critically appraising and evaluating research, feeling removed from knowledgeable partners, and the possible perceptions of the minimal benefits from EBP (Irvine, 2008).

Teaching EBP principles as foundational to undergraduate nursing students begins with the exposure to IS and practice. Active lectures, team and group projects, experiential learning through interactive assignments in the steps of the process, collaboration with interdisciplinary teams, and application in the clinical setting are all based on varying levels of research evidence. These implementation strategies are also important to advanced nursing practice. Doctor of nursing practice (DNP) projects are rooted in translational science (TS) and support evidence-based uptake. Improving quality of care, patient safety, and population health are cornerstones to the DNP inquiry project (Riner, 2015).

Riner (2015) provided her DNP program's journey of incorporating IS as core to their DNP projects. Including their clinical partners in this journey was important to their product because she and her colleagues elected to use IS as the framework for structuring the DNP project experience. According to Riner, "For DNP education, this emerging field provides the conceptual link between scientific knowledge and implementing this knowledge in practice" (p. 201). Riner and her faculty began this process through curriculum development course mapping. The author identified the courses in their DNP program and specifically described courses that support EBP uptake and IS. The program incorporated the American Association of Colleges of Nursing's doctoral essentials. Their inquiry courses were particularly focused on the DNP project and were built on combined epidemiology and statistics courses. The students also engaged in a course centered on data for decision making in which students used data, conducted analyses, and made decisions for clinical care. Riner (2015) described the integration of practicum and project courses in which the faculty adviser provides guidance through this process.

Riner (2015) provided an excellent table that outlines specific topics, artifacts, course competencies, program outcomes, and the corresponding American Association of Colleges of Nursing's doctoral essentials. For example, the topic implementation plan with the measurement and evaluation component is specific to how the student will implement the intervention, including a measurement and evaluation component with timelines. Riner goes through course modules and provides specific student examples. For example in the article "Module 4: Plans for Implementing the Intervention" outlines student assignments including the development of a practical framework of how the intervention is expected to work referring to the theory of implementation (Riner, 2015, p. 204). As part of this module, students also write a five- to six-page implementation plan and outline how critical aspects of the intervention are expected to work. Riner (2015) provided the outline for this assignment including aims and questions about the implementation process, elements of the local environment, and identifying specific methods. The example provided describes the student using the cycle of change model to design a project on the use of an evidence-based decision support algorithm for seizure management in the intellectually and developmental disability population living in community settings. Riner shared the importance of faculty development in going through the process. Overall, the DNP program's integration of IS was determined to be successful.

Boehm et al. (2020) reviewed IS programs, organizations, and literature to analyze the roles of nurses and nurse scientists in translating evidence into routine practice. Through this analysis, the authors provided a robust listing of organizations and institutions with websites and a brief description of the services and resources for each agency. The authors provided an excellent clinical example comparing quality improvement and IS. Addressing delirium from a quality improvement lens, the clinicians conduct real-time tracking of delirium assessment accuracy trends via a run chart. Clinicians noted improvement from 70% to 96%, motivating the team to spread to two other hospital units. This was accomplished through the implementation of specific evidence-based interventions, such as education and monitoring accuracy trends, to improve patients' outcomes. Following the quality improvement approach, the authors described how an implementation scientist would analyze current adherence and accuracy of delirium assessment in a practice setting, engaging a multidisciplinary team to investigate best strategies for implementation challenges and choosing relevant measures to determine the effectiveness of a strategy. Implementation strategies such as audit and feedback, dynamic training, and disincentives are some of the evidence-based strategies identified that implementation scientists may focus on to improve clinical outcomes. The implementation scientist may also focus on the nurses and their choice or preference of strategies and if the strategy was effective from a perspective of satisfaction, usefulness, utility, and feasibility. IS is also applicable to frontline nurses who may apply IS methods such as creating a unit advisory board, appraising the literature, and proposing strategies most appropriate for their clinical environment.

APPLICATION TO NURSE EDUCATION: UNDERGRADUATE NURSING STUDENTS

Introducing prelicensure students to IS is a natural evolution of EBP and quality improvement. As students are exposed to EBP models and begin asking the inquiry question, performing quality literature searches and evidence synthesis are essential to developing EBP competencies. IS through the introduction of theories, models, and frameworks and evidence-based implementation strategies can provide the groundwork for application and integration into clinical immersion experiences. Prelicensure students are readily applying EBP to their clinical practice experiences, aligning rigorous evidence to the delivery of nursing care. Exposure to how nursing care is performed through intervening in ways that promote quality and safe nursing care is integral to IS and practice. The following examples provide exemplars for prelicensure students.

Prelicensure Students

Assignment 1: Implementation Frameworks— Implications for Evidence-Based Practice

Students are exposed to a selected number of implementation models, primarily focused on the elements and processes of translating evidence into practice. Implementation models that are in the literature include the RE-AIM (Reach, Effectiveness, Adoption, Implementation, Maintenance) framework (Glasgow et al., 1999); PRECEDE-PROCEED (Green, 2015), the dynamic sustainability framework (Chambers et al., 2013); the Practical, Robust Implementation and Sustainability Model (Feldstein & Glasgow, 2008); the Consolidated Framework for Implementation Research (Damschroder et al., 2009); and Promoting Action on Research Implementation in Health Services (Kitson et al., 1998). Didactic content on the selected models provides foundational information for students to explore the origin of the model and the application to research and practice. With basic understanding about the various models, students are asked to find an article that applies the model in a real-world setting. Students are also given a list of research articles that apply the model in research and real-world settings. Faculty provides a list of selected research articles using implementation frameworks. Using critical appraisal skills, the students critique the article and share their work with peers. This can be done via an online discussion board (allowing for cross-posting) or in-class small group discussion. The overall aim for this assignment is to provide an opportunity for sharing the utility of the models, as well as reinforcing critical appraisal skills.

Assignment 2: Critical Appraisal of Research on Evidence-Based Implementation Strategies

This assignment builds on assignment 1. Armed with the knowledge and application of IS, the students have context to applying critical appraisal skills to research on evidence-based implementation strategies. Students are provided with didactic information on evidence-based implementation strategies. Building on implementation models and research that apply the models, the students are asked to identify evidence-based implementation strategies and the research evidence that support the use of these strategies. As part of their overall EBP content, critical appraisal skills have been introduced. This assignment will build on this content and will critique the research evidence. Using critical appraisal skills, the students critique the article and share their work with peers. This can be done via an online discussion board (allowing for cross-posting) or in-class small group discussion. The overall aim for this assignment is to provide an opportunity for sharing how the merit of the research evidence supports the implementation strategies. This assignment will also reinforce critical appraisal skills.

Assignment 3: Evidence-Based Implementation Strategies and Clinical Application

Through this assignment, students will continue their exploration and application of implementation models and evidence-based implementation strategies. This assignment will call on students' clinical practice experience as they begin to learn more about evidence-based nursing care. In this assignment, students will select a nursing intervention(s) that they are applying to a patient care encounter. The student will explore the evidence that provides rationale (support) for the steps in their nursing care delivery (policy/procedure). Working through the process of carrying out the steps (that are evidence-based), the student aligns (when possible) the evidence-based implementation strategy that supports the "how to" of the actual intervention plan. The student will also consider evaluation of the intervention and implementation strategies. This assignment works well during the student's clinical practicum experiences and is a good postconference interactive exercise.

Assignment 4: Quality and Safety Education for Nurses and Implementation Science

This assignment incorporates IS and the QSEN competencies. After reading the article titled "Implementation Science: New Approaches to Integrating Quality and Safety Education for Nurses Competencies in Nursing Education" by Dolansky et al. (2017), the student will discuss via a virtual discussion board or in-class meeting the overall aim of the article and the application to quality and safety patient care. Using their example of implementation strategies for quality and safety competency integration at program (organizational) and course (individual) levels, the student will draw on their leadership experience (final practicum) to relate QSEN competencies to implementation strategies. This may be done via an interview with organizational leaders involved in quality and safety education of nurses.

APPLICATION TO NURSE EDUCATION: GRADUATE NURSING STUDENTS

Graduate nursing students come armed to their advanced nursing programs with foundational knowledge and application of EBP and TS. Graduate students will gain a deeper understanding with the expectations that they will engage in quality and EBP projects, mentoring their peers, and interprofessional partners. Integrating models, advanced critical appraisal skills, and a fundamental understanding of evidence-based implementation strategies that are carried out with fidelity are what levels the educational expectations of advanced nursing practice. The following examples provide exemplars for graduate students.

Advanced Nursing Students

Assignment 1: Evidence-Based Implementation Strategies and Clinical Application

This assignment aligns with the assignment detailed in Riner's (2015) work on DNP projects and IS. Specifically, students are provided readings and resources on implementation models, theories, and frameworks. Implementation models that are in the literature include the RE-AIM framework (Glasgow et al., 1999); PRECEDE-PROCEED (Green, 2015); the dynamic sustainability framework (Chambers et al., 2013); the Practical, Robust Implementation and Sustainability Model (Feldstein & Glasgow, 2008); the Consolidated Framework for Implementation Research (Damschroder et al., 2009); and Promoting Action on Research Implementation in Health Services (Kitson et al., 1998). Students will critically appraise at least two implementation models and share their appraisals with peers virtually on a discussion board. From this initial appraisal, the student will do an in-depth critique of a model they select to guide their DNP project focus area. Students will also use their DNP project guidelines as they complete this assignment to begin to integrate IS into their beginning project planning.

Assignment 2: Improvement and Implementation Sciences

Building on IS models, theories, and frameworks, the student will be exposed to several improvement models through readings and resources. The student also completes the Institute of Healthcare Improvement Open School modules on improvement capability and patient safety. The student will select one to do an in-depth critique on that they would like to use to guide their DNP project focus area. The student will build on their IS framework and integrate the improvement science into their project planning process. Through improvement methodologies, the student will also begin to think through outcome measurement. Students will also use their DNP project guidelines as they complete this assignment to begin to integrate IS into their beginning project planning.

Assignment 3: Translational Science and Evaluation Models

This assignment builds on assignments 1 and 2, with the focus being on developing a logic model. Riner (2015) provided excellent information on the development of this assignment. Specifically, Riner shared the importance of providing a variety of logic model readings, including Kellogg (2000). Using these resources and armed with knowledge of TS, the student creates a visual program logic model that illustrates the connections among the situation, assumptions, activities, outcomes, and intended impact of the intervention and implementation strategies. Students will also use their DNP project guidelines as they complete this assignment to begin to integrate IS into their beginning project planning. The student begins to put the many facets of TS together through improvement, implementation, and evaluation sciences.

Assignment 4: Translational Science and Doctor of Nursing Practice Projects

This can be a series of assignments for completion of the final DNP project. This is the connecting the dots of all facets of TS and project management. Students use their DNP project guidelines (or SQUIRE 2.0 guidelines) as they complete this assignment to begin to integrate IS into their beginning project planning.

CONCLUSION

This chapter provided an overview of the basic principles and concepts from implementation and dissemination sciences and practice focused on translational nursing and application to undergraduate and graduate nursing. Content related to evidence-based implementation from the teaching–learning perspective was included and threaded through the various assignments provided as exemplars for faculty and student. Selected IS content was introduced and context offered related to best practice IS nursing models.

REFLECTIVE QUESTIONS

1. Using the RNAO Toolkit (https://rnao.ca/sites/rnao-ca/files/RNAO_ToolKit_2012_rev4_FA.pdf), consider the Knowledge to Action process (Figure 1, p. 12). Describe the major concepts of the framework and its clinical application.
2. Consider the Expert Recommendations for Implementing Change project's evidence-based implementation strategies. Select two strategies and describe how you would apply to a change project.

REFERENCES

André, B., Aune, A. G., & Brænd, J. A. (2016). Embedding evidence-based practice among nursing undergraduates: Results from a pilot study. *Nurse Education Practice, 18*, 30-35. https://doi.org/10.1016/j.nepr.2016.03.004

Boehm, L., Stolldorf, P., & Jeffery, A. (2020). Implementation science training and resources for nurses and nurse scientists. *Journal of Nursing Scholarship, 52*(1), 47-54.

Cader, R., Derbyshire, J., Smith, A. G., Gannon-Leary, P., & Walton, G. (2006). In search of evidence: A small-scale study exploring how student nurses accessed information for a health needs assignment. *Nurse Education Today, 26*, 403-408. https://doi.org/10.1016/j.nedt.2005.11.010

Chambers, D. A., Glasgow, R. E., & Stange, K. C. (2013). The dynamic sustainability framework: Addressing the paradox of sustainment amid ongoing change. *Implementation Science, 8*, 117. https://doi.org/10.1186/1748-5908-8-117

Chaudoir, S. R., Dugan, A. G., & Barr, C. R. (2013). Measuring factors affecting implementation of health innovations: A systematic review of structural, organizational, provider, patient, and innovation level measures. *Implementation Science, 8*, 22. https://doi.org/10.1186/1748-5908-8-22

Crookes, K., Crookes, P. A., & Walsh, K. (2013). Meaningful and engaging teaching techniques for student nurses: A literature review. *Nurse Educator Practice, 13*, 239-243.

Cullen, L. & Adams, S. (2012). An implementation model to promote adoption of evidence-based practice. *Journal of Nursing Administration, 42*(4), 222-230.

Cullen, L., Hanrahan, K., Farrington, M., DeBerg, J., Tucker, S., & Kleiber, C. (2018). *Evidence-based practice in action: Comprehensive strategies, tools, and tips from the University of Iowa Hospitals and Clinics.* Sigma Theta International.

Damschroder, L., Aron, D., Keith, R., Kirsh, S., Alexander, J., & Lowery, J. (2009). Fostering implementation of health services research findings into practice: A consolidated framework for advancing implementation science. *Implementation Science, 4*(1), 50.

Dolansky, M. A., Schexnayder, J., Patrician, P. A., & Sales, A. (2017). Implementation science: New approaches to integrating quality and safety education for nurses competencies in nursing education. *Nurse Educator, 42*(5S Suppl. 1), S12-S17. https://doi.org/10.1097/NNE.0000000000000422

Feldstein, A. C., & Glasgow, R. E. (2008). A practical, robust implementation and sustainability model (PRISM) for integrating research findings into practice. *Joint Commission Journal of Quality Patient Safety, 34*(4), 228-243.

Glasgow, R., Vogt, T., & Boles, S. (1999). Evaluating the public health impact of health promotion interventions: The RE-AIM framework. *American Journal of Public Health, 89*(9), 1322-1327.

Green, L. (2015). The Precede-Proceed model of health planning and evaluation. http://lgreen.net/precede.htm

Greenhalgh, T., Robert, G., Macfarlane, F., Bate, P., & Kyriakidou, O. (2004). Diffusion of innovations in service organizations: Systematic review and recommendations. *The Milbank Quarterly, 82*(4), 581-629.

Horntvedt, M. E., Nordsteine, A., Fermann, T., & Severinsson, E. (2018). Strategies for teaching evidence-based practice in nursing education: A thematic literature review. *BMC Medical Education, 18*(172), 1-33.

Iowa Model Collaboration. (2017). Iowa Model of evidence-based practice: Revisions and validation. *Worldviews on Evidence-Based Nursing, 14*(3), 175-182. https://doi.org/10.1111.wvn.12223

Irvine, F., Gracey, C., Jones, O. S., Roberts, J. L, Tamsons, R. E., & Tranter, S. (2008). Research awareness: Making learning relevant for pre-registration nursing students. *Nurse Educator Practice, 8*, 267-275. https://doi.org/10.1016/j.nepr.2007.09.006

Jordan, Z., Lockwood, C., Munn, Z., & Aromataris, E. (2019). The updated Joanna Briggs Institute Model of Evidence Based Healthcare. *International Journal of Evidence-Based Healthcare, 17*(1), 58-71. https://doi.org/10.1097/XEB.0000000000000155

Kellogg, W. K. (2000). Foundation: Using logic models to bring together planning evaluation and action: Logic model development guide. https://www.wkkf.org/resource-directory/resource/2006/02/wk-kellogg-foundation-logic-model-development-guide

Khan, K. S., & Coomarasamy A. (2006). A hierarchy of effective teaching and learning to acquire competence in evidenced-based medicine. *BMC Medical Education, 6*, 59.

Kitson, A., Harvey, G., & McCormack, B. (1998). Enabling the implementation of evidence-based practice: A conceptual framework. *Quality in Health Care, 7*, 149-158. https://doi.org/10.1136/qshc.7.3.149

Knowles, M. S. (1980). *The modern practice of adult education: From pedagogy to andragogy* (2nd ed.). Cambridge Books.

Malik, G., McKenna, L., &, Griffiths, D. (2017). Using pedagogical approaches to influence evidence-based practice integration–Processes and recommendations: Findings from a grounded theory study. *Journal of Advanced Nursing, 73*, 883-893. https://doi.org/10.1111/jan.13175

Powell, B. J., Waltz, T. J., Chinman, M. J., Damschroder, L. J., Smith, J. L., Matthieu, M. M., Proctor, E. K., & Kirchner, J. E. (2015). A refined compilation of implementation strategies: Results from the Expert Recommendations for Implementing Change (ERIC) project. *Implementation Science, 10*, 21. https://doi.org/10.1186/s13012-015-0209-1

Proctor, E., Silmere, H., Raghavan, R., Hovmand, P., Aarons, G., Bunger, A., Griffey, R., & Hensley, M. (2011). Outcomes for implementation research: conceptual distinctions, measurement challenges, and research agenda. *Administration and Policy in Mental Health, 38*(2), 65-76. https://doi.org/10.1007/s10488-010-0319-7

Registered Nurses' Association of Ontario. (2012). *Toolkit: Implementation of best practice guidelines* (2nd ed.). https://rnao.ca/sites/rnao-ca/files/RNAO_ToolKit_2012_rev4_FA.pdf

Riner, M. E. (2015). Using implementation science as the core of the doctor of nursing practice inquiry project. *Journal of Professional Nursing, 31*(3), 200-207.

Rogers, E. M. (1983). *Diffusion of innovations* (3rd ed.). Free Press.

Rogers, E. M. (2003). *Diffusion of innovations* (5th ed.). Free Press.

Rycroft-Malone, J., Harvey, G., Seers, K., Kitson, A., McCormack, B., & Titchen A. (2004). An exploration of the factors that influence the implementation of evidence into practice. *Journal of Clinical Nursing, 13*, 913-924.

Straus, S. E., Tetroe, J., Graham, I. D., Zwarenstein, M., Bhattacharyya, O., & Shepperd, S. (2010). Monitoring use of knowledge and evaluating outcomes. *Canadian Association Journal, 182*(2), E94-E98. https://doi.org/10.1503/cmaj.081335

Titler, M. G., & Everett, L.Q. (2001). Translating research into practice. Considerations for critical care investigators. *Critical Care Nursing Clinics of North America, 13*, 587-604.

Titler, M. G., Kleiber, C., Steelman, V., Rakel, B., Budreau, G., Everett, L. Q., Buckwalter, K. D., Tripp-Reimer, T., & Goode, C. J. (2001). The Iowa Model of evidence-based practice to promote quality care. *Critical Care Nursing Clinics of North America, 13*, 497-509.

van Achterberg, T., Schoonhoven, L., & Grol, R. (2008). Nursing implementation science: How evidence-based nursing requires evidence-based implementation. *Journal of Nursing Scholarship, 40*(4), 302-310. https://doi.org/10.1111/j.1547-5069.2008.00243. x

Waltz, T. P., Powell, B. J., & Matthieu, M. M. (2015). Use of concept mapping to characterize relationships among implementation strategies and assess their feasibility and importance: Results from the Expert Recommendations for Implementing Change (ERIC) study. *Implementation Science, 10*, 109. https://doi.org/10.1186/s13012-015-0295-0

IMPLEMENTATION SCIENCE AND PRACTICE

Entry Level of Practice

Janet E. Winter, DNP, MPA, FNAP, RN

CHAPTER OBJECTIVES

- Describe undergraduate curriculum perspective for content and context
- Integrate implementation science and practice into clinical rotations and simulation experiences
- Illustrate the implications for preceptorships and residencies for entry-level nursing students
- Explore principles of implementation and dissemination sciences in undergraduate student projects

KEY WORDS

- Accelerated second-degree nursing program
- Accreditation
- Baccalaureate nursing program
- Fidelity
- Implementation and dissemination sciences
- Implementation practice
- Preceptorships
- Residences
- Simulation experiences

Roussel, L. A., & Thomas, P. L. (Eds.). *Implementation Science in Nursing: A Framework for Education and Practice* (pp. 89-106).
© 2022 Taylor & Francis Group.

Requisite to sustained change in clinical practice is the acknowledgment that habits of nursing education drive the nurse graduate produced. The focus of this chapter is to describe how curriculum, accreditation, selection and interaction with practice partners, and nurse residencies or preceptorships can be leveraged strategically to influence future daily practice of entry-level nurses. Through deliberate and intentional identification, description, definition, and application of principles of implementation and translational science (TS), practitioners and educators can cultivate entry-level nurses poised for sustainable practice improvements.

BACCALAUREATE NURSING: EDUCATIONAL PATHWAYS

In general, there are three overarching educational pathways for an individual to consider when seeking to earn a bachelor of science (BS) or a bachelor of science in nursing (BSN) degree in the United States. Table 6-1 provides a brief overview of those educational pathways and highlights the distinction between prelicensure and postlicensure programming. The accelerated second-degree nursing program typically attracts someone seeking a second career choice, whereas the science further supporting the registered nurse (RN) to BSN or RN completion educational pathway was evidenced through the release of *The Future of Nursing: Leading Change, Advancing Health* report from the Institute of Medicine (IOM; 2011). This report highlighted the need for change in nursing education as a means to meet the increasing complexity in health care delivery by putting forth a goal to increase the number of RNs with a BSN degree to 80% by the year 2020 as "necessary to move the nursing workforce to an expanded set of competencies, especially in the domains of community and public health, leadership, systems improvement and change, research, and health policy" (IOM, 2011, p. 173).

At an individual level, there are a variety of reasons that compel associate degree–prepared RNs to return to school to earn a BSN degree. For example, earning a BSN degree affords additional career opportunities by opening avenues for promotion and advancement. In some cases, employers mandate the completion of a BSN degree within a certain time period. In recent decades, some acute care practice settings have incentivized their associate degree–prepared nurses to obtain their BSN degree within approximately 3 to 5 years of employment given the evidence of patient, clinical, and organizational outcomes when there is a higher proportion of BSN nurses (Altman et al., 2016). Nurses are lifelong learners who thoughtfully build on their credentials through degree achievements over time.

Each of these educational pathways (i.e., the traditional BSN, the accelerated second-degree BSN, and the RN to BSN or RN completion) depicts distinct student learner populations that all converge to achieve the outcome of earning a BS/BSN degree. Curricula designed for baccalaureate-prepared nurses hold notoriety in that "BSN nurses are prized for their skills in critical thinking, leadership, case management, and health promotion, and for their ability to practice across a variety of inpatient and outpatient settings" (American Association of Colleges of Nursing, 2019a, para. 1).

Casey et al. (2018) envisioned implementation science (IS) as "a way to ensure that evidence is translated into practice" (p. 1051). This definition, when viewed through the lens of BS/BSN programming, charges nursing faculty and administrators with ensuring that the nursing curriculum meets student learners where they are along their educational journey while transforming them to become BS/BSN-prepared professional nurses who are competent, relevant, safe, visionary, and influential in decisions regarding their profession and the delivery of health care at the individual, group, community, and population levels.

The application of different teaching modalities, such as reflective journaling, discussion boards, essay writing, testing, quizzing, and project-based work, promotes the nursing student's transformative journey toward professional practice. When done well, these teaching modalities can ultimately promote learning using a complement of activities that interface with an individual's

TABLE 6-1 **Three Pathways to the BS/BSN Degree**			
Prelicensure	Courses and complementary clinical experiences position the student to achieve legal authority to practice as a registered nurse through national board licensure Graduates of prelicensure programs take the National Council Licensure Examination for Registered Nurses	Traditional	• Direct admit into a nursing program after high school OR secondary application into a nursing program (usually during the sophomore year) • Full-time pace with an average 4-year time span • Didactic curricula may be delivered using a hybrid online format but are often delivered using a traditional in-seat format
		Accelerated second degree	• Individuals with a baccalaureate degree in another discipline • Full-time pace with an average time span between 11 to 18 months once prerequisite courses have been satisfied • Didactic curricula may be delivered using a hybrid online format
Postlicensure	Must have completed either an associate degree in nursing, an associate of applied science in nursing degree, or an associate of science in nursing degree	Registered nurse to bachelor of science in nursing or Registered nurse completion	• Proof of having earned the protected title of registered nurse either upon entry into the registered nurse to bachelor of science in nursing/registered nurse completion program or before graduation as stipulated by the bachelor of science in nursing program • Often at a part-time pace over an average time span of 1 to 2 years (sometimes less depending on prerequisites and program requirements) • Curricula are often designed using an online/hybrid or completely online delivery format inclusive of experiential learning that permits the learner to pace their coursework in consideration of work/life demands

visual, auditory, kinesthetic, and tactile senses. In combination, didactic coursework, real-life and simulated clinical experiences, and psychomotor skills acquired or reinforced in the laboratory setting comprehensively promote quality learning.

THE ROLE OF ACCREDITATION

Many BS/BSN programs seek national accreditation as a mechanism to ensure the quality of their programming. Table 6-2 offers an overview of some important functions of accreditation and the primary accrediting activities.

The process of accreditation allows for contextual relevance in that each program addresses the established accrediting body standards by creating, delivering, and revising its unique curricula in accordance with expected student outcomes that align with its university and college mission, vision, and core values. When vision, mission, and core value statements originate from environmental scanning that is inclusive of sociocultural, political, and economic factors, the curricula maintain relevance. Key elements such as professional nursing standards, guidelines, defined outcomes, and core competencies that are integrated across the curriculum and articulated through course objectives function to move the student toward proficiency in becoming an entry-level generalist baccalaureate nurse. These elements hardwire curricular consistency and constancy in maintaining evidence-based practices (EBPs) in baccalaureate nursing education. IS and TS principles can be introduced, reinforced, and woven into the curriculum to establish the foundation needed for execution in clinical rotations and eventual daily clinical practice.

BACCALAUREATE NURSING CURRICULUM

The curricular design and delivery of a baccalaureate nursing program have the power to accelerate or delay practice change that is based on research. The curriculum exerts its influence on nursing students as they progress through a program and continues its impact as they transition to nursing practice. Undergraduate courses that promote knowledge, skills, and abilities in areas such as research methodology, nursing research, EBP, critical appraisal, IS, informatics, analytics, systems, policy, interprofessional collaborative practice, change management, and leadership combine to position the nursing student to effectively make change where change is needed. Therefore, the curriculum not only equips the student to address present-day demands, but it also functions to pique the student's interest in continually seeking to understand the rationale for processes and procedures and appropriately challenge the status quo toward better outcomes.

Throughout the baccalaureate nursing student journey, there is continued cultivation of effective communication, clinical inquiry, critical thinking, clinical reasoning, and clinical judgment. The integration of didactic nursing education formulated on research and EBP is further applied into the practice setting through experiential clinical assignments.

The clinical rotation placements intentionally give the student entrance to a range of practice environments that support a generalist nursing education. Clinical placement rotations in prelicensure baccalaureate nursing programs commonly involve assignments in which faculty are responsible to oversee a predetermined number of students in the clinical setting for a specified number of hours over a definitive time frame. These faculty are employed by the teaching institution. Some faculty delivering the clinical rotation may be employed by the nursing school as tenure/tenure-track, affiliate, or visiting professors, whereas others may be hired on a part-time basis as a clinical instructor or adjunct professor. Many part-time clinical instructors work in the practice setting while they teach in a nursing program and teach the same clinical material over consecutive semesters. Familiarity with their organization's culture, policy, and procedures facilitates the student

TABLE 6-2

Important Functions of Accreditation and Primary Accrediting Activities

IMPORTANT FUNCTIONS OF ACCREDITATION	PRIMARY ACCREDITING ACTIVITIES
• Assess the quality of academic programs at institutions of higher education. • Create a culture of continuous improvement of academic quality at colleges and universities and stimulate a general raising of standards among educational institutions. • Involve faculty and staff comprehensively in institutional evaluation and planning. • Establish criteria for professional certification and licensure and for upgrading courses offering such preparation.	• Standards: The accreditor, in collaboration with educational institutions and/or programs, establishes standards. • Self-study: The institution or program seeking accreditation prepares an in-depth self-evaluation report that measures its performance against the standards established by the accreditor. • On-site evaluation: A team of peers selected by the accreditor reviews the institution or program on-site to determine firsthand if the applicant meets the established standards. • Decision and publication: Upon being satisfied that the applicant meets its standards, the accreditor grants accreditation or preaccreditation status and lists the institution or program in an official publication with other similarly accredited or preaccredited institutions or programs. Only public and private nonprofit institutions can qualify to award federal student aid based on preaccreditation. • Monitoring: The accreditor monitors each accredited institution or program throughout the period of accreditation granted to verify that it continues to meet the accreditor's standards. • Reevaluation: The accreditor periodically reevaluates each institution or program that it lists to ascertain whether continuation of its accredited or preaccredited status is warranted.

Data source: U.S. Department of Education. (2019, July 19). Overview of accreditation in the United States. https://www2.ed.gov/admins/finaid/accred/accreditation.html#Overview.

learning experience. Similarly, many tenure/tenure-track, affiliate, and visiting faculty maintain consistent clinical placements over time and foster similar organizational knowledge, in addition to their understanding of the curriculum and associated desired student learning outcomes. Faculty development and formal mentorships remain integral components to faculty preparation.

Depending on the size of the student cohort, there may be several faculty responsible at one time to deliver a portion of a specific clinical experience. By taking a team approach to this type of assignment configuration, faculty can share EBPs with each other and promote consistency in the delivery of the nursing education. For example, implementation practices include a collective review of the nursing program's curriculum, student learning outcomes, course objectives, relevant concepts, assignments, evaluation rubrics, the learning platforms, college resources, and university/college policy and procedures. Holding team meetings, especially at the beginning, middle, and end of a clinical rotation, can promote team cohesion and fuel synergistic efforts toward the implementation of relevant nursing education.

In addition to direct clinical faculty oversight, prelicensure and postlicensure students may also satisfy clinical requirements by being assigned to a preceptor in the clinical setting. In baccalaureate nursing education, clinical preceptors must be educated at or above the level of a BSN degree. The clinical preceptor is employed by the site where the baccalaureate nursing student is placed. The student works individually with the preceptor, often according to the preceptor's work schedule. "Preceptors facilitate the development of practical skills, professional socialization, report and documentation, prioritization, communication, and planning of daily activities" (Parker et al., 2012, as cited in McClure & Black, 2013, p. 338). In these assignments, the preceptor is oriented to the student's curriculum. A faculty member conducts regularly scheduled visits to ensure that the student learning experience is congruent with the course objectives. The faculty member also mentors the preceptor and supports the student throughout the experience.

Upon entry into practice, the preceptor plays a key role in the onboarding of a new graduate nurse. The preceptor is viewed by the health care organization as competent within "a specific area who serves as a teacher/coach, leader/influencer, facilitator, evaluator, socialization agent, protector, and role model to develop and validate the competencies of another individual" (Ulrich, 2012, p. 1). This role highlights an institutionalized approach by health care organizations to ensure quality and safety in the delivery of its health care services.

Similarly, many health care organizations offer a nurse residency program for their new graduate nurses. Outcomes stemming from nurse residency programs in alignment with IS include "increased decision-making competence and confidence, improved professional commitment and satisfaction, consistent use of evidence-based practices, stronger clinical nursing leadership and critical thinking skills" (American Association of Colleges of Nursing, 2019b, p. 2). The existence of preceptors and nurse residency programs signals opportunity for continued reinforcement of IS in the delivery of baccalaureate nursing education as a mechanism to ease some of the transitional challenges associated with entry into practice for new graduate nurses and the hiring health care organization.

Expanding the scope beyond the acute care setting is critical to making broadscale changes toward improved health care outcomes. "Entry-level nurses, for example, need to be able to transition smoothly from their academic preparation to a range of practice environments, with an increased emphasis on community and public health settings" (IOM, 2011, p. 164). At a macrolevel, the IOM's core competencies for health care providers include providing patient-centered care, working in interdisciplinary teams, using EBP, applying quality improvement, and using informatics (IOM, 2003, pp. 45-46). In alignment with the IOM, nursing education focuses on core competencies around quality and safety in education. The generalist baccalaureate nursing curriculum also integrates competencies associated with global, public, and community health. Overlapping categories between global and public health may be synthesized to include core competencies in "social justice, cultural competency, communication, assessment and management skills, environment, disease burden and epidemiology, ethics and professionalism, determinants of health, health

TABLE 6-3

Exercises in Promoting Vision, Mission, and Core Value Congruence Between Practice and Academic Partners

PRACTICE PARTNER EXERCISE	ACADEMIC PARTNER–CLINICAL INSTRUCTOR/STUDENT EXERCISE
• Review your employers' organizational core values. • Select one that you personally embrace. • Identify an action that you can take when interacting with nursing students that exemplifies this core value.	• Review the clinical placement site's vision, mission, and core value statements with your assigned students. • Have each student identify in a written reflection. • During a debriefing/postconference session, identify one way that the mission (purpose) of the organization was furthered by their actions.

systems/delivery, travel and migration, key players, research, and health promotion/illness prevention" (Clark et al., 2016, p. 179).

In transforming nursing education, various implementation practices can optimize learning among BS/BSN students in the clinical setting while ensuring high-quality, safe, person-centered outcomes within an array of practice environments. This premise shifts the notion of clinical placements as existing to solely fulfill student course requirements to one that partners over the student clinical placement in a way that is beneficial to the patients/clients, the placement site, the students, the faculty, the academic program, and the community at large. In seeking to enact the following implementation practices, the academic/practice partners support models of TS that recognize the necessity in gauging the readiness of the culture and climate to accept innovation.

IMPLEMENTATION PRACTICE: CONGRUENCY IN VISION, MISSION, AND CORE VALUES

Overall, practice partners should feel that nursing students placed in their clinical settings add value to their organization's vision, mission, and core values. This requires clinical staff and administrators to familiarize themselves with these foundational tenets and intentionally identify ways that students contribute, for example, to excellent care, integrity, and the preservation of dignity.

Similarly, nursing students aspire to be relevant through the application of their course content into the clinical setting in a way that positively influences patient/client and organizational outcomes. Therefore, before beginning a clinical rotation, the clinical instructor(s) and nursing students can review the placement site's organizational vision, mission, and core values to proactively consider their role in promoting the purpose of the organization within its espoused culture. Table 6-3 provides an example of exercises for practice and academic partners to consider in encouraging vision, mission, and core value congruence.

Implementation Practice: Advancing the Placement Site's Strategic Plan

In addition to integrating vision, mission, and core values, further application of IS occurs when the clinical instructor and students work with the clinical placement site to advance the organization's strategic plan. The strategic plan is a "future-oriented document that concisely depicts the priorities and desired outcomes deemed essential to achieving organizational viability over a stated period of time" (Thomas & Winter, 2020, p. 143). The strategic plan builds from the organization's vision, mission, and core values by identifying strategic priorities that take into consideration economic, environmental, political, technological, societal, and regulatory trends.

The desired outcomes within the strategic plan move the organization from its current state to its desired future state and are often determined through organizational assessments of internal and external supporting and mitigating forces. Objectives bridge the organizations' strategic priorities and outcomes by conveying incremental measurable results that need to occur in order to get to the desired state. Units or departments within organizations often have responsibility to identify tactics or action steps that help achieve objectives under specific strategies to affect the desired outcomes.

Practice partners and clinical instructors who intentionally incorporate clinical placement site strategic priorities, objectives, and tactics into the learning experience provide nursing students with a greater sense of the context in which IS is championed as well as the methodology involved in translating research findings into clinical practice change or program initiatives. Table 6-4 provides an example of exercises that academic and practice partners can undertake to achieve strategic priorities.

Implementation Practice: Indicator Performance Practices in the Clinical Experience

In addition to strategic plan initiatives, a clinical placement site may also monitor its performance on various indicators, many of which are reviewed by accreditation agencies and tied to financial reimbursement from Medicare and other insurers. Indicator dashboards trend performance and, when benchmarks are not being achieved, serve as a gauge to prompt quality improvement initiatives. Much like the strategic plan, indicator performance provides the clinical instructor and nursing student with additional context in terms of what is a priority to the clinical placement site, how evidence-based protocols are implemented and hardwired into the decision-making processes, and what measurable outcomes result from effective IS practices. Table 6-5 provides examples of exercises that promote contextual understanding of the clinical setting.

> Implementation fidelity is the degree to which an intervention is delivered as intended and is critical to successful translation of evidence-based interventions into practice. Diminished fidelity may be why interventions that work well in highly controlled trials may fail to yield the same outcomes when applied in real life contexts. (Breitenstein et al., 2010, p. 164)

Exercises such as these reinforce the understanding that "context matters and is widely acknowledged as an important influence on implementation outcomes" (Titler, 2018, p. 11). Clinical placements within the BS/BSN curriculum that embrace this type of collaboration between academic and practice partners ultimately serve to reinforce the importance of context in IS.

TABLE **6-4**

Exercises in Enhancing the Organization's Strategic Plan Between Practice and Academic Partners

PRACTICE PARTNER EXERCISE	ACADEMIC PARTNER–CLINICAL INSTRUCTOR/STUDENT EXERCISE
• Review your organization's strategic plan. • Select one strategic priority/objective/outcome that your clinical placement site is working to address and share this information with the clinical instructor and students. • In doing so, identify the action steps that have been or are being taken to achieve the desired outcome. • Identify supporting and mitigating aspects to implementing the practice change.	• Review the clinical placement site's strategic plan. Meet with the clinical placement site practice partner and identify a strategic priority/objective/outcome that the nursing students could work on that would also complement course objectives. • Within the clinical placement site's strategic plan, review a measurable objective with complementing tactics as a mechanism to better understand the steps involved in implementing a practice change. Have the students reflect on what surprised them about the implementation process. What might they suggest to expedite the adoption of evidence-based practices into the clinical setting? • Perform a portion of an environmental scan by having students visit credible websites to identify economic, environmental, political, technological, societal, and regulatory trends affecting health care delivery. Identify how these trends are or are not reflected in the clinical placement site's strategic plan.

TABLE **6-5**

Exercises in Indicator Performance Practices in the Clinical Experience Between Academic and Practice Partners

PRACTICE PARTNER EXERCISE	ACADEMIC PARTNER–CLINICAL INSTRUCTOR/STUDENT EXERCISE
• Share core unit or organizational performance indicator findings and evidence-based interventions with the clinical instructor and students to ensure optimum outcomes.	• Review the clinical site's performance indicator dashboard. • Together with the practice partner, select one indicator that aligns with the course focus. • Have the students perform a literature review to further inform and/or confirm that the intervention is based on current evidence.

ADDRESSING THE BARRIERS TO ENSURE ENTRY-LEVEL IMPLEMENTATION SCIENCE PRACTICES

Various limitations to the implementation of EBP exist. These include the following:

> . . . barriers to successful research such as: lack of awareness or understanding of (... EBP); lack of association with researchers; lack of ability to locate or find relevant research; lack of ability to understand the language of research; lack of recognition of the value of research in nursing practice; lack of availability of computer databases; lack of basic knowledge of information technology; and lack of time to obtain research information. (Godshall, 2015, p. 144)

After conducting a comprehensive search of contemporary literature from 2010 to 2015, Mallion and Brooke (2016) noted the following:

> . . . the traditionally acknowledged barriers of a lack of time, knowledge, and skills remained; however, nurses' beliefs toward EBP were more positive, but positive beliefs did not affect the intentions to implement EBP or the knowledge and skills of EBP. Nurses in hospital and community settings reported similar barriers and facilitators. (p. 148)

These barriers provide opportunity for the academic setting to partner with the clinical practice setting in codesigning nursing curricula that more intentionally prepare new graduate nurses in their ability to inform practice through critical appraisal and synthesis of research findings. From a didactic perspective, the nursing baccalaureate generalist education traditionally provides course content on research design and methodology, nursing research and theory, informatics, EBP frameworks and models, critical appraisal, PICOT (Population, Intervention, Comparison, Outcome, Time) question formation, and formative and summative evaluation. In addition, project work often requires the nursing student to work collaboratively in identifying an evidence-based intervention to address a clinical problem. However, the limitations to the implementation of EBP noted previously trigger a need for academic/practice partners to collectively review the relevance of current educational content and teaching modalities to optimize student acquisition of knowledge, skills, and attitudes in achieving student learning outcomes. The notion that nurses' beliefs toward EBP have become more positive serves as the medium to nurture growth in further implementing EBP. In forging academic/practice partnerships to codesign curricular content and exemplars, strategies could include the following:

- Inviting community partners into the classroom or clinical pre- and postconference sessions to share EBPs and processes
- Providing a platform for students to determine evidence-based interventions to clinical issues posed by practice partners
- Actively recruiting nursing students in the phases of faculty research, such as research design, methodology, problem identification, literature review, data collection, analysis, or dissemination
- Providing a mechanism that communicates faculty and/or practice partner scholarly activities
- Supporting students in conducting honors projects and independent research studies that have clinical significance to nursing practice
- Inviting university librarians into the classroom (physical or virtual) to serve as a resource for students conducting literature searches; this can include posting of online resources to facilitate knowledge and skill acquisition in assessing the strength and quality of the literature

Although it is important to drive toward greater proficiency in the student's capacity to implement EBP, nursing baccalaureate curricula should distinguish between this and TS or IS. Titler (2018) noted the following:

EBP and translation science, though related, are not interchangeable terms. EBP is the actual application of evidence in practice (the "doing of" EBP), whereas translation science is the study of implementation interventions, factors, and contextual variables that effect knowledge uptake and use in practices and communities. (p. 3)

The senior capstone project in baccalaureate nursing education offers the student the opportunity to collaborate with individuals in the practice setting to improve patient outcomes through a cocreated and codesigned project. In cocreation, the value between the academic and practice partner is contextualized, whereas in the project codesign a relevant issue can be addressed through critical appraisal of research to identify an evidence-based intervention that thoughtfully considers the elements of TS.

Thus, baccalaureate nursing education that builds awareness of theories and frameworks specific to IS advantages the new graduate to more readily contribute to transformative practices when in the clinical setting. These theories, models, and frameworks largely originate from the social sciences where humans or organizations are examined as a mechanism to explain and understand behavioral responses at the individual, group, organizational, or population level. The completion of courses in the social sciences, such as psychology, sociology, or anthropology, are often required early in the student's journey to become a baccalaureate-prepared nurse. They provide the nursing student with a critical element of a liberal education that builds on a foundation of the arts, sciences, humanities, and social sciences. The Association of American Colleges and Universities described liberal education as follows:

An approach to learning that empowers individuals and prepares them to deal with complexity, diversity, and change. It provides students with broad knowledge of the wider world (e.g., science, culture, and society) as well as in-depth study in a specific area of interest. A liberal education helps students develop a sense of social responsibility as well as strong and transferable intellectual and practical skills such as communication, analytical and problem-solving skills, and a demonstrated ability to apply knowledge and skills in real-world settings. (2011, p. 3)

In nursing, these intellectual and practical skills broaden to include the capacity to apply critical thinking, clinical reasoning, and clinical judgment to ensure that interventions are evidence-based and result in improved outcomes.

The general education portion of the nursing student's liberal education provides opportunity for students from a wide array of arts and sciences disciplines to examine and apply subject matter and "forms the basis for the development of important intellectual, civic, and practical capacities. General education can take many forms, and it increasingly includes introductory, advanced, and integrative forms of learning" (Association of American Colleges and Universities, 2011, p. 3). Examples within a nursing curriculum that further enhance the interdisciplinary experience gained through general education include those that promote knowledge, skills, and attitudes around interprofessional collaborative practices. For example, course content on the Core Competencies for Interprofessional Collaborative Practice focuses on helping to "prepare future health professionals for enhanced team-based care of patients and improved population health outcomes" (Interprofessional Education Collaborative [IPEC], 2016, p. 1).

In 2016, the IPEC Board updated its 2011 seminal report and, in reaffirming the value and influence of the core and subcompetencies, reconceptualized the original domains of values and ethics, roles and responsibilities, interprofessional communication, and teams and teamwork to become topics under the one singular domain of interprofessional collaboration. Their intention to create shared taxonomy among the health professions was to do the following:

... streamline and synergize educational activities and related assessment and evaluation efforts (and ultimately) broaden the interprofessional competencies to better achieve the Triple Aim (improve the patient experience of care, improve the health of populations, and reduce the per capita cost of health care), with particular reference to population health. (IPEC, 2016, p. 1)

Current attempts in baccalaureate nursing education to deliver content on interprofessional collaboration range from independent courses to separate modular offerings and may be facilitated by one or several disciplines involving in-seat, synchronous or asynchronous learning platforms. Overall, the offerings build from the multidisciplinary approach experienced in general education by giving students from various disciplines the opportunity to "learn about, from and with each other to enable effective collaboration and improve health outcomes" as originally envisioned in instances where "two or more professions" gather (World Health Organization, 2010, p. 13). The topics under the singular domain of interprofessional collaboration (values and ethics, roles and responsibilities, interprofessional communication, and teams and teamwork) may further contribute to the veracity of IS for new graduate nurses, physicians, and allied health professionals when considering additional opportunities to collectively engage over relevant subject matter through capstone projects and research. "The expectation that accompanies the idea of co-negotiated knowledge or engaged scholarship is that collaborative action in knowledge production is positively associated with knowledge implementation" (Salter & Kothari, 2016, p. 7). By being equipped while in the academic setting with the tools necessary to ensure effective interprofessional collaboration, students can move to gain greater proficiency in collectively evaluating implementation strategies in consideration of supporting and mitigating factors. The question for those designing and delivering curricula is to determine when it is best to introduce and re-emphasize interprofessional collaboration into the students' journey to heighten knowledge, skills, and attitudes around IS.

Similar consideration should be given to the integration of practice experiences across the nursing student's program of study that provides the student with a broad understanding of how knowledge is operationalized in context of the organization. In baccalaureate nursing education, this may begin with exposure to clinical decision support (CDS) in the practice setting. The Agency for Healthcare Research and Quality conveyed the following:

. . . the main purpose of CDS is to provide timely information to clinicians, patients, and others to inform decisions about health care. Examples of CDS tools include order sets created for particular conditions or types of patients, recommendations, and databases that can provide information relevant to particular patients, reminders for preventive care, and alerts about potentially dangerous situations. (2019, para. 3)

In addition to point-of-care products, exposure to quick reference guides or signage to support implementation of EBPs can also add to the nursing students' understanding of tactics that organizations put in place to ensure the consistent delivery of quality services. For example, evidence-based fall prevention interventions can be supported by offering the fall risk assessment on a quick reference guide, whereas a whiteboard in a patient's room identifying the individual's level of fall risk or level of required mobility assistance further standardizes evidence-based care to achieve safe outcomes. Fostering awareness on the purpose and application for these types of tools and aids can then be strengthened through deliberate clinical experiences that help the student understand how the tool or aid was selected, implemented, and sustained. Through this lens, the nursing student would learn about the practice sites' goals, objectives, and outcomes around fall prevention; would perhaps attend a multidisciplinary fall prevention committee meeting; might learn about the decision making that supported the selection of the fall risk assessment tool; would review the literature supporting the fall prevention interventions; and would meet with the marketing team that assisted in the development of the fall prevention signage. These are only a few examples that support student awareness of how organizations apply knowledge in context of their surroundings.

IMPLEMENTATION SCIENCE AND PRACTICES INTO SIMULATION-BASED EXPERIENCES

Despite efforts to gain consistency when implementing EBPs, opportunities to address barriers in maintaining implementation fidelity in the practice setting continue. Breitenstein et al. (2010) noted that barriers included the following:

Local adaptations of interventions, individual variations in practitioner adherence and competence, lack of available training and technical support, limited resources for supporting the intervention at the site level, and competing demands for the practitioners' time that can diminish their commitment or effectiveness (Botvin, 2004; Dévieux, et al., 2005; Hill, Maucione, & Hood, 2007). (p. 3)

One solution to mitigate these barriers around issues of implementation consistency could logically be found through the supplementation of undergraduate nursing clinical experiences in the practice setting with simulation-based experiences (SBEs). In the United States, state boards of nursing regulate the percentage of clinical experiences that can be attributed to SBEs in nursing program curricula. SBEs provide activities through thoughtfully designed scenarios that emphasize the achievement of desired student learning outcomes. According to the Agency for Healthcare Research and Quality Patient Safety Network, "the goal of simulation-based training is to enable the accelerated development of expertise, both in individual and team skills, by bridging the gap between classroom training and real-world clinical experiences in a relatively risk-free environment" (2019, para. 2).

In baccalaureate nursing education, IS is optimized when uniformity over the application of best practices can be achieved. The International Nursing Association for Clinical Simulation and Learning (INACSL) Standards of Best Practice provide faculty and staff with "an evidence-based framework to guide simulation design, implementation, debriefing, evaluation, and research" (2016, p. S12). The INACSL standards are expanded through specific criterion aimed at ensuring effective assessment of the participant and the participant's ability to achieve the identified objectives or expected outcomes as well as the efficient use of resources associated with the design of the SBE (p. S5). Simulation affords the student learner the opportunity to demonstrate delivery of the intervention as intended when specific simulation design elements are incorporated into SBEs to replicate real-world behaviors or situations. Congruent with clinical experiences in the practice setting, "context matters" when considering the impact on implementation outcomes through the lens of clinical simulation in undergraduate nursing education. According to the INACSL, this perception of realism requires attention to physical (or environmental), conceptual, and psychological aspects of fidelity. Table 6-6 features key factors related to each design element.

By using the appropriate types of fidelity, participants will be in a better position to engage in a relevant manner (INACSL, 2016, p. S7). Consequently, new nurses entering into practice who have been educated through modalities that promoted relevant engagement throughout their baccalaureate nursing educational journey will likely be nimbler in acclimating to their role as a professional nurse. This includes the implementation of EBPs.

Table 6-7 provides a brief overview of the methods and applications of simulation-based training that are more commonly integrated into nursing curricula to enhance student learning and promote the implementation of EBPs when in the practice setting. Nursing programs often use a combination of simulation methodologies.

Upon entry into practice, nurses may find themselves engaging in simulations that are physically integrated into the actual clinical environment with the providers who work in that location. Commonly referred to as in situ simulation, these SBEs may involve the use of part-task trainers or full-scale simulators. In situ simulation is viewed as an important part of training to improve reliability and safety in the delivery of health care.

TABLE 6-6
Realism in Simulation-Based Experiences: Aspects of Fidelity

ASPECT OF FIDELITY	DESCRIPTOR	FACTORS
Physical or environmental	How realistically the physical context of the simulation-based activity replicates the actual environment in which the situation would occur in real life.	The patient(s), simulator/manikin, standardized patient, environment, equipment, embedded actors, and related props.
Conceptual	All elements of the scenario or case relate to each other in a realistic way so that the case makes sense as a whole to the participant(s).	Cases or scenarios should be reviewed by subject matter expert(s) and pilot tested before use with participants.
Psychological	Maximizes the simulation environment by mimicking the contextual elements found in clinical environments. Works synergistically with physical and conceptual fidelity to promote participant engagement.	An active voice for the patient(s) to allow realistic conversation, noise and lighting typically associated with the simulated setting, distractions, family members, other health care team members, time pressure, and competing priorities.

Data source: International Nursing Association for Clinical Simulation and Learning Standards Committee (2016, December). INACSL standards of best practice: Simulation^sm Simulation Design. *Clinical Simulation in Nursing, 12*(S), S5-S12. https://doi.org/10.1016/j.ecns.2016.09.005.

To further promote a culture of safety through evidence that is translated into practice, academic and practice partners have continued to focus on the assessment of clinical competence among students within baccalaureate nursing programs. Obizoba (2018) noted that "Objective Structured Clinical Examination (OSCE), widely used in nursing education internationally has limited utilization in undergraduate nursing programs in the United States" (p. 71), whereas, its application in evaluating medical student and advanced practice nursing clinical competence is well documented. "A well-designed and implemented OSCE as a method of assessing students' clinical competencies provides students with opportunities to demonstrate interpersonal and interview skills, problem-solving abilities, teaching, assessment skills, and application of basic clinical knowledge" (McWilliam & Botwinski, 2012, p. 35). In addition, "with appropriate SP [standardized patient] selection and training, the utilization of appropriate tools and good data collection, OSCE can offer a valid and reliable means of testing student competencies" (McWilliam & Botwinski, 2012, p. 39).

However, baccalaureate nursing programs do assess their students' clinical competence using a standardized environment that is conducive to formal testing. Standardization in this sense is more commonly achieved through high-fidelity simulation that places the student in a true-to-life patient milieu through interactions with a sophisticated lifelike manikin. The high-fidelity manikin is operated from a control room by a simulation technologist who adjusts the manikin's responses throughout the event while faculty apprised of the course objectives direct the educational aspect of the student experience. Additional "guides" may interface with the student during the SBE. The guide serves as an embedded participant who brings more context to the scenario. Evaluation associated with simulation in undergraduate nursing curricula is often formative in nature in that the SBE results in the student receiving constructive feedback on how to improve in performance. Furthermore, the element of briefing and debriefing as part of the student's SBE promotes student

TABLE 6-7	Simulation Methodologies	
SIMULATION METHODOLOGY	APPLICATION	EXAMPLES
Part-task trainers	Train specific clinical skills through simulation	Anatomically correct limb models for the demonstration of phlebotomy skills or placement of intravenous catheters
Full-scale simulators	To teach the physical examination and other fundamental clinical skills	Full-body manikin, which, in addition to anatomic landmarks, can offer realistic physiological simulation (such as heart sounds and respirations)
Virtual reality	Learners physically interact with the environment as they would in real life using systems that are increasingly complex and technologically sophisticated	Immersion into a highly realistic clinical environment, such as an operating room or intensive care unit
Standardized patients	Employing trained actors to simulate real patients	Teach basic history taking and physical examination skills or teach patient safety skills, such as error disclosure

Data source: Agency for Healthcare Research and Quality Patient Safety Network. (2019). Simulation training. https://psnet.ahrq.gov/primer/simulation-training.

reflection and knowledge transformation. In contrast, the assessment of student competencies in associated health care activities in which a judgment is rendered requires the integration of summative or high-stakes evaluation methods. In summative evaluation, a grade determination may be conferred, whereas high-stakes evaluation occurs at a discreet point in time and connotes a significant outcome or consequence, such as a pass/fail determination (INACSL, 2016).

Movement toward the integration of competency-based assessment in undergraduate nursing curricula requires intentionality around SBEs that align with identified competencies in nursing education. Continued dialogue with practice partners to identify competencies that can be achieved through simulation will further ensure new graduate nurses' successful transition to practice. This approach has implications for the future design of nurse residency programs and the conceptualization of the role of the preceptor with new graduate nurses.

Simulation training of faculty, technology staff, and standardized patients serves as an implementation practice to ensure collective proficiency in the execution of competency-based outcome measurement. Lewis et al. (2017) noted the following:

On one end of the continuum, in high stakes assessment, SPs (standardized patients) may be trained to behave in a highly repeatable or standardized manner in order to give each learner a fair and equal chance and are often referred to as standardized patients. It is important to note that in this context, SPs are individuals whose behavior has been standardized. In formative educational settings, where standardization may not play an important part in the session design, carefully trained SPs can respond with more authenticity and flexibility to the needs of individual learners and are referred to as simulated patients. (para. 9)

When using a standardized approach in the SBE, there is some opportunity for implementation fidelity if there is attention to whether the evidence-based intervention was delivered as intended. Without applying context in the standardized SBE, it might be more challenging for the student to implement the evidence-based intervention once in the practice setting.

Moving forward, it will be important for baccalaureate nursing education to consider coordinating SBEs across the curricula by introducing and building on unfolding case studies through simulated scenarios that reinforce knowledge uptake. For example, curricula that are designed to provide the student with opportunities to interact with the patient over the course of their projected illness may serve to cultivate the student's capacity to "use clinical forethought to predict what could happen next" (Moench, 2019, para. 4). Guided reflective prompting that requires the student to consider interventions that *could* have been implemented with regard to core competencies, such as patient preference/patient-centered care, gives the learner "a glimpse of the power of informed prediction to prevent adverse outcomes" (Moench, 2019, para. 4). Interventions retrospectively identified by the student should also speak to the elements of TS. For example, guided reflective prompts could include specific questions on student nurse preparation, implementation, and ideas for sustainability when considering contextual factors related to a patient's social determinants of health.

Conclusion

The curricular design and delivery of a baccalaureate nursing program have the power to accelerate or delay practice change that is based on research. To position new baccalaureate-prepared graduate nurses to effectively and efficiently translate evidence into practice requires the integration of knowledge, skills, and attitudes specific to IS across the nursing curriculum. Governing influences through accreditation, state board regulation, professional nursing standards, guidelines, outcomes, and core competencies are integrated across the curriculum and articulated through course objectives that move the student toward proficiency in becoming an entry-level generalist baccalaureate nurse. These elements hardwire curricular consistency in maintaining EBPs in baccalaureate nursing education. Moreover, curricula that are codesigned between academic and practice partners provide further context and intentionality in preparing new graduate nurse capacity to inform practice through critical appraisal and synthesis of research findings. Strategies to ensure that nursing education is consistently delivered as intended by faculty and preceptors are achieved through orientation, training, and mentoring. Didactic nursing education formulated on research and EBP and interprofessional education are further applied into the practice setting through experiential clinical assignments. Shared implementation practices between academic and practice partners can optimize learning among BS/BSN students while ensuring high-quality, safe, person-centered outcomes within an array of practice settings where students are placed. Furthermore, strategies to ensure that the nursing intervention is delivered as intended bring consistency to student learning through simulated experiences and guided reflective prompting that explore the factors affecting implementation.

Reflective Questions

1. Using Table 6-4, select one academic partner–clinical instructor exercise and develop a plan of action.
2. Identify at least two barriers that may impact successful IS practices and describe ways that these challenges can be overcome.
3. Consider a recent simulated clinical experience that you have participated in and describe the implementation plan (with rationale) that was integrated into the assignment.

REFERENCES

Agency for Healthcare Research and Quality. (2019). Clinical decision support. https://www.ahrq.gov/cpi/about/otherwebsites/clinical-decision-support/index.html

Agency for Healthcare Research and Quality Patient Safety Network. (2019). Simulation training. https://psnet.ahrq.gov/primer/simulation-training

Altman S., Butler A., & Shern L. (2016). Assessing Progress on the Institute of Medicine Report *The Future of Nursing*. Committee for Assessing Progress on Implementing the Recommendations of the Institute of Medicine Report The Future of Nursing: Leading Change, Advancing Health; Institute of Medicine; National Academies of Sciences, Engineering, and Medicine. National Academies Press. https://www.ncbi.nlm.nih.gov/books/NBK350161/

American Association of Colleges of Nursing. (2019a). The impact of education on nursing practice. https://www.aacnnursing.org/News-Information/Fact-Sheets/Impact-of-Education

American Association of Colleges of Nursing. (2019b). Vizient/AACN nurse residency program. https://www.aacnnursing.org/Portals/42/AcademicNursing/NRP/Nurse-Residency-Program.pdf

Association of American Colleges and Universities. (2011). The LEAP vision for learning: Outcomes, practices, impact, and employers' views. https://leap.aacu.org/toolkit/wp-content/uploads/2010/12/LEAP-Vision_Summary.pdf

Breitenstein, S., Gross, D., Garvey, C., Hill, C., Fogg, L., & Resnick, B. (2010). Implementation fidelity in community-based interventions. *Research in Nursing & Health, 33*,164-173. https://doi.org/10.1002/nur.20373

Casey, M., O'Leary, D., & Coghlan, D. (2018). Unpacking action research and implementation science: Implications for nursing. *Journal of Advanced Nursing, 74*, 1051-1058. https://doi.org/10.1111/jan.13494

Clark, M., Raffray, M., Hendricks, K., & Gagnon, A. (2016). Global and public health core competencies for nursing education: A systematic review of essential competencies. *Nurse Education Today, 40*, 173-180. https://doi.org/10.1016/j.nedt.2016.02.026

Godshall, M. (2015). Barriers to disseminating the evidence. In M. Godshall (Ed.), *Fast facts for evidence-based practice in nursing* (2nd ed., pp. 143-160). Springer Publishing Company.

Institute of Medicine. (2003). *Health professions education: A bridge to quality*. The National Academies Press. https://www.ncbi.nlm.nih.gov/books/NBK221519/

Institute of Medicine. (2011). *The future of nursing: Leading change, advancing health*. The National Academies Press. https://doi.org/10.17226/12956

International Nursing Association for Clinical Simulation and Learning Standards Committee (2016, December). INACSL standards of best practice: Simulation^sm Simulation Design. *Clinical Simulation in Nursing, 12*(S), S5-S12. https://doi.org/10.1016/j.ecns.2016.09.005.

Interprofessional Education Collaborative. (2016). *Core competencies for interprofessional collaborative practice: 2016 update*. Interprofessional Education Collaborative.

Lewis, K. L., Bohnert, C. A., Gammon, W. L., Hölzer, H., Lyman, L., Smith, C., Thompson, T. M., Wallace A., & Gliva-McConvey, G. (2017). The Association of Standardized Patient Educators (ASPE) standards of best practice (SOBP). *Advances in Simulation, 2*(10), 1-8. https://doi.org/10.1186/s41077-017-0043-4

Mallion, J., & Brooke, J. (2016). Community- and hospital-based nurses' implementation of evidence-based practice: Are there any differences? *British Journal of Community Nursing, 21*(3), 148-154. https://doi.org/10.12968/bjcn.2016.21.3.148

McClure, E., & Black, L. (2013). The role of the clinical preceptor: An integrative literature review. *Journal of Nursing Education, 52*, 335-341. https://doi.org/10.3928/01484834-20130430-02

McWilliam, P. L., & Botwinski, C. A. (2012). Identifying strengths and weaknesses in the utilization of objective structured clinical examination (OSCE) in a nursing program. *Nursing Education Research, 33*(1), 35-39. https://doi.org/10.5480/1536-5026-33.1.35

Moench, B. (2019). Using unfolding case studies to develop clinical forethought in novice nursing students. QSEN Institute. https://qsen.org/using-unfolding-case-studies-to-develop-clinical-forethought-in-novice-nursing-students/

Obizoba, C. (2018). Mitigating the challenges of objective structured clinical examination (OSCE) in nursing education: A phenomenological research study. *Nurse Education Today, 68*, 71-74. https://doi.org/10.1016/j.nedt.2018.06.002

Salter, K. L., & Kothari, A. (2016). Knowledge 'translation' as social learning: Negotiating the uptake of research-based knowledge in practice. *BMC Medical Education, 16*(76), 1-10. https://doi.org/10.1186/s12909-016-0585-5

Thomas, P., & Winter, J. (2020). Strategic practices in achieving organizational effectiveness. In L. Roussel, P. Thomas, J. Harris (Eds.), *Management and leadership for nurse administrators* (8th ed., pp. 135-154). Jones & Bartlett Learning.

Titler, M. G. (2018). Translation research in practice: An introduction. *The Online Journal of Issues in Nursing, 23*(2), 1-15. https://ojin.nursingworld.org/MainMenuCategories/ANAMarketplace/ANAPeriodicals/OJIN

Ulrich, B. (2012). *Mastering precepting: A nurse's handbook for success*. Sigma Theta Tau International.

U.S. Department of Education. (2019, July 19). Overview of accreditation in the United States. https://www2.ed.gov/admins/finaid/accred/accreditation.html#Overview

World Health Organization. (2010). *Framework for action on interprofessional education & collaborative practice*. Health Professions Network Nursing and Midwifery Office Within the Department of Human Resources for Health. https://apps.who.int/iris/bitstream/handle/10665/70185/WHO_HRH_HPN_10.3_eng.pdf;jsessionid=BC90102389D898860B390AC66BCAA804?sequence=1

Exemplar 6-1

Interprofessional Collaboration

Margaret Moore-Nadler, DNP, RN

The College of Nursing at the University of South Alabama collaborates with Allied Health, University of South Alabama Family Medicine, Auburn Harrison School of Pharmacy, and previous students to introduce health care preprofessionals to IPEC, TeamSTEPPS, and Motivational Interviewing and Mindfulness. Undergraduate nursing students were involved in this collaborative effort. Team and TS were frameworks integrated into the IPEC. The purpose is to increase students' knowledge, skills, and ability to apply these concepts when providing patient-centered care that is safe and increases patient and provider satisfaction while decreasing the cost of health care.

The methodology developed is teaching interprofessional health care student teams in three phases throughout the curriculum. Developing a curriculum using a multifaceted approach was the evidence-based implementation strategy undertaken to increase collaboration among preprofessionals. This intervention was developed in three phases with evaluation measures built into each phase (Moir, 2018). Phase 1 focuses on building a foundation of knowledge base upon course concepts. Phase 2 promotes developing skills of all concepts, and Phase 3 is applying the knowledge and skills with a vulnerable patient population attending a behavioral health clinic. Data collected includes students' attitudes of IPEC core competencies, quizzes in all phases, and forum discussions. The final project is an evidence-based poster presentation related to learned concepts applied to a vulnerable population seen at the behavioral health clinic.

The results from the data collected reflect that the students' attitudes improve after learning the concepts of IPEC; furthermore, the threaded discussions strongly support learning TeamSTEPPS, motivational interviewing, and mindfulness (the multifaceted approach selected). This was noted to be relevant to improving students' learning and improving the health of patients.

In conclusion, the IPEC faculty believe health care preprofessionals must have a solid foundation of the theory and evidence-based research to improve the quality of health care globally. Using a multifaceted approach and IS, the IPEC team was armed with tools to enhance collaboration and team learning. Organizations and professionals must value, respect, and include all health care staff in the stages of changing a process or intervention. Without employee involvement in planning and designing a change or intervention, it is less likely that the implementing will achieve the desired outcome.

Reference

Moir, T. (2018). Why is implementation science important for intervention design and evaluation within educational settings? *Frontiers in Education, 3*, 61. https://doi.org/10.3389/feduc.2018.00061

IMPLEMENTATION AND DISSEMINATION SCIENCES AND PRACTICE
Graduate Nursing Education and Advanced Practice

Cynthia Peltier Coviak, PhD, RN, FNAP

CHAPTER OBJECTIVES

- Outline key differences between the doctor of philosophy/doctor of nursing science/doctor of the science of nursing and practice-focused degrees at the doctoral or master's level in nursing relating to the understanding and use of research and the roles that graduates will undertake in relation to research

- Explore practice-focused graduate students' differentiation between translational science and evidence-based practice and how this advanced knowledge prepares them to lead change in clinical areas

- Identify experiences that foster the development of knowledge and skills in translational science and evidence-based practice for research-focused doctoral and doctor of nursing practice students

- Describe doctor of philosophy and doctor of nursing practice collaboration in education for translational science and the impact on population health and health care system change

- Apply master of science in nursing student competencies and application for translational science and evidence-based practice

Roussel, L. A., & Thomas, P. L. (Eds.). *Implementation Science in Nursing: A Framework for Education and Practice* (pp. 107-131).

KEY WORDS

- Dissemination science
- Doctor of nursing practice
- Doctor of philosophy–doctor of nursing practice collaboration
- Implementation science
- Master of nursing competencies

- Nursing practice
- Nursing research
- Research-focused doctorate
- Translational science
- Translational science competencies

In this chapter, the challenges of educating master's-prepared nurses, advanced practice nurses from doctor of nursing practice (DNP) programs, and nurse scientists in relation to translational science (TS) and evidence-based practice (EBP) are discussed. The competencies desired for leadership and practice in EBP and the field of TS that overlap with the expectations for research-focused and practice-focused nurses are examined. Courses, content, and experiences in the curriculum for both doctoral and master's-level students that can foster the development of both nursing and TS competencies are considered, and suggestions for leveling the competencies for master's-level and doctoral students are presented. Appropriate EBP and TS scholarly endeavors that can be important culminating projects, products of these activities, and venues for their dissemination are described.

In many of their clinical experiences as students or in the first positions of their careers, many nurses of the baby boomer generation and those who came before were likely to hear from "seasoned" nurses that the procedures they were to do had "always been done that way." Often, this statement was accompanied by admonishments from the seasoned nurses, or if the new professional's work presented too great a deviation from the norm, comments were included on professional evaluations from supervisors indicating that the new staff member needed to adhere to policies—however outdated and lacking of evidence the policies might be. Fortunately, nurses and other health care professionals have since learned that what we "always" did was not always the right or safe thing to do. Research and reports completed after publication of the Institute of Medicine's report *To Err Is Human: Building a Safer Health System* (2000), along with theoretical and opinion papers, have documented that often provider actions have been wrong. As this chapter is being written, 20 years after this report was published, the reasons for errors and poor health care outcomes are under scrutiny, and improvements designed to mitigate the factors that lead to many mistakes and tragedies are being sought.

Innovation can be a wonderful thing, but it too does not always result in the most appropriate or efficient solution to a dilemma. After all, often what the seasoned nurses presented as tradition was at one time someone's novel approach or improvement to the practices of the period or setting. The difference is that nurses now have the capacity to design and test innovation in systematic ways to generate confidence in an approach, including when it should be used, how it should be performed, what the results should be from its usage, and when the results should be apparent.

Nurses of any educational level with any degree of expertise can devise innovative approaches to care. Views of nursing as both art and science bring opportunities for ingenuity in interventions, and there is pride in nursing's perseverance and creativity when resources are scarce. Nurses may use esthetic as well as empirical patterns of knowing to guide actions (Carper, 1978). Nevertheless, it is a nurse with a graduate education who must use scientific processes and procedures to test an innovation's efficacy, effectiveness, safety, and efficiency in the real-life contexts where care is provided in order to ascertain its usefulness for broad use. In nursing, both research and practice experts are being prepared in graduate programs, and practice-focused nurses are educated at both the master's and doctoral levels. The potential exists for more widespread and cost-effective deployment of nursing and health care innovations. For this to occur, not only are the traditional skills of a scientist needed in the nursing workforce, but also the capabilities of a practice expert.

TS in health care, as a field that focuses on dissemination and implementation of innovations among health professionals, provides evidence to highlight processes and outcomes of a discipline's improvements when they are applied to the care environment. The complementary talents of nurse scientists and advanced nursing practice experts are needed for the conduct of TS in nursing. For TS efforts to be successful, graduate programs in nursing must provide courses and experiences in research that are suitable for students' chosen roles. Students also need a foundation in dissemination science (DS) and implementation science (IS) that prepares them to be successful in their future distinct roles in TS.

Nursing Research, Nursing Practice, and Translational Science

Graduate nursing education and the roles that nurses with various degrees assume in relation to EBP as well as the conduct and use of research have been evolving rapidly in the last 50 years. In the mid-1970s to early 1990s, it was not uncommon for students achieving a master's degree in nursing (MN or MSN) to complete a thesis that involved a small-scale or pilot research project usually limited to settings likely to have unique characteristics and clients. The findings from their work were unlikely to have generalizability to guide practice in substantive ways. The roles that master's program graduates would take were often in education or administration; as time went on, they entered advanced nursing practice as nurse practitioners and clinical nurse specialists. The research experiences of these nurses while in educational programs provided preparation that was practical for a general understanding of research methods. However, because of the limitations of their projects, there was often little to guide practice in those roles.

Some major changes in the health care system prompted reassessment of nursing education. In the mid-1980s, with the enactment of diagnostic-related groupings (Mistichelli, 1984), cost containment became a priority and challenge. During the 1990s, information accessibility became ubiquitous as the Internet matured and was used by increasing numbers of health care providers (Grol & Grimshaw, 2003). With these dynamics in place, what was happening in health care was stressing the system. Quality and safety issues documented in *To Err Is Human: Building a Safer Health System* (Institute of Medicine, 2000) then spurred urgency for responses from health care professionals. Members of the American Association of Colleges of Nursing (AACN) urged reconsideration of the types and forms of graduate education. By 2000, the AACN was advocating a shift in the focus of master's education from the traditional specialties to the development of a new role—the clinical nurse leader (CNL; AACN, 2004b). The educational preparation for this role was conceptualized as that of an "advanced generalist," a nurse whose expertise is developed beyond those of a baccalaureate degree–prepared nurse to include skills in risk assessment and anticipation, collaboration and coordination of care within a microsystem of patients, introduction of EBP initiatives, and other competencies fostering quality and safety practices at the point of care (Ott et al., 2006).

At the same time, AACN was engaging with its members and other stakeholders to explore and eventually endorse the DNP degree as the appropriate graduate preparation for the advanced nursing practice roles of nurse practitioner, clinical nurse specialist, nurse anesthetist, and nurse midwife (AACN, 2004a). This practice degree was to have an "emphasis on scholarly practice, practice improvement, innovation and testing of interventions and care delivery models, evaluation of health care outcomes, and expertise to inform health policy and leadership in establishing clinical excellence" (Marion et al., 2003, as cited in AACN, 2004a, p. 6). It was specifically noted that any research experiences in the degree program should emphasize practice contexts, that theory and research methodology content should be less than in research-focused doctorates, and that the evaluation and use of research should be the focus rather than conducting research (AACN, 2004a). This was in contrast to the doctor of philosophy (PhD) in nursing and the doctor of the science of nursing (DSN) or the doctor of nursing science (DNS/DNSc) degrees, which were often modeled after the research-focused doctorates in the natural and social sciences. The research-focused doctoral programs in nursing have embraced the roles for its graduates that the Carnegie Foundation for the Advancement of Teaching identified in its report *The Formation of Scholars: Rethinking Doctoral Education for the Twenty-First Century* (Walker et al., 2008). These were the maintenance and development of nursing science, stewardship of the nursing discipline, and education of the next generation of scholars (AACN, 2001, 2010).

With the differentiation of the practice-focused and research-focused doctoral degrees in their purposes and goals, there have been ongoing deliberations about master's- and doctoral-level research expectations and competencies and experiences in advanced nursing practice. *The Essentials of Master's Education in Nursing* (AACN, 2011) and *The Essentials of Doctoral Education for Advanced Nursing Practice* (AACN, 2006) guide curricula for practice-focused degree programs, whereas research-focused doctoral programs strive to demonstrate quality as described in *The Research-Focused Doctoral Program in Nursing: Pathways to Excellence* (AACN, 2010) and the earlier document, *Indicators of Quality in Research-Focused Doctoral Programs in Nursing* (AACN, 2001). The *Essentials* documents do not consistently address competencies for graduates of the programs. Instead, because degrees are not the same as roles and competencies are focused on the ability to fulfill particular roles (Leung, 2002; Nodine, 2016), distinct guidance papers have been developed such as *Competencies and Curricular Expectations for the Clinical Nurse Leader Education and Practice* (AACN, 2013), *Clinical Nurse Specialist Core Competencies* (National CNS Competency Task Force, 2010), *Nurse Practitioner Core Competencies Content* (National Organization of Nurse Practitioner Faculties NP Core Competencies Work Group, 2014), and *Common Advanced Practice Registered Nurse Doctoral-Level Competencies* (AACN Common APRN Doctoral-Level Competencies Work Group, 2017). From these documents and others, student knowledge, skills, and attitudes (KSAs) appropriate for their future roles are outlined, and curricula that will prepare them with competencies for those roles can be developed.

Task force reports address the competencies for many of the graduate programs and assist faculty in choosing content and clinical experiences. Examples of these statements include *Recommended CNL Practice Experiences* (AACN, 2017) and *The Doctor of Nursing Practice: Current Issues and Clarifying Recommendations* (AACN, 2015). In the documents to develop competencies related to clinical use of a scientific foundation, most of the practice degree programs are urged to require culminating projects that involve the use and implementation of EBPs in a clinical situation, often within a quality improvement (QI) context (AACN, 2015, 2017). The literature provides many examples of methods used to provide these experiences (Brown & Crabtree, 2013; Buchholz et al., 2015; Graves et al., 2018; Melnyk, 2013; Moore & Watters, 2013).

Simultaneously, faculty of research-focused programs are exhorted to design curricula that include foundations in "emerging" science, including TS and rigorous theoretical and methodological coursework updated to account for these new sciences (Breslin et al., 2015; Henly et al., 2015; Melnyk, 2013). However, for many reasons, practical and appropriate ways to provide training in TS to research-focused doctoral students in nursing are needed, as well as experiences in collaborative TS projects. The barriers to training include a lack of funding for TS, few nursing faculty with expertise in TS, and the newness of TS itself (Breslin et al., 2015; Buchholz et al., 2015; Henly et al., 2015; Lusk & Marzilli, 2018; Melnyk, 2013; Santacroce et al., 2018).

However, the paucity of expertise in TS is not confined to nursing. Several of the National Institutes of Health, as well as the Canadian Institutes of Health Research, have sponsored training programs to prepare translational scientists and "practitioners" (Chambers et al., 2017; Meissner et al., 2013; Moore et al., 2018; Proctor & Chambers, 2017; Santacroce et al., 2018; Straus et al., 2011). The content of the programs initially offered was based on the opinions of the IS experts of the time (Meissner et al., 2013; Proctor et al., 2013; Straus et al., 2011). Through initial and follow-up evaluations of the original trainings, ongoing expansion of the TS field, and advancement of various research methodologies, preliminary competencies for individuals involved in scientific or practice roles in EBP and TS were developed (Melnyk et al., 2014; Moore et al., 2018; Padek et al., 2015; Proctor & Chambers, 2017; Tabak et al., 2017).

Although in most cases the identified competencies represent a single level of ability to execute role expectations, some authors have begun the process of differentiating several levels of competency because "practitioners" (people who would be responsible for enacting EBPs in a particular context) were sometimes included in training programs (Moore et al., 2018; Proctor & Chambers, 2017). For instance, Padek et al. (2015) used an online card sorting methodology with DS and IS experts to identify 43 competencies that were then categorized as beginning, intermediate, or advanced skills. Mallidou et al. (2018) conducted a scoping review of 210 studies and gray literature to develop a comprehensive list of 19 "core" competencies for roles in research and practice in "knowledge translation" (the Canadian term for TS or IS). Additionally, Melnyk et al. (2014) identified competencies for practicing registered nurses involved in EBP and built on those to create competencies appropriate for advanced practice nursing. From the work of these TS leaders from multiple disciplines, a set of competency domains that encompass both research and practice roles is now available for planning education in DS and IS.

With competencies now identified, the challenge arises of integrating the proficiencies for both the graduate nursing and TS fields in coherent curricula that account for their science and practice. One factor that is favorable to this undertaking is that TS has been considered by experts in the field to be "inherently" multidisciplinary and requiring a team science approach (Chambers et al., 2017; Meissner et al., 2013). This observation parallels the existing expectations for practice-focused doctoral- and master's-level nursing curricula described in the *Essentials* documents that call for "Interprofessional collaboration for improving patient and population health outcomes" (AACN, 2006, p. 14, 2011, p. 22). For the research-focused programs (PhD, DSN, DNS, and DNSc), these interprofessional or multidisciplinary experiences are recommended to enhance the understanding of theories and the science of other disciplines, as well as to acquire skills in team science (AACN, 2010). Because both TS and nursing have recommended multidisciplinary, team, or interprofessional coursework and field (clinical) experiences, the interprofessional/multidisciplinary areas of competency can be evaluated for their suitability for each field's curricular needs. Also, because some leveling of competencies for TS has been attempted as well as the differentiation of practice and scientific role expectations, TS and nursing competencies can be linked at various points of research- or practice-focused curricula.

An exhaustive mapping of TS and graduate nursing competencies is beyond the scope of this chapter, particularly because there is as yet no universal agreement about the competencies for TS, and for nursing programs the contexts in which a curriculum must be delivered will determine emphases for the programs and the student experiences required to achieve program outcomes. However, several of the KSAs identified by Mallidou et al. (2018) in their literature review of TS competencies can be considered for applicability in nursing research- and practice-focused degree programs. If applicable, then appropriate nursing courses and curricular expectations can be identified to build toward these KSAs.

Previous discussions in this chapter have made it clear that key differences between the PhD/DNS/DSN and practice-focused degrees at the doctoral or master's level in nursing relate to the understanding and use of research and the roles that graduates will undertake in relation to research. Through a Delphi study, Melnyk et al. (2014) identified competencies applicable to practice, addressing registered nurse and advanced practice nurse use of EBP. Many of these overlap with the competencies identified by TS educators. Mallidou et al. (2018) extracted six knowledge, eight skills, five attitudes, and three competencies categorized as "other" from the TS literature. This research team included studies that addressed competencies for both research-focused and practice-focused TS participants. Because of the broader focus of the roles reflected in the competencies identified by Mallidou et al. (2018) compared with Melnyk et al. (2014), the competencies found in the TS review are used for our discussion. Table 7-1 provides a partial listing of the KSAs identified by Mallidou et al. (2018). These KSAs were chosen for their relationships to practice-based research (in contrast to bench research) to allow comparisons between expectations of research- and practice-focused doctoral nursing students. Attitudes about TS among research- and practice-focused graduates should be parallel, but for knowledge and skills the suggested emphases for a scientist compared with a practice expert are evident.

Table 7-2 displays possible leveling of practice-focused competencies for graduates of master's programs. Some of the leveled competencies overlap those of practice-focused doctoral graduates; this is because at the current time there are still many advanced practice registered nurse (APRN) roles that can be achieved through the completion of an MSN degree. However, with the growing number of postbaccalaureate DNP programs focusing on nurse practitioner roles (AACN, 2019), it is likely that what is suggested as an MSN competency now may be expanded or modified to apply to doctoral-level practice in a few years if the AACN's recommendation is realized for entry to advanced practice nursing at the DNP level (Auerbach et al., 2014).

TRANSLATIONAL SCIENCE COMPETENCY DEVELOPMENT IN GRADUATE NURSING EDUCATION

Doctoral Nursing Program Content

For graduate students to achieve their desired competencies, their education should include coursework and experiences that provide practice in the areas to be mastered. One of the competencies identified by Mallidou et al. (2018) for the field of TS that overlaps with nursing's concerns is an understanding of TS and EBP processes. This competency is particularly relevant to a practice discipline such as nursing that has both research- and practice-focused doctoral degrees. We use this competency as an example for our discussion of curriculum planning because there are both unique and common concerns about TS for research- and practice-focused students at the doctoral level. The overall design and management of TS projects will be a primary responsibility of PhD/DSN/DNS/DNSc graduates, whereas nurses with a DNP degree will lead teams in using EBP in the health care system.

For research-focused graduate students in nursing, it will be essential that they are able to differentiate between TS and EBP activities. TS is fundamentally concerned with the conduct of research and the formation of theories and frameworks about translation processes. EBP is the enactment of the process in the actual delivery or management of care. TS requires formal research methods for investigation of the implementation and dissemination processes, and the implementation of EBP involves the use of change methodologies in ways that best foster the incorporation of existing research. The education of research-focused graduate students should be designed to prepare them to lead the scientific aspects of TS.

Practice-focused graduate students must also fully comprehend the differences between TS and EBP, but they must do so because they will lead change in clinical areas. They must hone skills in assessing health system processes and practices, eliciting stakeholder opinions and needs, and performing other activities of a change agent so that practice modifications can proceed. These differences in the role between future researchers and practice experts illustrate that to prepare doctoral nursing students for engagement in TS, educators must consider not only that some responsibilities will overlap, such as clearly differentiating theories and activities for TS and EBP, but also that each student group will have unique duties that will shape the curriculum they will need.

In many aspects, the traditional education of a research-focused doctoral nursing program will be adaptable for a student preparing for a career in TS. Courses that focus on theory development, critique, concept development, and so on can be altered to include the examination of several relevant frameworks of IS and DS, such as the Promoting Action on Research Implementation in

TABLE 7-1

Differences in Selected Knowledge, Skills, and Attitudes for Implementation Science in Research-Focused and Practice-Focused Doctoral-Level Nursing Graduates

TRANSLATIONAL SCIENCE COMPETENCIES	RESEARCH-FOCUSED GRADUATES	PRACTICE-FOCUSED GRADUATES
Knowledge Competencies		
1.1 Understand context	• Identifies and uses stakeholder involvement to assess context • Determining reasonable procedures for research context that maintain rigor	• Uses knowledge of stakeholder interests and practice expertise to inform translational science efforts
1.2 Understand the research process	• Articulates well-framed questions, steps to successful project completion, data collection, and data analysis • Interprets findings in light of translational practice	• Recognizes importance of rigorous procedures for translational science validity • Articulates suitability/unsuitability of specific research procedures for context
1.5 Understand translational science and evidence-based practice processes	• Critiques frameworks, models, and theories for utility in translation science/evidence-based practice efforts • Identifies levels of fidelity of translational science/evidence-based practice to original research	• Explains processes of change and seven steps of evidence-based practice in clinical areas; knows intended outcomes of translational science and evidence-based practice • Evaluates outcomes of evidence-based practice
1.6 Understand translation and dissemination activities	• Using frameworks, theories and models, creates plans and procedures for translation and dissemination that maintain rigor while appropriate to context	• Articulates practice rationale for changes in procedures • Uses theories, models, and/or frameworks to lead translational science and dissemination activities
Skills		
2.1 Collaboration and teamwork	• Engages stakeholders in project methodology, data collection, and determining ethical procedures	• Leads translational science practice team members in procedures at setting

(continued)

TABLE 7-1 (CONTINUED)

Differences in Selected Knowledge, Skills, and Attitudes for Implementation Science in Research-Focused and Practice-Focused Doctoral-Level Nursing Graduates

TRANSLATIONAL SCIENCE COMPETENCIES	RESEARCH-FOCUSED GRADUATES	PRACTICE-FOCUSED GRADUATES
2.2 Leadership	• Mentors practice experts in literature critique, finding knowledge gaps; coaches in translational science procedures	• Coaches translational science practice team members during change process
2.3 Sharing knowledge	• Communicates findings from translation to scientific community and relevant stakeholders in formats appropriate to targeted audiences	• Provides prompt and relevant updates to members of translational science team • Presents findings from translational science efforts to relevant local, regional, and national audiences
2.7 Foster innovation	• Creates novel approaches to translate evidence and collect data about translation process	• Incorporates practice-based knowledge in novel translation approaches
Attitudes		
3.1 Confidence	• Displays expertise and flexibility in conducting translational science	• Demonstrates expertise in guiding practice activities in translational science efforts
3.2 Having trust	• Relies on team to act ethically, obtain and secure data from translational science efforts, and fulfill responsibilities	• Exhibits conviction that all members of translational science team, including research-focused, have client welfare orientation
3.3 Valuing research	• Shows commitment to research endeavors as a life occupation	• Relies on research evidence as a primary source of knowledge for practice
3.4 Self-directed lifelong commitment to learning	• Continually participates in opportunities to advance skills in methodology, practice advances, analytic methods, etc.	• Seeks knowledge about practice improvement, scientific methods, and theories underlying translational science approaches

(continued)

TABLE 7-1 (CONTINUED)

Differences in Selected Knowledge, Skills, and Attitudes for Implementation Science in Research-Focused and Practice-Focused Doctoral-Level Nursing Graduates

TRANSLATIONAL SCIENCE COMPETENCIES	RESEARCH-FOCUSED GRADUATES	PRACTICE-FOCUSED GRADUATES
3.5 Valuing teamwork	• Seeks practice input from early stages of translational science projects and involves team throughout processes	• Seeks nurse scientists as well as practice experts as mentors and consultants in translational science
Other Competencies		
4.1 Knowledge of quality improvement methods and tools, communication strategies, and health policy and systems	• Assesses and critiques quality improvement methods in light of frameworks and research rigor • Aligns research methods to systems • Identifies health policy implications of evidence	• Facile in operationalizing current quality improvement methods • Evaluates suitability of quality improvement methods to clinical problems • Communicates realistic quality improvement processes for context
4.2 Skills related to project planning, management, information technology use, sound judgment, discretion/tact/ diplomacy/ resourcefulness	• Plans research procedures fostering rigor; uses information technology efficiently for data collection, management, and analysis	• Identifies short-term, intermediate, and long-term outcomes realistic to plan; efficiently uses information technology and system knowledge to allow for plan changes
4.3 Attributes such as integrity, commitment to professional work ethic, commitment to high standards of professionalism, and interest in latest developments in communications	• Demonstrates all characteristics of professional researcher, allowing for leadership in field of translational science	• Demonstrates all characteristics of practice expert, allowing for practice leadership in field of translational science

Competencies adapted from Mallidou, A. A., Atherton, P., Chan, L., Frisch, N., Glegg, S., & Scarrow, G. (2018). Core knowledge translation competencies: A scoping review. *BMC Health Services Research, 18*, 502 and Melnyk, B. M. (2013). Distinguishing the preparation and roles of doctor of philosophy and doctor of nursing practice graduates: National implications for academic curricula and health care systems. *Journal of Nursing Education, 52*(8), 442-448.

TABLE 7-2

Selected Knowledge, Skills, and Attitudes for Implementation Science in Master's-Level Nursing Graduates

TRANSLATIONAL SCIENCE COMPETENCIES	MASTER'S-LEVEL COMPETENCIES
Knowledge Competencies	
1.3 Understand context	• Contributes knowledge of microsystem and/or defined populations of responsibility to inform translational science efforts
1.4 Understand the research process	• Recognizes place of research as "best available evidence" in resolving practice issues • Appraises suitability of specific research procedures for context with attention to intervention fidelity as a factor in effectiveness
1.7 Understand translational science and evidence-based practice processes	• Differentiates rapid-cycle and other quality improvement procedures from formal research and translational science processes • Articulates seven steps of evidence-based practice process
1.8 Understand translation and dissemination activities	• Fosters culture of inquiry in microsystem while evaluating rationale for changes in care • Participates in the uses of theories, models, and/or frameworks as member of translational science and dissemination teams
Skills	
2.1 Collaboration and teamwork	• Participates in interprofessional team at point-of-care to advance translational science
2.2 Leadership	• Leads change processes in microsystems and for designated populations of responsibility
2.3 Sharing knowledge	• Provides practice team with information gleaned from relevant sources to support translational science and evidence-based practice
2.7 Foster innovation	• Uses data and practice evidence to promote change
Attitudes	
3.1 Confidence	• Displays poise in presenting information to colleagues and in proposing plans of action for practice changes
3.2 Having trust	• Demonstrates expectations of success and team fulfillment of responsibilities
3.3 Valuing research	• Provides research findings as foundation for change processes and evidence-based practice

(continued)

TABLE 7-2 (CONTINUED)
Selected Knowledge, Skills, and Attitudes for Implementation Science in Master's-Level Nursing Graduates

TRANSLATIONAL SCIENCE COMPETENCIES	MASTER'S-LEVEL COMPETENCIES
3.4 Self-directed lifelong commitment to learning	• Seeks opportunities for enhancement of knowledge of research, translational science, and quality improvement processes
3.5 Valuing teamwork	• Convenes team members in huddles and other appropriate communication situations to address care issues
Other Competencies	
4.1 Knowledge of quality improvement methods and tools, communication strategies, and health policy and systems	• Chooses appropriate quality improvement methods and strategies for practice changes with specified populations
4.2 Skills related to project planning, management, information technology use, sound judgment, and discretion/tact/diplomacy/resourcefulness	• Plans quality improvement projects that include appropriate stakeholders and use of information technology
4.3 Attributes such as integrity, commitment to professional work ethic, commitment to high standards of professionalism, and interest in latest developments in communications	• Models dedication to ongoing improvement in practice, fulfilling obligations in relation to quality improvement and client-centered practice while supporting translational science and general research endeavors

Competencies adapted from Mallidou, A. A., Atherton, P., Chan, L., Frisch, N., Glegg, S., & Scarrow, G. (2018). Core knowledge translation competencies: A scoping review. *BMC Health Services Research, 18,* 502 and Melnyk, B. M. (2013). Distinguishing the preparation and roles of doctor of philosophy and doctor of nursing practice graduates: National implications for academic curricula and health care systems. *Journal of Nursing Education, 52*(8), 442-448.

Health Services framework (Kitson et al., 1998) or Rogers' diffusion of innovations theory (Rogers, 2003). In courses focused on developing skills in various research methods and designs, emphasis can be placed on intervention designs; decisions about issues of efficacy, effectiveness, and maintaining intervention fidelity in practice settings when creating protocols; designing pragmatic trials; creating protocols that use cluster sampling or phased interventions; and analytical techniques for these new methods. Although there must be concentrated attention to building skills for critiquing studies, the techniques of rapid appraisal of studies should also be presented as one of the steps of EBP. Depending on the background of the research-focused doctoral student and the intended area of the dissertation project, there might also be a need for coursework in the areas of health care systems research and theory, quality assurance methodologies, policy formation, and various courses in sociology or public health that could further inform the practice issues that an IS or DS project might address. These courses might include additional study of theories and methods useful in the TS field such as community-based participatory research.

One of the issues that faculty designing an overall curriculum for research-focused doctoral students will need to consider is whether an immersion, field, or laboratory experience (such as bench science) should be a requirement for all students or considered solely for students seeking to complete TS for dissertation projects. Research-focused doctoral programs in nursing do not always incorporate such experiences unless a student's interests and intended project demand them. For instance, doctoral students in a research-focused nursing program would not usually be expected to study in a mentor's bench or applied science laboratory unless their intended dissertation topics require it. However, TS is recognized as an area for which there is a need for future nursing scientists (Henly et al., 2015). TS inherently requires that a researcher be familiar with the context in which knowledge is to be applied. Therefore, given the need to move toward greater nursing involvement in emerging areas of science such as TS, it is logical that a laboratory course or field work in settings similar to those in which they may engage in TS might be required of students in research-focused programs. This would ensure that even those who are not undertaking a TS project for their dissertations will have a practical grounding in the matters that surround the adoption of any research contributions they intend to provide to professional nursing practice during their careers.

With their solid preparation in interprofessional advanced practice nursing, population health, and QI methods, students in practice-focused DNP programs will be the leaders in clinical settings to enact the changes that are at the center of TS efforts. In the literature, much attention has been directed to defining the scope of responsibilities of nurses who hold a DNP degree, their practice competencies, the types of scholarship appropriate for their educational projects and following graduation, their roles as leaders in nursing practice, and their engagement in QI through practice change (AACN, 2015; AACN Common APRN Doctoral-Level Competencies Work Group, 2017; Bleich, 2019; Brown & Crabtree, 2013; Melnyk, 2013). These are salient issues for considering what will be needed in DNP students' education to assure that they will be able to use EBP in their roles in advanced nursing practice and contribute to TS as a valued team member.

Table 7-3 provides a listing of some of the experiences suggested for students by leaders in DNP education that can foster the development of knowledge and skills in EBP. Previous discussions in this chapter have noted the curricular experiences that research-focused students need, including framework or model critique and development, literature review and critique, development of procedures for a TS project, engagement of stakeholders, and other points of the TS process. These experiences overlap many of the experiences listed in Table 7-3 that are important for DNP students. Although there is overlap, it is important to differentiate the emphases and focus of the content each degree requires.

First, in the area of literature review, preparing students in a DNP program for EBP and participation in TS should include developing their abilities to obtain appropriate literature for an area of practice. They need to also critique that literature in terms of its overall design, methodological soundness, relevancy to the desired population and clinical context, and strength for dissemination in general clinical practice (Dawes et al., 2005; Melnyk et al., 2014; Moore & Watters, 2013; Padek et al., 2015; Riner, 2015; Straus et al., 2011). The process of rapid appraisal of evidence is the central focus of the research coursework DNP students need to achieve competencies (Melnyk, 2013; Melnyk et al., 2014). To be able to do this, students may need coursework covering research methodology content, especially if they have not had such a foundation in their prior education. However, the coursework in research methods should use as its foundation the context of practice and scholarly application of research concepts to practice rather than a science (discovery) framework and approach. For instance, students may need to have an introduction to various types of qualitative research as a means of being able to review the available evidence. However, to explore in detail the philosophies that underlie qualitative methods is not appropriate.

TABLE 7-3
Experiences for Developing Evidence-Based Practice Competencies in Practice-Focused Doctoral Programs

SUGGESTED EXPERIENCE	AUTHORS IDENTIFYING EXPERIENCE
Conduct literature review of practice issue/problem	Buchholz et al. (2015)
	Graves et al. (2018)
	Melnyk (2013)
	Moore & Watters (2013)
	Riner (2015)
Identify and use frameworks for evidence-based practice, practice changes, and/or quality improvement	Graves et al. (2018)
	Moore & Watters (2013)
	Riner (2015)
Evaluate external (research) evidence and translate evidence to practice or policy	Brown & Crabtree (2013)
	Melnyk (2013)
	Moore & Watters (2013)
	Riner (2015)
Immersion in clinical setting, leading to practice change or policy development	Brown & Crabtree (2013)
	Edwardson (2010)
	Moore & Watters (2013)
	Riner (2015)
Completing coursework/course content for quality improvement methods: benchmarking, statistical control, trend analysis, six sigma, and interviewing and focus group skills	Brown & Crabtree (2013)
	Graves et al. (2018)
Organizational assessment/context assessment for barriers or facilitators of evidence-based practice/practice change	Brown & Crabtree (2013)
	Melnyk (2013)
	Riner (2015)
Generating internal (practice site) evidence through quality improvement, outcomes management, and evidence-based practice projects	Brown & Crabtree (2013)
	Melnyk (2013)
Evaluating practice change in setting	Brown & Crabtree (2013)
	Melnyk (2013)
Participate in and take leadership in transdisciplinary/multidisciplinary/interprofessional project teams	Brown & Crabtree (2013)
	Buccholz et al. (2015)
	Moore & Watters (2013)
Mentoring and leading others in evidence-based practice	Brown & Crabtree (2013)
	Melnyk (2013)
	Moore & Watters (2013)
Professional assessments of or by peers	Edwardson (2010)

Many educators may question the need to address qualitative research at all. To further illustrate how certain areas of qualitative research methods are relevant, let us consider the example of grounded theory. What is important about having some knowledge of grounded theory is that (a) in some areas of practice, grounded theory or other qualitative research may be the only available external research evidence that can inform practice; (b) several types of research reviews include qualitative studies, notably metasummaries; (c) qualitative studies are included in the Joanna Briggs Institute database (The Joanna Briggs Institute, 2017), which is an important resource concerned with nursing interventions; and (d) a particular qualitative method, such as grounded theory, might be used for a TS project to describe the implementation or dissemination processes and/or to evaluate outcomes with stakeholders. Therefore, having overall knowledge of grounded theory's principles and methods would not only expand the DNP student's knowledge and skill in critique for EBP but also add value to contributions as a team member in TS projects.

Some measurement concepts are also areas of research methodology content that will be important to include in a DNP curriculum. Rationale for this will be discussed further in relation to the needed coursework about theory, frameworks, and models. Additional research method content important to a DNP student's engagement in TS and EBP includes concepts of internal and external validity, efficacy, and effectiveness, as well as the concept of effect size. DNP graduates need to understand the balance between internal and external validity as an important aspect of determining how quickly a new intervention can be moved to general practice (Dawes et al., 2005; Tabak et al., 2017). Studies judged to be more internally valid should be understood as being done in a more artificial context, whereas a study with greater external validity is usually closer to real-world uses. Practices or programs that have only been tested in efficacy trials emphasizing internal validity are not likely to be ready to be implemented in care settings and, therefore, may not be ready for TS investigations or EBP implementation. Also, if an intervention has been seen to have only a small effect in a trial focused on efficacy testing, its potential for use in the context of usual nursing practice may be slight because it is usually not possible to maintain high levels of experimental control once a new procedure is put into general use. In clinical practice, techniques that are easily integrated into existing care processes without major disruptions of workflow or interference with stakeholder practices are more readily adopted (Grol & Grimshaw, 2003). The more a procedure must be modified for a particular population or setting, the more likely it will be that some of its effect will be diminished. If its effect was small in the original efficacy trials, positive effects may be completely lost when it is modified. Additional efficacy testing after modifications of the innovation may be needed before its effect is great enough to maintain its benefits in general practice contexts (Zoellner & Porter, 2017). Understanding these important research concepts will be needed by DNP students to balance judgments about the costs and benefits of practice change and to effectively implement EBP for their own personal practices as well as those of their care settings.

As previously noted, an understanding of basic measurement theory is research content that is also important to the DNP student. The field of psychometric research is outside the areas of competency of DNP-prepared nurses. They might participate as practice experts who judge the face validity of a measure's items or as team members who might collect data for research led by colleagues who are health care and nurse scientists. DNP-prepared nurses should understand that measures should accurately reflect an abstract concept; otherwise, they do not capture what they are intended to measure. Because they evaluate EBP, which may involve capturing abstract perceptions such as stakeholder attitudes or effects of an intervention on client or staff knowledge, beliefs, or emotions, they need to understand the validity and reliability of measures. Choosing an appropriate measure is an undertaking that would ideally be a collaborative endeavor done in partnership with colleagues who have intensive research training in psychometrics. However, this is not always possible because many DNP graduates practice in settings where this type of assistance is not available. Therefore, coursework that assists DNP students to understand the importance of the reliability and validity of a psychometric measure, as well as to insist on the reliability of biophysiological instruments that may be used in judging client outcomes, is important to their future roles as leaders in EBP, as well as members of a TS team (Chambers et al., 2017; Dawes et al., 2005).

The understanding of measurement theory needed by practice-focused doctoral students overlaps with the foundational knowledge they need about theory, frameworks, and models. A DNP-educated nurse is not intended to be a theorist in the formal sense of the term but can use esthetic, personal, and ethical ways of knowing to contribute practice (internal) evidence to nursing, to EBP in health care, and to TS. To facilitate these processes of knowledge generation, the DNP student should be supported in developing skills of reflective practice (Riner, 2015). Learning about the seminal works of early nursing theorists and philosophers and the study of middle-range theories from nursing and other disciplines are activities that can foster these skills. While the theories and frameworks are studied, the skills of concept analysis should be introduced, which can assist the student in understanding how the measurement of concepts is linked to their meanings. As with research-focused students, IS and DS frameworks can be included in courses that provide the theoretical and scientific foundation for doctoral work in nursing (Chambers et al., 2017; Riner, 2015; Straus et al., 2011). As noted previously, the focus for these topics with DNP students should be application and critique rather than creation and integration of diverse theories or concepts. These latter undertakings will be responsibilities of the nurse scientist.

There are many other experiences listed in Table 7-3 that will assist DNP students to achieve competencies for their practice roles in TS and EBP. Health policy is an area in which DS is very important to influence institutions and governmental stakeholders regarding practice issues. Besides formal course experiences, attendance at conferences designed to assist nurses to convert health care evidence to policy, such as the AACN policy summits (AACN, 2020b), or involvement in the American Nurses Advocacy Institute (American Nurses Association, n.d.), should be encouraged. The competencies in QI models, QI methods, organizational assessment, outcomes management, and other areas of practice improvement can be developed in coursework with a focus on QI in a health care context, and they are areas of concern to TS. These policy and QI topics are consistent with AACN's guidance for preparing DNP graduates who will practice with aggregates (AACN, 2006). Statistical methods that are used for QI should supplement content about detecting changes in outcomes, and content such as epidemiology, which is needed to intervene to address population health, should accompany the subject matter dealing with these interventions (Anderson et al., 2019; Riner, 2015).

Doctoral Nursing Program Clinical and Simulation Experiences

The Essentials of Doctoral Education for Advanced Nursing Practice (AACN, 2006) provides direction regarding the types and amount of clinical experiences that DNP students should complete in their programs. This document states the following:

> In order to achieve the DNP competencies, programs should provide a minimum of 1,000 hours of practice post-baccalaureate as part of a supervised academic program. Practice experiences should be designed to help students achieve specific learning objectives related to the *DNP Essentials* and specialty competencies. These experiences should be designed to provide systematic opportunities for feedback and reflection. Experiences include in-depth work with experts from nursing as well as other disciplines and provide opportunities for meaningful student engagement within practice environments. (AACN, 2006, p. 19)

The guidance set forth in this statement provides a structure useful for creating curricula for DNP students that integrate TS and EBP competencies. The directive for work with various experts, both from nursing and from other disciplines, as well as a need for environments that foster engagement in practice, are specific requisites for developing skills in leadership, practice roles within team science, and organizational dynamics. The 1,000 hours needed in the program include the number for achieving advanced practice competence. In most cases, the APRN hours will be a minimum of 500 to 600 clinical hours (American Nurses Credentialing Center, n.d.) accompanied by at least another 400 to 500 for immersion experiences that will include the scholarly project (AACN, 2006). At first glance, a curriculum planner might assume that practice hours used to develop TS skills would occur in the immersion experiences. However, there are many ways that the early specialty practice hours can be used for developing TS competencies.

One of the factors to be considered is that the clinical experiences of the DNP student should "provide systematic opportunities for feedback and reflection" (AACN, 2006, p. 19) and that the student should be interacting with experts and members of other professions and disciplines. The clinical hours a student spends being closely mentored by an experienced clinician should not only be spent in learning things like "how to" do assessments, procedures, charting, and so on, but also (and these are just as important) techniques of effective interaction with peers as a member of a team; efficient ways to complete one's workload and, as a clinical leader, to assess the workload of those team members who report to oneself; the real-time costs of various decisions made in the clinical area; and, always, consideration of the best available evidence to address clinical and organizational issues. When these aspects of practice are addressed from the start of their clinical experiences, DNP students are likely to identify many areas of practice appropriate for their scholarly projects. Moreover, these activities can promote a mindset of continuous improvement, questioning of entrenched work processes, and judicious balancing of the benefits and costs of changes in clinical practices. These are experiences and behaviors that are assets in TS as well as in leading others in EBP.

It is not an easy task to find clinical settings where the previously described activities will be available. The increasing numbers of DNP programs in the United States (AACN, 2018) and difficulties in obtaining clinical placements for DNP students create problems for locating them in settings where the opportunities enumerated earlier will be available or encouraged. Preceptors who share the values of a specific nursing program are invaluable resources, particularly those who educate students to embrace a scholarly approach to clinical practice. Faculty aiming to develop these attributes in their students will need to maintain involvement and a regular presence in their students' clinical settings (Brown & Crabtree, 2013). Faculty roles in clinical conferencing with students that include providing feedback about students' observations about potential practice changes and possible immersion projects can be enhanced by preceptors who embrace mentorship of new clinicians.

Simulation can also be used, even in low-fidelity formats, to develop TS competencies. Written case studies are one of the forms of simulation most readily adaptable and available to programs with limited resources. Not only can care of clients be examined and critiqued through the use of case studies, but also organizational issues can be deliberated by students, either individually or in groups. Organizational case studies have been used by the Harvard Graduate School of Business in course offerings over many years (Harvard Business Publishing Education, 2020). They stimulate reflection and respect for peer contributions and practical application of theoretical content such as the use of models to devise solutions to problems at hand. Depending on the type and complexity of other resources available to a program, simulations can be adapted to more realistically portray clinical scenarios. Examples include videotaping of simulated client and team interactions, communication among project team members in a TS meeting situation, use of standardized patients in laboratory sessions wherein discussions are occurring of untested therapies to be considered for adoption in their care, presentations of proposals to organizational administrators or to governmental officials, and simulated staff meetings where evidence is presented with the goal of adoption. Simulations will not always consist solely of verbal interactions among students and their mentors. Rather, they can also be used for training students in data collection procedures for a TS project; for the evaluation of EBP via interviews, focus groups, or physical examinations; or for training students for measurement involving new equipment or unique procedures.

Doctor of Philosophy and Doctor of Nursing Practice Collaboration in Education for Translational Science

In our discussion of suggested courses and experiences for DNP students, opportunities presented by TS for collaboration with research-focused graduate students were not yet addressed. This is because the number of colleges and universities having both practice- and research-focused doctoral programs is small relative to the overall student populations in these degree programs. In the fall of 2017, there were 336 DNP programs in the United States compared with only 136 research-focused doctoral programs (AACN, 2018). The overall number of students in the same survey year was 29,093 DNP students compared with 4,632 pursuing a PhD. This means that the vast majority of DNP programs in the country have limited opportunities to foster collaboration experiences among research- and practice-focused doctoral students and that too few PhD students are available to collaborate with DNP students. One option is to establish consortia with universities that offer a PhD in nursing (Breslin et al., 2015). Unfortunately, if a DNP program seeks to create a consortium agreement with a PhD program, the opportunities for partnership experiences are still likely to be limited. This is because the DNP students in any one university are likely to greatly outnumber the PhD nursing students, and research-focused students wishing to collaborate are likely to find a partner among their home institution's practice-focused students quite readily. An alternative may be to engage the DNP students in projects with faculty members who hold a PhD. However, although it is very important to a student's development to have a mentor, a faculty–student relationship is not one of peers, and, with this arrangement, it will be more difficult to replicate typical team interactions.

When a PhD–DNP student partnership can be created to enable engagement in TS and EBP as a team, assignments and experiences that can be completed together include (a) identifying a practice issue that would improve practice and/or efficiency in a setting; (b) completing an exhaustive literature review; (c) proposing a TS project; (d) completing a limited project or initial phase of a project using DS or IS frameworks and procedures; and (e) conducting the evaluation, including evaluation research methods where applicable. These activities can include areas of practice in which an evidence gap exists, requiring original research by the PhD student. Alternately, because of intervention or context complexity, activities might involve testing of an approach designed by the PhD student followed by DNP student projects to ascertain stakeholder perceptions regarding the intervention's potential for further dissemination and adoption in a similar setting or population (Buchholz et al., 2015; Cygan & Reed, 2019). Various other assignments throughout programs can connect research and practice perspectives. Examples include research–practice teams in theory courses to assess the practical utility of frameworks or models, group assignments to conduct concept analysis, exercises among DNP and PhD students to conduct rapid appraisals of evidence, and teams considering organizational theories and/or change theories from the standpoint of concepts that can guide TS or EBP efforts.

In research-focused programs, the traditions of dissemination of dissertation work are long established (Anderson et al., 2019). The usual processes of completing proposals, data collection, data analysis, writing findings, and presenting them to a committee of advisors and the research community can be revised readily for student projects that are embedded in TS. Modifications in the project itself may include differences in sampling, such as cluster sampling and intervention assignment; measures that may mix qualitative and quantitative phases or data collection; analyses to account for the adaptations; and presentations to scientific audiences. However, an element that should be added would be presentation of the work to the institution, agency, or clinical site that hosted the study.

For DNP students, the expectations of the culminating work for their degrees are continuing to evolve (AACN, 2015; Anderson et al., 2019; Brown & Crabtree, 2013). What is agreed on is that a scholarly project for the DNP should reflect the integration of coursework and clinical experiences in a program (AACN, 2006). The project should address a practice or organizational change that focuses on health care outcomes of clients or a system (AACN, 2015). Whether the project will be reviewed by other mentors besides one or two faculty members will vary from school to school. Similarly, whether or not a formal presentation at the conclusion of the project is required also may not be a universally required practice. However, because projects in TS are expressly designed to illuminate processes of dissemination and implementation of research evidence, the DNP project that arises from TS should be expected to culminate with one or more presentations to stakeholders involved in the practice or organizational changes as well as representatives of the scientific community. That is not to say that a defense, as it is known in research traditions, is necessary. However, presentations should include some accounting of the procedures, findings, lessons learned or implications, and steps that should be taken in the future. This can be done orally, by an executive summary, or a formal report; through the creation of policy or procedure manuals or tool kits; or through other products such as cost-benefit analyses.

It has been noted that DNP-prepared nurses can generate practice (internal) knowledge (Melnyk, 2013). Because of this, the dissemination of project findings to the broader health practice and research communities is important to facilitate transferability (not generalizability) of project methods and findings more broadly, as appropriate. All of TS is context dependent (i.e., stakeholders, the setting's standard practices, and clientele are unique for any TS effort). Nevertheless, various processes and other aspects of a practice setting may bear similarities to others. This is the reason TS is salient as a research field. So that the field of TS may expand its science (frameworks, models, methods, etc.), a DNP's project that reflects participation in TS should be disseminated.

The recognition of DNP scholarship has resulted in the broadening of venues for dissemination that are open to PhD student presentations as well. Organizations that welcome reports of TS include major professional nursing organizations, such as the American Nurses Association and Sigma Theta Tau International, and those dedicated to nurse practitioners, nurse midwives, and nurse anesthetists; research societies (Midwest Nursing Research Society, Eastern Nursing Research Society, Western Institute of Nursing, etc.); and the Doctors of Nursing Practice, Inc. In addition, projects that address quality improvement can be presented at the annual American Nursing Credentialing Center's National Magnet Conference or at the Academy Health Annual Research Meeting, among other events. There are also many conferences associated with the health informatics field, such as those sponsored by the American Nursing Informatics Association, the Health Information and Management Systems Society, and the University of Maryland School of Nursing. In some of these organizations, student projects can be considered for special awards; many will fund projects that are proposed or in progress. All of these examples show that TS is becoming established as a form of scholarship for nursing doctoral study.

Master of Science in Nursing Student Competencies and Curriculum for Evidence-Based Practice

The experiences needed by MSN/MN students to develop TS and EBP competencies cannot be forgotten. We have noted previously that many APRN specialties have not eliminated master's-level eligibility for certification examinations. As the APRN certification eligibility process moves to requiring the DNP degree, the CNL will become the major role prepared at the MSN level. CNLs are expected to put "evidence-based practice into action to ensure that patients benefit from the latest innovations in care delivery" (AACN, 2004c, para. 7). Also, the CNL role was explicitly designed to "improve the quality of patient care outcomes" (AACN, 2020a, para. 1). To accomplish these goals, the MSN curriculum should have three major components: (a) a graduate nursing core, (b) a direct care core, and (c) functional area content (AACN, 2011, pp. 7-8).

One of the three components, the direct care core, is already stipulated by AACN to be composed of advanced physiology/pathophysiology, health assessment, and pharmacology. The other components, master's graduate core and functional area content, are the elements in which content to support the development of TS and EBP competencies can be included. For the MSN student, the content and experiences of the graduate nursing core will usually include opportunities to study and apply theoretical foundations to nursing practice, particularly middle-range and practice theories, leadership and role performance theory, effective communication among members of the health team, health systems and organizational theory, health policy, ethical foundations of practice at an advanced level, quality improvement theory, and methods to enable EBP (e.g., data collection, statistical analysis, and the effective use of technology for these efforts). Functional area content is then focused on specific role competencies. An APRN student would progress in diagnostic and intervention skills to enhance health, focus on specific populations (e.g., older adults, children and adolescents, communities, women), assume leadership in teams devoted to the care of individuals and families in the population, advocate for these populations including attention to the cost and quality of care, and implement EBP to address the health needs of the population. Most of the content needed to participate in TS and implement EBP can be integrated into these courses required for the functional area. A minimum of 500 hours of clinical practice are required for APRN certification, so the skills for TS and EBP can be practiced in the clinical setting. Although students seeking to complete MSN degrees to enter practice as an APRN are not required by AACN to complete a clinical scholarly project, preceptors and environments similar to those desired for DNP students are important for the development of TS skills.

For the CNL, who is an "advanced generalist," less emphasis will be placed on the specific health care needs of a particular population, but more will be directed toward health care delivery in microsystems, change in processes, improvement and systems theory and methods, budgeting for microsystems, evaluation of EBP including performance measures for a team, analytics and risk assessment, and the use of safety analysis tools such as failure mode and effects analysis and root cause analysis (AACN, 2013). Expectations that will be common across all roles among MSN graduates will be the use and facilitation of EBP for fulfilling responsibilities in the client population or microsystems of care. However, the obligations in these areas will differ in their depth and breadth. APRNs prepared at the MSN level will place more focus on the evidence aligned with the care of clients for whom they have personally provided or directed care. CNLs bear accountability for the clients of a microsystem such as a hospital unit, a clinic, or special service department, like discharge or transition planning. Therefore, the experiences planned for these different roles at the MSN level will require different foci.

MSN students preparing for APRN roles must complete a minimum of 500 clinical hours to be eligible to take certification examinations required for licensure for practice in a state. The clinical hours are often designed to focus first on uncomplicated, routine health concerns of well individuals or individuals with temporary, acute alterations in health. As the students advance through the curriculum, the care of individuals with chronic conditions is addressed. In culminating experiences, students can shift to population-based care, such as individuals with a specific long-term condition or other complex health management challenges (e.g., individuals who are homeless). To develop competencies in EBP and processes, phases, or elements of TS, concentrated efforts should be made to incorporate experiences of appraising evidence, applying change theories and frameworks in a care process context, collecting evaluation data about the patient outcomes of the change, and dissemination of the work that was completed. What was learned can be integrated in assignments for these clinical courses. A culminating project could be included in the curriculum plan whereby a specific client's health concern is addressed through EBP and processes of change, or a population health concern, such as opiate use, overuse of antibiotics, pre- or postoperative workups, transitions to primary care after hospitalization, and so on can be addressed in a novel way. Processes of change that were applied could be documented.

Students preparing for CNL roles will require a broad array of experiences to develop competencies. Their accountability is to a microsystem that demands continual leadership in the assessment, and the evaluation of care processes among members of care teams is a major characteristic of their future roles. These students are required to complete 400 clinical hours, 300 of which should be dedicated to an immersion experience (AACN, 2017). They should be mentored during clinical practice by an experienced CNL, a clinical nurse specialist, or another professional dedicated to care

---

TABLE 7-4

Recommended Clinical Nurse Leader Curriculum Experiences to Develop Translational Science and Evidence-Based Practice Competencies

CLINICAL NURSE LEADER RECOMMENDED EXPERIENCES
Conduct a microsystem analysis
Identify clinical and cost outcomes and their relationship to clinical/patient outcomes
Assess a microsystem's resources, perform a gap analysis, prioritize the needs, and communicate to stakeholders
Develop and conduct a change process to implement a new or revised evidence-based practice
Participate in the assessment of a practice guideline or practice process
Analyze actual and potential risks for a patient cohort within a specific care environment/ setting
Communicate to an audience in an informal setting ideas/information about a practice issue
Observe role models engaging in communication and conflict resolution
Analyze interprofessional patterns of communication and chain of command
Present to leaders or other stakeholders outside of the academic setting
Use and aggregate data set to prepare report(s) and justify needs for patient care improvements
Evaluate practices and outcomes of care for potential cost savings
Present a recommendation for use or implementation of existing or new healthcare technology

Adapted from American Association of Colleges of Nursing. (2017, May). *Recommended CNL practice experiences.* Author. https://www.aacnnursing.org/Portals/42/CNL/AACN-CNL-Clinical-Experiences-2017.pdf.

---

quality in a clinical area (AACN, 2017). The settings for clinical experience should value EBP and continuous QI as inherent to its mission of care.

An expert panel was convened by AACN to prepare recommendations for CNL students' practice experiences. In 2017, the expert panel presented its report that outlined recommendations for 24 "critical" practice experiences and the strong recommendation that students complete an "evidence-based quality improvement" (AACN, 2017, p. 3). If a curriculum is designed with this improvement project, many experiences for achieving competency in EBP and applying skills required to facilitate TS as a practice partner can be accomplished. If not, however, many of the "critical" practice experiences recommended by the expert panel can provide the foundations for TS and EBP competencies. The experiences suggested by the panel that are most related to TS and EBP are listed in Table 7-4.

An ideal preceptor for an MSN student preparing to be an APRN or CNL would be a DNP-prepared nurse in the practice area. However, if this is not possible, a faculty member who has extensive experience with health system and/or practice change can be an effective role model for the student. Because these students will be practicing with a small group of team members, the interpersonal communication skills they obtain will be some of the most critical areas needed for their participation in TS and EBP activities. If they are perceived as too overbearing or, conversely, too passive or weak, they are not likely to engender confidence among team members. Because their roles will be that of a facilitator or agent of change, they will need to put forward a perception of competency and confidence in their actions that will inspire others to follow. Whether the MSN student completes a formal practice change project or has other experiences in which processes linked to practice change and EBP were enacted, some form of dissemination should be expected. The type of dissemination should be appropriate to the experience. APRNs can present case studies from their practice change to peers or organizational representatives. If they participated in or led a larger effort, some venues we have previously suggested for DNP project presentations, such as nurse practitioner conferences or poster sessions at regional research society conferences, might be appropriate. CNL students may have experiences amenable to presentation at health system conferences, Magnet conferences, or the American Nursing Informatics Association conference, as well as national and regional CNL conferences. Whether these broad venues are used to disseminate or not, their work should be presented to the appropriate health system constituency (i.e., the microsystem team, a group of higher level of administrators, or nursing practice committees in an organization). Oral presentations, executive summaries, or tool kits are all appropriate ways to communicate student work.

CONCLUSION

EBP is central to the delivery of safe, quality, and efficient services to health care consumers. TS focuses on the processes and outcomes of incorporating evidence into the contexts of real-world health care practice. Nursing graduate programs awarding doctoral or master's degrees can use identified competencies of both nursing and TS to plan and execute curricula that prepare graduates capable of leading TS projects and modeling EBP while enacting their roles.

In this chapter, competencies were summarized that are applicable to practice at the MSN and DNP levels, as well as for nurses preparing for a research career as translational scientists. Curriculum experiences suitable for the development of competencies were outlined. Venues for the dissemination of student TS and EBP projects were described.

REFLECTIVE QUESTIONS

1. Guided by TS knowledge competencies aligned with master's competencies in Table 7-2, describe a variety of activities and experiences that will enhance skill development.
2. Using Table 7-3, select one of the suggested experiences and provide examples that can be used to advance competencies and skills in TS.

REFERENCES

American Association of Colleges of Nursing. (2001). *Indicators of quality in research-focused doctoral programs in nursing.* Author. https://www.aacnnursing.org/Portals/42/News/Position-Statements/Doctoral-Indicators.pdf

American Association of Colleges of Nursing. (2004a). *AACN position statement on the practice doctorate in nursing.* Author. https://www.aacnnursing.org/Portals/42/News/Position-Statements/DNP.pdf

American Association of Colleges of Nursing. (2004b). *Dialogue with the board. AACN Clinical Nurse Leader Project.* Author. https://www.aacnnursing.org/Portals/42/CNL/Spring04Dialogue.pdf

American Association of Colleges of Nursing. (2004c). *Talking points.* Author. https://www.aacnnursing.org/CNL/About/Talking-Points

American Association of Colleges of Nursing. (2006). *The essentials of doctoral education for advanced nursing practice.* Author. https://www.aacnnursing.org/Portals/42/Publications/DNPEssentials.pdf

American Association of Colleges of Nursing. (2010). *The research-focused doctoral program in nursing: Pathways to excellence.* Author. https://www.aacnnursing.org/Portals/42/Publications/PhDPosition.pdf

American Association of Colleges of Nursing. (2011). *The essentials of master's education in nursing.* Author. https://www .aacnnursing.org/Portals/42/Publications/MastersEssentials11.pdf

American Association of Colleges of Nursing. (2013). *Competencies and curricular expectations for Clinical Nurse Leader^sm education and practice.* Author. https://www.aacnnursing.org/Portals/42/AcademicNursing/CurriculumGuidelines /CNL-Competencies-October-2013.pdf

American Association of Colleges of Nursing. (2015). *The doctor of nursing practice: Current issues and clarifying recommendations.* Author. https://www.aacnnursing.org/Portals/42/DNP/DNP-Implementation.pdf

American Association of Colleges of Nursing. (2017, May). *Recommended CNL practice experiences.* Author. https://www .aacnnursing.org/Portals/42/CNL/AACN-CNL-Clinical-Experiences-2017.pdf

American Association of Colleges of Nursing. (2018). *Annual report 2018.* Author. https://www.aacnnursing.org/Portals /42/Publications/Annual-Reports/2018-AACN-Annual-Report.pdf

American Association of Colleges of Nursing. (2019). *Fact sheet: The doctor of nursing practice (DNP).* Author. https:// www.aacnnursing.org/Portals/42/News/Factsheets/DNP-Factsheet.pdf

American Association of Colleges of Nursing. (2020a). *Clinical nurse leader (CNL).* https://www.aacnnursing.org/CNL

American Association of Colleges of Nursing. (2020b). *2020 student policy summit this March: Register and sponsor today!* https://www.aacnnursing.org/Students/Student-News/View/ArticleId/24548/Student-Policy-Summit-2020

American Association of Colleges of Nursing Common APRN Doctoral-Level Competencies Work Group. (2017). *Common advanced practice registered nurse doctoral-level competencies.* Author. http://www.aacnnursing.org/Portals /42/AcademicNursing/pdf/Common-APRN-Doctoral-Competencies.pdf

American Nurses Association. (n.d.). *The American Nurses Advocacy Institute.* https://www.nursingworld.org/practice-policy/advocacy/

American Nurses Credentialing Center (n.d.) FAQs. https://www.nursingworld.org/certification/faqs/

Anderson, K. M., McLaughlin, M. K., Crowell, N. A., Fall-Dickson, J. M., White, K. A., Heitzler, E. T., Kesten, K. S., & Yearwood, E. L. (2019). Mentoring students engaging in scholarly projects and dissertations in doctoral nursing programs. *Nursing Outlook, 67,* 776-788. http://doi.org/10.1016/j.outlook.2015.04.002

Auerbach, D. I., Martsolf, G., Pearson, M. L., Taylor, E. A., Zaydman, M., Muchow, A., Spetz, J., & Dower, C. (2014). *The DNP by 2015: A study of the institutional, political, and professional issues that facilitate or impede establishing a post-baccalaureate doctor of nursing practice program.* Rand Corporation. https://www.aacnnursing.org/Portals/42/DNP /DNP-Study.pdf

Bleich, M. R. (2019). Implementation science as a leadership and doctor of nursing practice competency. *The Journal of Continuing Education in Nursing, 50*(11), 491-492. https://doi.org/10.3928/00220124-20191015-03

Breslin, E., Sebastian, J., Trautman, D., & Rosseter, R. (2015). Sustaining excellence and relevance in PhD nursing education. *Nursing Outlook, 63,* 428-431. http://dx.doi.org/10.1016/j.outlook.2015.04.002

Brown, M. A., & Crabtree, K. (2013). The development of practice scholarship in DNP programs: A paradigm shift. *Journal of Professional Nursing, 29*(6), 330-337. https://doi.org/10.1016/j.profnurs.2013.08.003

Buchholz, S. W., Yingling, C., Jones, K., & Tenfelde, S. (2015). DNP and PhD collaboration: Bringing together practice and research expertise as predegree and postdegree scholars. *Nurse Educator, 40*(4), 201-206. https://doi.org/10.1097 /NNE.0000000000000141

Carper, B. (1978). Fundamental patterns of knowing in nursing. *Advances in Nursing Science, 1*(1), 13-23.

Chambers, D. A., Proctor, E. K., Brownson, R. C., & Straus, S. E. (2017). Mapping training needs for dissemination and implementation research: Lessons from a synthesis of existing D & I research training programs. *Translational Behavioral Medicine, 7,* 593-601. https://doi.org/10.1007/s13142-016-0399-3

Cygan, H. R., & Reed, M. (2019). DNP and PhD scholarship: Making the case for collaboration. *Journal of Professional Nursing, 35,* 353-357. https://doi.org/10.1016/j.profnurs.2019.03.002

Dawes, M., Summerskill, W., Glasziou, P., Cartabellotta, A., Martin, J., Hopayian, K., Porzslot, F., Burls, A., Osborne, J., & Second International Conference of Evidence-Based Health Care Teachers and Developers. (2005). Sicily statement on evidence-based practice. *BMC Medical Education, 5,* 1. https://doi.org/10.1186/1472-6920-5-1

Edwardson, S. (2010). Doctor of Philosophy and Doctor of Nursing Practice as Complementary Degrees. *Journal of Professional Nursing, 26*(3), 137-140, https://doi.org/10.1016/j.profnurs.2009.08.004

Graves, B. A., O'Neal, P. V., Roussel, L., & Polancich, S. (2018). EBP design and translation: Teaching how to begin a scholarly practice project. *Worldviews on Evidence-Based Nursing, 15*(2), 152-154. https://doi.org/10.1111/wvn.12270

Grol, R., & Grimshaw, J. (2003). From best evidence to best practice: Effective implementation of change in patients' care. *The Lancet, 362*(9391), 1225-1230. https://doi.org/10.1016/S0140-6736(03)14546-1

Harvard Business Publishing Education (2020). Cases. https://hbsp.harvard.edu/cases/

Henly, S. J., McCarthy, D. O., Wyman, J. F., Stone, P. W., Redeker, N. S., McCarthy, A. M., Alt-White, A. C., Dunbar-Jacob, J., Titler, M. G., Moore, S. M., Heitkemper, M. M., & Conley, Y. P. (2015). Integrating emerging areas of nursing science into PhD programs. *Nursing Outlook, 63,* 408-416.

Institute of Medicine. (2000). *To err is human: Building a safer health system.* National Academies Press. https://doi.org /10.17226/9728

The Joanna Briggs Institute. (2017). *Checklist for qualitative research.* Author. https://joannabriggs.org/sites/default/files /2019-05/JBI_Critical_Appraisal-Checklist_for_Qualitative_Research2017_0.pdf

Kitson, A., Harvey, G., & McCormack, B. (1998). Enabling the implementation of evidence based practice: A conceptual framework. *Quality in Health Care, 7*(3), 149-158.

Leung, W. (2002). Competency based medical training: review. *BMJ, 325*, 693-695. https://doi.org/10.1136/bmj.325.7366.693

Lusk, M. D. & Marzilli, C. (2018). Innovation with strengths: A collaborative approach to PhD/DNP integration in doctoral education. *Nursing Education Perspectives, 39*(5), 327-328. https://doi.org/10.1097/01.NEP.0000000000000393

Mallidou, A. A., Atherton, P., Chan, L., Frisch, N., Glegg, S., & Scarrow, G. (2018). Core knowledge translation competencies: A scoping review. *BMC Health Services Research, 18*, 502. https://doi.org/10.1186/s12913-018-3314-4

Meissner, H.I., Glasgow, R.E., Vinson, C.A., Chambers, D., Brownson, R. C., Green, L. W., Ammerman, A. S., Weiner, B. J., & Mittman, B. J. (2013). The U.S. training institute for dissemination and implementation research in health. *Implementation Science, 8*, 12. https://doi.org/10.1186/1748-5908-8-12

Melnyk, B. M. (2013). Distinguishing the preparation and roles of doctor of philosophy and doctor of nursing practice graduates: National implications for academic curricula and health care systems. *Journal of Nursing Education, 52*(8), 442-448. https://doi.org/10.3928/01484834-20130719-01

Melnyk, B. M., Gallagher-Ford, L., Long, L. E., & Fineout-Overholt, E. (2014). The establishment of evidence-based practice competencies for practicing registered nurses and advanced practice nurses in real-world clinical settings: Proficiencies to improve healthcare quality, reliability, patient outcomes, and costs. *Worldviews on Evidence-Based Nursing, 11*(1), 5-15. https://doi.org/10.1111/wvn.12021

Mistichelli, J. (1984). Diagnosis related groups (DRGs) and the prospective payment system: Forecasting social implications. *Scope Note, 4*, 1-10. https://repository.library.georgetown.edu/bitstream/handle/10822/556896/sn4.pdf?sequence=1&isAllowed=y

Moore, E. R., & Watters, R. (2013). Educating DNP students about critical appraisal and knowledge translation. *International Journal of Nursing Education Scholarship, 10*(1), 237-244. https://doi.org/10.1515/ijnes-2012-0005

Moore, J. E., Rashid, S., Park, J. S., Khan, S., & Straus, S. E. (2018). Longitudinal evaluation of a course to build core competencies in implementation practice. *Implementation Science, 13*(1), 106. https://doi.org/10.1186/s13012-018-0800-3

The National CNS Competency Task Force. (2010). *Clinical nurse specialist core competencies. Executive Summary 2006-2008.* Author. https://www.nacns.org/wp-content/uploads/2017/01/CNSCoreCompetenciesBroch.pdf

National Organization of Nurse Practitioner Faculties NP Core Competencies Content Work Group. (2014). *Nurse practitioner core competencies content.* Author. https://cdn.ymaws.com/www.nonpf./resource/resmgr/competencies/2014npcorecompscontentfinaln.pdf

Nodine, T. R. (2016). How did we get here? A brief history of competency-based higher education in the United States. *Competency-Based Education, 1*, 5-11. https://doi.org/10.1002/cbe2.1004

Ott, K. M., Haase-Herrick, K., & Harris, J. (2006). *American Association of Colleges of Nursing working statement comparing the Clinical Nurse Leader and nurse manager roles: Similarities, differences and complementarities.* Author. https://www.aacnnursing.org/Portals/42/CNL/CNL-Manager-Roles.pdf

Padek, M., Colditz, G., Dobbins, M., Koscielniak, N., Proctor, E. K., Sales, A. E., & Brownson, R. C. (2015). Developing educational competencies for dissemination and implementation research training programs: An exploratory analysis using card sorts. *Implementation Science, 10*, 114. https://doi.org/10.1186/s13012-015-0304-3

Proctor, E., Landsverk, J., Baumann, A. A., Mittman, B., Aarons, G. A., Brownson, R. C., Glisson, C., & Chambers, D. (2013). The implementation research institute: Training mental health implementation researchers in the United States. *Implementation Science, 8*, 105. https://doi.org/10.1186/1748-5908-8-105

Proctor, E., & Chambers, D. (2017). Training in dissemination and implementation research: A field-wide perspective. *TBM Translational Behavioral Medicine, 7*, 624-635. https://doi.org/10.1007/s13142-016-0406-8

Riner, M. E. (2015). Using implementation science as the core of the doctor of nursing practice inquiry project. *Journal of Professional Nursing, 31*(3), 200-207. http://dx.doi.org/10.1016/j.profnurs.2014.11.002

Rogers, E. M. (2003). *Diffusion of innovations* (5th ed.). Free Press.

Santacroce, S. J., Leeman, J., & Song, M.-K. (2018). A training program for nurse scientists to promote intervention translation. *Nursing Outlook, 66*(2), 149-156. https://doi.org/10.1016/j.outlook.2017.09.003

Straus, S. E., Brouwers, M., Johnson, D., Lavis, J. N., Légaré, F., Majumdar, S. R., McKibbon, K. A., Sales, A. E., Stacey, D., Klein, G., Grimshaw, J., & KT Canada Strategic Training Initiative in Health Research (2011). Core competencies in the science and practice of knowledge translation: Description of a Canadian strategic training initiative. *Implementation Science, 6*, 127. https://doi.org/10.1186/1748-5908-6-127

Tabak, R.G., Padek, M. M., Kerner, J. F., Stange, K. C., Proctor, E. K., Maureen J. Dobbins, M. J., Colditz, G. A., Chambers, D. A., & Brownson, R. C. (2017). Dissemination and implementation science training needs: Insights from practitioners and researchers, *American Journal of Preventive Medicine, 52*(3), S322-S329. https://doi.org/10.1016/j.amepre.2016.10.005

Walker, G. E., Golde, C. M., Jones, L., Bueschel, A. C., & Hutchings, P. (2008). *The formation of scholars: Rethinking doctoral education for the twenty-first century.* Carnegie Foundation for the Advancement of Teaching. Jossey-Bass.

Zoellner, J. M., & Porter, K. J. (2017). Translational research: Concepts and methods in dissemination and implementation research. In A. M. Coulston, C. J. Boushey, M. G. Ferruzzi, & L. M. Delahanty (Eds.), *Nutrition in the prevention and treatment of disease* [Digital edition version] (4th ed., pp. 125-143). Elsevier. http://dx.doi.org/10.1016/B978-0-12-802928-2.00006-0

Exemplar 7-1

Evidence-Based Best Practice for Pediatric Patient/Family Education in a Cardiovascular Intensive Care Setting

Tedra S. Smith, DNP, CRNP, CPNP-PC, CNE, CHSE

Andrew Loehr, BSN, MSN, CNP

Background

At ABC Children's Hospital, the cardiovascular intensive care unit (CVICU) is a patient care area providing complex postsurgical care for critically ill pediatric patients. The environment is primarily filled with machines that create frequent beeping sounds, with children on ventilators and inundated with tubes and wires. Pediatric patients traditionally admit to the CVICU after a critical surgical encounter at a time when parents/guardian (i.e., caregivers) are highly stressed and potentially emotional.

The Problem

Staff nurses in the CVICU must orient and educate patients/caregivers in an environment that is overwhelming and can aggregate anxiety and stress in grieving caregivers and other family members. An additional challenge for the CVICU staff registered nurse is assessing and modifying education because of the health literacy of the caregiver. Each patient/caregiver family situation is unique and requires a flexible approach to education and an environment that is conducive to the health literacy and emotional status of the learner while ensuring that standardized and necessary education is delivered.

Evidence-Based Application

The pediatric CVICU is a setting where caregivers may benefit from patient discussions and education being provided in a more private and less stimulating environment (Hill et al., 2019). Approximately 36% of adult individuals in the United States are estimated to have low basic health literacy skills (Mahadevan, 2013). Visual and digital patient educational tools with written text maximize the usability by those with low health literacy skills (Choi et al., 2010).

IMPROVEMENT INTERVENTION

The project team developed a concept idea that consisted of having a picture of a patient with the most common medical devices attached to their person and text descriptions of the medical devices. The most effective way to educate patients and caregivers with literacy levels of varying degrees is by using a number-labeling system on the picture that coordinated with the medical term, layman's term, and basic definitions. The project team developed a list of the 12 most common medical devices that are seen on a postoperative patient in the CVICU and wrote a basic definition for each of the medical devices. The educational tool provided a visual image on one side and a written color-coded guide on the other side to meet the needs of individuals with different learning preferences. The color code depicted which device was safe to be touched or not touched by the patient/caregiver. The improvement team received consent from a patient's family to capture a picture that best depicted the use of medical devices on a patient postsurgery for the educational tool.

DATA COLLECTION AND FINDINGS

Data were derived from pre- and postsurveys completed by the participant as well as a postintervention focus group with CVICU staff registered nurses. From August through December 2019, 12 patients met the inclusion criteria. Of the 12 participants 70% were able to identify all 12 medical devices after implementation compared with 25% before the intervention. All 12 patient caregivers reported that they would like more information related to the medical devices their child will have before the intervention. It is important to note that 100% of participants reported an increase in confidence related to providing care for their child postintervention.

CONCLUSION

Using an evidence-based approach to improvement is an effective method to improve the delivery of education in a pediatric intensive care unit environment. The project team was able to implement a standardized postoperative caregiver education process using an educational tool that created a sense of comfort for caregivers. Furthermore, the standardized process created a dedicated time for caregiver education in a low-stress environment, which led to an increase in family involvement in the care of the patient.

REFERENCES

Choi, J., Bakken, S., Choi, J., & Bakken, S. (2010). Web-based education for low-literate parents in neonatal intensive care unit: Development of a website and heuristic evaluation and usability testing. *International Journal of Medical Informatics, 79*(8), 565-575. https://doi.org/10.1016/j.ijmedinf.2010.05.001

Hill, C., Knafl, K. A., Docherty, S., & Santacroce, S. J. (2019). Parent perceptions of the impact of the paediatric intensive care environment on delivery of family-centered care. *Intensive and Critical Care Nursing, 50*, 88-94. https://doi.org/10.1016/j.iccn.2018.07.007

Mahadevan, R. (2013). Health literacy fact sheet. Center for health care strategies, Inc. Published October 2013. Accessed July 13, 2020. https://www.chcs.org/resource/health-literacy-fact-sheets/

ORGANIZATIONAL SYSTEMS AND LEADERSHIP
Impact on Translational Nursing

Linda A. Roussel, PhD, RN, NEA-BC, CNL, FAAN
Patricia L. Thomas, PhD, RN, FAAN, FACHE, FNAP, NEA-BC, ACNS-BC, CNL

CHAPTER OBJECTIVES

- Describe change management responses on a continuum and the effectiveness of using a framework to enhance successful implementation
- Outline implications for team and engagement science concepts that facilitate exemplar work with interprofessional teams
- Delineate a variety of research strategies (qualitative, quantitative, mixed methods, and community action research) that support leadership and organizational systems assessments
- Discuss the impact of influence and messaging to enhance implementation, dissemination, and sustainability
- Describe implications using evidence-based organizational assessment tools and strategies to improve health systems outcomes

---

Roussel, L. A., & Thomas, P. L. (Eds.). *Implementation Science in Nursing: A Framework for Education and Practice* (pp. 133-144).

> **KEY WORDS**
>
> - Change management
> - Change responses
> - Health systems thinking
> - Influence
> - Message
> - Organizational assessment tools
> - Organizational systems
> - Systems thinking
> - Team and engagement sciences

This chapter focuses on systems thinking, leadership, and change management from an implementation and dissemination sciences and practice perspective. Team and engagement sciences have implications for rigorous implementation and dissemination. Exploring organizational dynamics and their application to promoting positive health care outcomes and community outreach will be advanced as implementation science and practice impact organization culture and readiness for change. Specific tools and assessment guides are described because they impact entry and advanced nursing practice and education. This chapter incorporates a strong translational nursing practice perspective and includes implications for academic–clinical–community partnership. Building on implementation, dissemination, and translational science provides foundational content in which to address concepts of organizational systems, leadership, team building, and change management.

Organizational systems and leadership are essential to any sustained improvement in health care. Executives and managers in health care address leadership challenges in evidence-based practice (EBP) implementation as they convey the need to ensure the efficient use of resources and to prioritize what quality services are provided. Health systems thinking provides a framework for context and perspectives that are the larger view of problems, issues, and gaps. We know that context and frameworks are pivotal to successful implementation practice as well as to strengthen translational nursing practice with implications for academic–clinical–community partnership. Understanding systems thinking and health systems thinking provides a foundation for a deeper reflection on implementation and dissemination sciences.

ORGANIZATIONS AND SYSTEMS THINKING

Johnson and Anderson (2017) offered a perspective on systems thinking that describes a way of thinking that is a new language focused on whole systems vs. individual components. This way of thinking encourages health professionals and system leaders to search for root causes, bottlenecks, and constraints that are barriers to workable and innovative solutions. The emphasis is on measurable, sustainable outcomes. A systems thinking framework invites proactive approaches that are open and circular vs. a linear, reductionist approach (Johnson & Anderson, 2017). Senge (1990) provided the concept of mental models, which goes hand in hand with systems thinking and offers a language on restructuring the way we think. Johnson and Anderson (2017) offered principles that underpin systems thinking and, subsequently, health systems thinking. These principles include reframing the conversation to enhance seeing the whole vs. isolated silos. In doing so, organizational leaders help others to recognize patterns, inter-relationships, and boundaries that may not be apparent when "breaking down" the parts of a problem or issue. To that end, seeing the whole offers a larger context that resists breaking down concerns and issues into smaller (possibly irrelevant) components. This second principle facilitates multiple viewpoints and perspectives, and all stakeholders are expected to share their personal lens encouraging interconnectedness, which is critical to sustainable options and solutions. The third principle considers systems thinking as a transformational way of understanding and addressing community-based remedies. Interconnectedness and transformational approaches can accelerate the visualization of trends, interactions, and connections at all levels (individual, team, organizational, and community), underscoring the need to consider systemic approaches to solve problems from a larger scale vs. isolated solutions. The fourth and final principle promotes the importance of examining complex challenges using systems thinking tools, such as feedback loops, balancing feedback loops, and behavior over time diagrams (Johnson & Anderson, 2017). More tools and strategies are described by Johnson and Anderson (2017).

With a systems thinking perspective guiding health systems thinking, Powell and Stone (2015) offered excellent insights from a patient safety lens. In their work, Powell and Stone described the working model/framework of Emanuel et al. (2008) on patient safety as a system. This well-thought-out model considers recipients of care, systems for therapeutic action, and workers (teams trained to rescue from or manage failure). Methods such as continuous quality improvement, including technology (hardware), the physical environment (plant), and advocacy (policy), as well as competence, communication, and teamwork provide ways to intervene within the components of the patient safety system (Powell & Stone, 2015). In addition to the model described, Powell and Stone (2015) also considered multiteams, including a coordinating team, a core team, and ancillary and support services. Microsystems thinking as the basic building block is also discussed in relationship to meso-systems and macrosystems. For example, microsystems are the smallest replicable units that provide care to patients, mesosystems bind these units, and macrosystems are the "vessels" that hold the micro- and mesosystems together. This provides a holistic perspective to what might be considered a more compartmentalized, siloed approach to the inner workings of health care systems (Powell & Stone, 2015). Patient safety and high-reliability organizations (HROs) are also included from a health systems thinking perspective. Leadership, culture, and dynamic process improvement are key principles of HROs (Chassin & Loeb, 2013). These principles are incorporated into the health care system's organizational culture and consider strategies such as just culture (Marx, n.d.), staff engagement, coaching and mentoring, and well-designed data systems that capture patient harm and near misses. Contextualizing organizational systems and how leaders can access these tools and strategies is key to the successful implementation and dissemination of critical health systems and population outcome (Powell & Stone, 2015). These concepts are foundational to translational nursing practice and have implications for academic–clinical–community partnerships.

We know that patient safety is front and center in organizational strategic initiatives and required in best practices to meet regulatory requirements. Working in HROs adds further complexity to our health care system given the high degree of medical errors ending in fatal events. Along with basic standards of care, innovation must also be at the forefront of exploring ways to improve health care and system outcomes of safe, effective, efficient, and equitable care. Leadership is important to sustainable organizational change, achieving an engaging climate for implementation, and assuring more positive attitudes toward EBPs. There are limited leadership development models that highlight specific strategies that organizations and leaders can use to improve the climate for EBP uptake and implementation in health care systems. Culture, contextual, and individual factors must be a major focus when facilitating EBP implementation. Leaders who do not pay attention to these factors often end up with poor or failed fidelity of implementation strategies, fragmented service delivery, compromised patient care, and decreased population health outcomes (Aarons et al., 2014).

When considering organizational context from team and engagement science perspectives, the leader is mindful of systems dynamics such as culture, climate, communication channels, and structure. Readiness for change assessment involves all components of organizational dynamics. Organizational readiness for change is considered a critical precursor to the successful implementation of complex changes in health care settings (Armenakis et al., 1993). Some authors have shared that failure to establish sufficient readiness accounts for one half of all unsuccessful, large-scale organizational change efforts (Cassidy, 1994; Hardison, 1998; Schein, 2010). Considering Lewin's (1951) three-stage model of change, change management experts have prescribed various strategies to create readiness by "unfreezing" existing mental models and creating motivation for change. Health systems thinking can also be useful here, providing underlying principles for pattern recognition and interconnectedness with key stakeholders and organizational leaders. Readiness for change strategies includes highlighting the differences between current and desired performance levels, investigating dissatisfaction with the status quo, creating an engaging vision of a bright future, and facilitating confidence that this future state is achievable with current organizational stakeholders (Kotter, 1996). Although the evidence base for these strategies may be limited, this guidance can be considered reasonable to health systems leaders. Unlike individual readiness for change, organizational readiness for change has not been extensively studied compared with individual readiness for change. A desire for more research is inadequate at best, particularly given the limited evidence on the reliability or validity regarding measuring organizational readiness for change. More basic to reliability or validity is the conceptual ambiguity about the meaning of organizational readiness and limited theoretical grounding in determining outcomes of organizational readiness (Aarons et al., 2015). Further exploration and greater clarity are necessary and, if not addressed, will halt a deeper understanding of organizational readiness, particularly because it is critical to successful implementation and dissemination practices (Aarons et al., 2015). This has a significant impact on the organization's ability to influence outcomes and create meaningful messages for sustained best practices and innovations.

Birken et al. (2017) described organizational theory for dissemination and implementation research. Specifically, the authors outlined the importance of using organizational theories in strategically planning research efforts. Discussing their research on SafeCare, an EBP for preventing child abuse and neglect, the authors described the following organizational theories that framed their study: transaction cost economics, resource dependency theory, institutional theory, and contingency theories. Integrating these four well-known organizational theories, the researchers applied these concepts into their efforts to implement SafeCare. Specifically, the transaction cost economics theory predicted how uncertain processes frequently applied for contracting SafeCare may have generated inefficiencies, possibly compromising implementation among private child welfare organizations. The institutional theory described how child welfare systems were likely motivated to implement SafeCare because this may have aligned with the expectations of key stakeholders within child welfare system professional communities. The contingency theories delineated efforts such as interagency collaborative teams that promoted SafeCare implementation by facilitating adaptation to child welfare agency internal and external contexts. The resource dependency theory explained how interagency relationships supported by contracts, memoranda of understanding, and negotiations advanced SafeCare implementation by balancing autonomy and dependence on funding agencies and SafeCare developers. Along with the retrospective application of the organizational theories described previously, the researchers advocated for the robust use of organizational theories to design implementation research. Specifically, the researchers posited that implementation strategies should be determined based on minimizing the transaction costs, promoting and maintaining congruence between organizations' dynamic internal and external contexts over time, and at the same time attending to organizations' financial needs while preserving their autonomy. This study provided an excellent example of implications for integrating organizational theory in implementation research for implementation strategies, the evaluation of implementation efforts, measurement, research design, theory, and practice. The researchers offered context to organizational system leaders for exploring strategies to advance learning, engagement, and professional development in health care systems. The perspectives offered by these authors can enhance a stronger organizational system approach to translational nursing practice.

ORGANIZATIONAL SYSTEMS, CHANGE MANAGEMENT, AND CHANGE RESPONSES

According to the Society for Human Resource Management, change management can be described as the systematic approach and application of knowledge, tools, and resources used to address change. Specifically, change management integrates defining and adopting corporate strategies, structures, procedures, and technologies to confront changes in external conditions and within the organization's culture. Change management that is effective reaches beyond logistics, technical tasks, and project management to enact organizational changes and involves the human side of major change within an organization. To be successful, change management includes positive implementation of new processes, products, and business strategies while minimizing negative responses and mediating barriers to overcome resistance to change. Resistance to change responses introduced by Coch and French (1948) were the first approaches when considering the best ways to manage successful change. The evolution of change goes beyond the resistance to change to incorporate various degrees of acceptance (or readiness) for change and creating a continuum of change responses. Coetsee (1999) outlined seven forms of change responses moving from aggressive resistance, active resistance, and passive resistance to indifference, support, involvement, and commitment. According to Coetsee's framework, a change response can be conceptualized as a tridimensional attitude. These three components include cognitive (opinions about changes, their usefulness, advantages, and disadvantages), affective (feelings about changes), and intentional/ behavioral (actions already taken or that will be taken for or against changes). Elizur and Guttman's (1976) conceptualization of the three components includes cognitive (opinions about changes, their usefulness, advantages, and disadvantages, etc.), affective (feelings about changes), and intentional/behavioral (actions already taken or that will be taken for or against changes). This expanded Coetsee's continuum of change responses. Using Coetsee's framework, Nilsen et al. (2019) applied an inductive approach when conducting interviews using a semistructured interview guide with 30 health care professionals (physicians, registered nurses, and assistant nurses) employed in the Swedish health care system. The authors used Coetsee's analytical framework to analyze the informants' change responses in which change responses were perceived as a continuum spanning from a strong acceptance of change to strong resistance to change (using the seven forms of change responses). Additionally, the change response was conceptualized as a tridimensional attitude composed of three components (cognitive, affective, and intentional/behavioral) as described by Elizur and Guttman (1976). The data revealed 10 types of change responses, which were mapped onto five of the seven response categories of Coetsee's framework. It is noteworthy that the participants did not report change responses that aligned with the two most extreme forms of responses in the framework (i.e., commitment and aggressive resistance). Specifically, most change responses were classified as either indifference or passive resistance to changes. The authors reported that they could not find any change responses that were not aligned with the framework. When health care professionals initiated the change themselves, or when there was active input that was well founded and well communicated, there was greater engagement of the participants. Overall, the authors found the framework to be a useful way of understanding how stakeholders respond to change (vs. only addressing resistance to change). Additionally, this framework also proved to be a productive way to manage change and for efforts to achieve positive implementation of EBPs in health care.

Organizational Systems and Team Science: Implication for Implementation Science

Incorporating team science into organizational systems offers real hope for ensuring that research is translated into evidence-based policy and practice. We know that interventions often fall short of expectations or worsen the problems and issues, often due to a limited or faulty understanding of real-world structures, dynamic complexity, and HROs. Systems science can provide principles and insights into solving major challenges in public health. As we described previously, systems-based approaches may contribute to changing the language (vocabulary) and methods for conceptualizing and acting within challenging, complex systems. Improving the modeling used in dissemination and implementation research by applying best principles of systems science can provide greater insights (Northridge & Metcalf, 2016). The modeling process as reported by Northridge and Metcalf (2016) is described as an iterative sequence of steps, beginning with problem definition and concluding with policy analysis. Specifically, Step 1 (problem identification) involves boundary setting. Steps 2 (dynamic hypothesis) and 3 (model formulation) focus on causal mapping and specifying equations and algorithms. Steps 4 (model testing) and 5 (policy analysis) center on identifying boundaries of logical behaviors and creating what-if scenarios and sensitivity testing. This model can provide a frame of reference for bringing teams together to do the work of the organization through systems science principles. Team and engagement sciences can provide additional context to modeling and successful team collaboration. Northridge and Metcalf (2016) proposed four best principles derived from ongoing systems science research and scholarship that may guide and incentivize implementation scientists in their own thinking and research initiatives. A focused theme of these best principles involves meaningfully informing the modeling process. Considering dissemination, the authors purported that implementation research mandates an intentional objective to mindfully reflect and confront the complex and challenging problems that may be barriers to the adoption and integration of evidence-based health interventions and changing practice patterns within specific settings. The following four principles provide further conceptualization of systems science within complex health care organizations (Northridge & Metcalf, 2016):

- Best principle #1: Model the problem, not the system; trying to model the system rather than the problem often leads to confusion and futility. Formative research and interdisciplinary collaboration are critical to guiding implementation scientists toward modeling the problem, not the system.

- Best principle #2: Pay attention to what is important, not just what is quantifiable; not everything that we count or measure is most impactful when considering implementation and dissemination. We know that studies of dissemination and implementation are often based on strategies by which health information, evidence-based interventions, and best clinical practices are adopted and embedded in community and public health and health care services across the continuum. We also know that a broad range of methodological approaches are used and include both traditional designs (randomized controlled trials) and newer approaches such as hybrid effectiveness–implementation designs (Northridge & Metcalf, 2016). A mixed methods design is becoming more popular and encouraged in implementation research. There continues to be a need for greater clarity around connectedness across program levels and components. Thinking contextually as described in systems science models expands the way we think about the system; thus, we are not limited to constructs that can only be quantifiable. We must deeply think and reflect on multiple (interrelated) perspectives that open us up to what is relevant and important and not just what can be quantifiably measured.

- Best principle #3: Leverage the utility of models as boundary objects; Black (2013) described a boundary object as a representation that may include a model, diagram, sketch, or prototype that assists individuals in effectively collaborating across boundaries by reconciling differences in knowledge, training, or objective. This helps research and practice teams to develop a shared language about engaging in problem solving more efficiently. Consideration must be given to the utility of the representation of the boundary objects and how readily modifiable and perceptible representations are to the team. If there is adequate representation and a shared local knowledge, there is greater opportunity for sharing across networks. Thus, there is greater cooperation, which enhances team learning and sustained initiatives.

- Best principle #4: Adopt a portfolio approach to model building; according to Northridge and Metcalf (2016), the portfolio approach provides a collaborative way of interacting through multiple entry points and checkpoints to the modeling process. This enhances input from different team members, which allows for separate work to come together, particularly if team members are working in parallel. When they come together, they often note related models in diverse ways; thus, greater collaboration can occur. Through the portfolio approach to model building, along with greater collaboration and flexibility to the modeling process, multiple opportunities are provided for the input and adjustment of models by different members of the team. This is an iterative modeling process and facilitates exploration and discovery with a variety of models that may or may not be workable; however, they may be modified, useful, and adapted by the implementation team.

ORGANIZATIONAL SYSTEMS, INFLUENCE, AND MESSAGING: IMPLICATIONS FOR IMPLEMENTATION SCIENCE

We have explored the importance of organizational context, culture, and communication to successful implementation and dissemination. Health systems thinking offers principles that underpin how organizational leaders can ready their environments for sustainable change and innovations. Team and engagement science further expand thinking and practices that enhance interprofessional teamwork and collaboration. Aarons et al. (2012) provided extensive research evidence on implementation-specific organizational factors including implementation climate, implementation leadership, and implementation citizenship behavior. Specifically, they defined implementation climate as a shared perception among associates of the extent to which EBP implementation is expected, supported, and provides an incentive within the organization. Implementation leadership is described as the attributes and behaviors of leaders who support effective implementation. Defining implementation citizenship behavior includes going beyond the "call of duty" to enhance implementation. The authors noted that most studies are generally limited to single organizations, and although studies of multiple organizations are available, they do not always examine alignment across organizations, which is often critical to interconnectedness and network analysis. Aarons et al. (2015) posited that the focus on single organizations does not always align with the fundamental nature of integrated care, often bringing together very different health care service systems with the objective of increasing access to care with the provision of effective health services.

BEST PRACTICE ASSESSMENT TOOLS AND STRATEGIES

Organizational systems and leadership skills are crucial to creating an environment in which EBPs can be implemented and sustained. Consideration needs to be given to leader behaviors, implementation leadership, organizational context, and implementation outcomes (Aarons et al., 2015). Specifically, these authors focused on the role of first-level leaders, who are critical to organizational effectiveness. Building on the work of Avolio and Bass (1991), Aarons et al. (2015) considered the full-range leadership model focused on transformational leadership, including context, facilitation, and evidence to support theory concepts.

Aarons et al. (2012, 2015) created their Leadership and Organizational Change for Implementation (LOCI) team, which developed a leadership training curriculum that is tailored specifically for health, behavioral health, and social service agencies and programs (Beidas & Kendall, 2010). The training is a scaffolded approach and incorporates well-established leadership and management strategies to integrate the development of positive team climate and organizational supports for EBPs. This training is comprehensive with the intent of incorporating real-time educational sessions and mentoring.

Combining leadership development with targeted organizational strategies, the LOCI team purport to create an organizational climate supportive of EBP. The LOCI program developed at the University of California, San Diego provides curricula, training, and coaching to support the implementation of EBPs. More effective leadership in community behavioral health programs is associated with more positive staff attitudes toward the adoption of EBP and lower staff turnover (Aarons et al., 2015). Effective leadership has also been correlated with higher consumer satisfaction, implementation climate, and implementation success and sustainability (Aarons et al., 2015; Shuman et al., 2020).

The LOCI team provides several valid and reliable assessment tools that have been developed and researched. Their website describes several scales/instruments that practitioners can access and use with permission. The assessment tools available are described in the following section.

The Implementation Citizenship Behavior Scale

The Implementation Citizenship Behavior Scale is a pragmatic six-item measure that identifies critical behaviors employees perform to go beyond the call of duty to support EBP implementation. The Implementation Citizenship Behavior Scale can be used to gain insight on key employee behaviors that should assist in the probability of implementation success.

The Implementation Leadership Scale

The Implementation Leadership Scale (ILS) is a brief 12-item measure assessing leaders' support for EBP implementation. The ILS can be used for leader and organizational development to improve EBP implementation.

Shuman et al. (2020) tested the ILS with frontline managers. Specifically, the authors described that frontline manager implementation leadership is a critical contextual factor influencing EBP implementation. Their study provided strong evidence supporting the validity and reliability of the ILS to measure implementation leadership behaviors of nursing frontline managers in acute care. The ILS can help clinicians, researchers, and leaders in nursing contexts assess frontline manager implementation leadership, deliver interventions to target areas needing improvement, and improve the implementation of EBP.

The Implementation Climate Scale

The Implementation Climate Scale is a brief 18-item measure assessing the extent to which an organization prioritizes and values the successful implementation of EBPs. The Implementation Climate Scale can be used to evaluate and better understand their current climate as they consider how to improve the likelihood of implementation success.

The Evidence-Based Practice Attitude Scale

The Evidence-Based Practice Attitude Scale is an empirically validated measure assessing mental health provider attitudes toward the adoption of EBP. This scale has two options: one with 15 items and one with 50 items. With permission, practitioners and researchers can adopt these tools to obtain baseline information on their teams in order to better focus interventions and training opportunities.

Another important resource that provides a viable implementation model with evidence-based implementation strategies is the University of Iowa Hospitals and Clinics' framework named Implementation Strategies for Evidence-Based Practice. Each phase provides a robust list of implementation strategies for clinicians, organizational leaders, and key stakeholders, as well as an organizational system focus. For each of the phases (i.e., create awareness and interest, build knowledge and commitment, promote action and adoption, and pursue integration and sustained use), strategies are tailored for practitioners and researchers.

Using the University of Iowa Hospitals and Clinics' framework from an organizational systems and leadership perspective, topical areas such as change agents, link practice change and power holder/stakeholder priorities, change agents: EBP change champion, change agents: opinion leader, and change agents: thought leaders are but a sampling of strategies. As you drill down on specific strategies (and strategies can be combined), the authors of the framework provide further detail to include the phase within the model and the focus. The strategy is defined and describes the benefits, outlines a procedure, provides examples, and identifies citations.

For example, using the change agents: opinion leader implementation strategies, the practitioner learns that this is a viable strategy in Phase 2 (i.e., build knowledge and commitment) with the focus of connecting with clinicians, organizational leaders, and key stakeholders. This strategy is defined with benefits. The procedure further advances this implementation strategy to include outlining that different or multiple opinion leaders may need to be selected, as well as the need to consider discipline specifics and the need to change over time.

It is important to combine opinion leadership with other effective strategies for the greatest impact. How to select an opinion leader and how to define the specific role are also detailed for further action. The strategies provide practitioners and researchers detailed implementation strategies that can be explored and used with confidence, knowing that much work has been done to provide this robust listing (Cullen et al., 2017). Chapter 5 provides a copy of the model with greater details as to the various phases.

CONCLUSION

This chapter focused on systems thinking, leadership, and change management from an implementation and dissemination sciences and practice perspective. Specific tools and assessment guides were described because they impact entry and advanced nursing practice and education. This chapter incorporated a strong translational nursing practice perspective.

REFLECTIVE QUESTIONS

1. Describe the importance of organizational context in successful implementation in an interprofessional change project.
2. Discuss team science and its application to implementation science and practices.
3. Select two assessment tools and apply them to your practice. Discuss your experience with using the tools and the benefits of using valid tools to assess readiness for implementing EBP.

REFERENCES

Aarons, G. A., Ehrhart, M. G., Farahnak, L. R., & Sklar, M. (2014). Aligning leadership across systems and organizations to develop a strategic climate for evidence-based practice implementation. *Annual Review of Public Health, 35*, 255-274. https://doi.org/10.1146/annurev-publhealth-032013-182447

Aarons, G. A., Ehrhart, M. G., Farahnak, L. R., & Hurlburt, M. S. (2015). Leadership and organizational change for implementation (LOCI): A randomized mixed method pilot study of a leadership and organization development intervention for evidence-based practice implementation. *Implementation Science, 10*, 11.

Aarons, G. A., Glisson C., Green, P. D., Hoagwood, K., Kelleher, K. J., Landsverk, J. A., Research Network on Youth Mental Health; Weisz, J. R., Chorpita, B., Gibbons, R., Glisson, C., Green, E. P., Hoagwood, K., Jensen, P. S., Kelleher, K., Landsverk, J., Mayberg, S., Miranda, J., Palinkas, L., & Schoenwald, S. (2012). The organizational social context of mental health services and clinician attitudes toward evidence-based practice: A United States national study. *Implementation Science, 7*, 56.

Armenakis, A. A., Harris, S. G., & Mossholder, K. W. (1993). Creating readiness for organizational change. *Human Relations, 46*, 681-703. https://doi.org/10.1177/001872679304600601

Avolio, B. J., & Bass, B.M. (1991). *Manual for the full range of leadership.* Bass, Avolio & Associates.

Beidas, R. S., & Kendall, P. C. (2010). Training therapists in evidence-based practice: A critical review of studies from a systems-contextual perspective. *Clinical Psychology Science and Practice, 17*, 1-30.

Birken, S. A., Bunger, A. C., Powell, B. J., Turner, K., Clary, A. S., Klaman, S. L, Yu, Y., Whitaker, D. J., Self, S. R., Rostad, W. L., Chatham, J. R. S., Kirk, M. A., Shea, C.M., Haines, E., & Weiner, B. J. (2017). Organizational theory for dissemination and implementation research. *Implementation Science, 12*(1), 62. https://doi.org/10.1186/s13012017-0592-x

Black, L. J. (2013). When visuals are boundary objects in system dynamics work. *Systems Dynamic Review, 29*(2), 70-86.

Cassidy, J. (1994). System analyzes readiness for integrated delivery. *Health Progress, 75*, 18-20.

Chassin, M. R., & Loeb, J. M. (2013). High-reliability health care: Getting there from here. *The Milbank Quarterly, 91*(3), 459-490. https://doi.org/10.1111/1468-0009.12023

Coch, L., & French, J. P. R. (1948). Overcoming resistance to change. *Human Relations, 1*(4), 512-532.

Coetsee, L. (1999). From resistance to commitment. *Public Administration Quarterly, 23*, 204-22.

Cullen, L., Wagner, M., Matthews, G., & Farrington, M. (2017). Evidence into practice: Integration within an organizational infrastructure. *Journal of PeriAnesthesia Nursing, 32*(3), 247-256. https://doi.org/10.1016/j.jopan.2017.02.003

Elizur, D., & Guttman, L. (1976). The structure of attitudes toward work and technological change within an organization. *Administration Science Quarterly, 21*, 611-622.

Emanuel, L., Berwick, D., Conway, J., Combes, J., Hatlie, M., Leape, L., Reason, J., Schyve, P., Vincent, C., & Walton, M. (2008). What exactly is patient safety? In K. Henriksen, J. B. Battles, M. A. Keyes, et al. (Eds.), *Advances in patient safety: New directions and alternative approaches* (Vol. 1: Assessment). Agency for Healthcare Research and Quality. https://www.ncbi.nlm.nih.gov/books/NBK43629/

Hardison, C. (1998). Readiness, action, and resolve for change: Do health care leaders have what it takes? *Quality Management in Health Care, 6*, 44-51.

Johnson, J. A., & Anderson, D. E. (2017). *Systems thinking for health organizations, leadership, and policy.* Sentia Publishing.

Kotter, J. P. (1996). *Leading change.* Harvard Business Press.

Lewin, K. (1951). *Field theory in social science: Selected theoretical papers.* Harper.

Marx, D. (n.d.). Just culture. https://justculture.com/

Nilsen, P., Schildmeijer, K., Ericsson, C., Seing, I., & Birken, S. (2019). Implementation of change in health care in Sweden: A qualitative study of professionals' change responses. *Implementation Science, 14*(1), 51. https://doi.org/10.1186/s13012-019-0902-6

Northridge, M. E., & Metcalf, S. S. (2016). Enhancing implementation science by applying best principles of systems science. *Health Research Policy Systems, 14*, 74. https://doi.org/10.1186/s12961-016-0146-8

Powell, S., & Stone, R. (2015). *The patient survival handbook: Avoid being the next victim of medical error.* Book Logix Publishing Services.

Schein, E. H. (2010). *Organizational culture and leadership.* Wiley.

Senge, P. (1990). *The fifth discipline: The art and practice of the learning organization.* Doubleday.

Shuman, C. J., Ehrhart, M. G., Torres, E. M., Veliz, P., Kath, L. M., VanAntwerp, K., Banaszak-Holl, J., Titler, M. G., & Aarons, G. A. (2020). EBP implementation leadership of frontline nurse managers: Validation of the Implementation Leadership Scale in acute care. *Worldviews on Evidence-Based Nursing, 17*(1), 82-91.

Exemplar 8-1

A STRATEGY FOR ENHANCING STAFF CONFIDENCE IN DE-ESCALATING A CRISIS SITUATION

Donna Copeland, DNP, RN, NE-BC, CPN, CPON, AE-C

Workplace violence is described as any physical threat or assault directed toward health care personnel while they are on duty (Occupational Safety and Health Administration, n.d.). Hospitals are supposed to be places of healing and comfort; however, they are the least safe place in America when it comes to violent assaults against health care workers. Furthermore, many nurses report that workplace violence is just the nature of the job (Evans, 2017). Therefore, to address workplace violence, it is critical that nurse managers and organizational leadership adopt a zero tolerance for workplace violence and support a formal training program to reduce incidences of workplace violence.

Considering evidence-based implementation strategies, an interprofessional team developed a crisis prevention program for staff called the Nonviolent Crisis Intervention training program within a 152-bed children's and women's hospital. Using well-established implementation interventions, a training program was offered and consisted of didactic learning and simulated practice, including de-escalation skills, and personal safety techniques to prepare staff to recognize early warning signs of potential crisis that could result in violence or assault. The goal was to reduce reports of physical and verbal assaults of health care workers by 10% over 6 months (Cullen et al., 2017).

Staff members were notified of the Nonviolent Crisis Intervention training program during staff meetings, daily huddles, and the health system email system, and flyers were distributed to all departments and posted in key locations throughout the hospital. Participation was voluntary and confidential, and each participant was asked to complete a pretest and a post-test with an evaluation at the completion of the training. Results indicated that staff members felt more confident and better prepared to respond to a crisis. The implications of this study are that the knowledge gained will help nurse managers and organizational leaders develop future programs to ensure the safety and welfare of staff and promote a healthy working environment.

REFERENCES

Cullen, L., Wagner, M., Matthews, G., & Farrington, M. (2017). Evidence into practice: Integration within an organizational infrastructure. *Journal of PeriAnesthesia Nursing, 32*(3), 247-256. https://doi.org/10.1016/j.jopan.2017.02.003

Evans, G. (2017). Enough is enough: OSHA to issue regulation on violence. *Case Management Advisor, 28*(9), 43-45.

Occupational Safety and Health Administration. (n.d.). Fact sheet. https://www.osha.govOshDoc/data_General_Facts/factsheet-workplaceviolence.pdf

Exemplar 8-2

IMPLEMENTATION OF THE BRADEN SCALE FOR PREDICTING PRESSURE INJURY RISK IN THE EMERGENCY DEPARTMENT

Tiffany Tscherne, RN, DNP, MBA, FACHE

Donna Copeland, DNP, RN, NE-BC, CPN, CPON, AE-C

The emergency department (ED) is the initial point of patient access, and the patient often remains in the ED for prolonged periods without the assessment and implementation of pressure injury prevention measures. Pressure injuries are considered a never event and preventable through the application of evidence-based guidelines.

As a result, a quality improvement project was developed in a 401-bed community hospital to align pressure injury risk assessment and communication between the ED and inpatient units, thereby reducing the time of initiation of pressure injury prevention strategies (Agency for Healthcare Research and Quality, 2014). Considering the implementation of this project, an evidence-based implementation strategy, forming a multidisciplinary team for expertise, resource allocation, and dissemination of information, was undertaken (Cullen et al., 2017). Further implementation strategies/interventions developed by the team included the alignment of the initial pressure injury assessment and interventions in the ED with that of the inpatient units and consistent staff documentation of standard pressure injury assessment and intervention (Health Research & Educational Trust, 2017). The aim was to reduce Stage III and Stage IV pressure injuries by 20% by the end of a 90-day period.

The implementation of the Braden Scale in a 48-bed ED was initiated for patients placed in an observation or inpatient status by a physician order. Working with our multidisciplinary team, we learned the importance of maintaining the fidelity of our interventions. Because the Braden Scale was not part of the ED registered nurse workflow, standardized mandatory education was delivered via the existing electronic education platform. Aligning evidence-based implementation practices of a proactive skin and pressure injury risk assessment between the ED and inpatient units demonstrated a patient safety impact as evidenced by a decrease in the time to initiate prevention protocols by 50% from 15 hours 25 minutes to 7 hours 46 minutes.

REFERENCES

Agency for Healthcare Research and Quality. (2014). Preventing pressure ulcers in hospitals. http://www.ahrq.gov/professionals/systems/hospital/pressureulcertoolkit/index.html

Cullen, L., Wagner, M., Matthews, G., & Farrington, M. (2017). Evidence into practice: Integration within an organizational infrastructure. *Journal of PeriAnesthesia Nursing, 32*(3), 247-256. https://doi.org/10.1016/j.jopan.2017.02.003

Health Research & Educational Trust. (2017). Preventing hospital-acquired pressure ulcers/injuries. https://patientcare-link.org/wp-content/uploads/2017/10/2017-hapu_change_package_508.pdf

THE APPLICATION OF IMPROVEMENT SCIENCE
Quality Improvement, Change Management, and Sustainability

David H. James, DNP, MSHQS, RN, CCNS, NPD-BC
Patricia L. Thomas, PhD, RN, FAAN, FACHE, FNAP, NEA-BC, ACNS-BC, CNL

CHAPTER OBJECTIVES

- Appreciate continuous quality improvement is an essential part of the daily work of all health care professionals
- Analyze the strengths and limitations of common quality improvement methods
- Design, implement, and evaluate tests of change in daily work using an experiential learning method such as Plan-Do-Study-Act
- Describe the alignment of improvement science with implementation science
- Recognize principles of change management to successfully lead teams

KEY WORDS

- Change management
- Implementation science
- Improvement science
- Plan-Do-Study-Act
- Quality improvement

Roussel, L. A., & Thomas, P. L. (Eds.). *Implementation Science in Nursing:*
A Framework for Education and Practice (pp. 145-161).
© 2022 Taylor & Francis Group.

TABLE 9-1	

Key Terms to Know

TERM	DEFINITION
Implementation science	Study of "How and How well systems adopt existing evidence into practice" (Granger, 2018)
Science of improvement	Study of which processes are best suited to achieve quality outcomes in complex health care systems (Granger, 2018)
Theory	Provides an explanation of observed phenomena and allows for prediction (Nilsen, 2015)
Model	Closely related to theories; may not be a true representation of the phenomena and lacks the explanatory features of theory (Nilsen, 2015)
Framework	Does not provide explanation, only describes observations within the context of set criteria (Nilsen, 2015)

The Institute of Medicine (IOM) reports in the early 2000s made the necessity to redesign the nation's health care system clear. Despite groundbreaking reports in *To Err Is Human: Building a Safer Health System* (IOM, 2000), *Crossing the Quality Chasm: A New Health System for the 21st Century* (IOM, 2001), *Health Professions Education: A Bridge to Quality* (IOM, 2003a), and *Patient Safety: Achieving a New Standard for Care* (IOM, 2003b), today's health care system continues to be plagued by unsafe practices, ineffectiveness, provider-centric care, slow responsiveness, inefficiencies, and unequitable care (Agency for Healthcare Research and Quality, 2018). Equipping health care professionals with the knowledge, skills, and attitudes to redesign systems can improve quality and safety across disciplines. Specifically, Quality and Safety Education for Nurses (QSEN) seeks to equip nurses in practice and academe with the knowledge and skills needed to address the quality and safety gaps in our health care system (QSEN, 2020). A review of the literature related to addressing these gaps is rife with terms, concepts, and jargon (Table 9-1; Bauer et al., 2015; Nilsen, 2015). The focus of this chapter is to discuss how health care providers can apply improvement science to lead change initiatives in practice.

A PHILOSOPHICAL PERSPECTIVE ON IMPROVING HEALTH CARE

"There are more things in heaven and earth, Horatio, than are dreamt your philosophy."—
Hamlet (Shakespeare, 1599/1992, 1.5.167-8)

Philosophy or "love of wisdom" is the rational investigation of truths related to being, knowledge, or conduct (dictionary.com). For clinicians, the abstract notions of philosophy often do not fit within the busy workflow of modern health care. However, despite our frantic pace and commitment to patient-centered care, we remain vexed by both new and old problems. Although solutions to these problems are unknown and the focus of ongoing research, many are well researched with best practice recommendations available. Unfortunately, the uptake of best practices into clinical practice can take up to 17 years (Morris et al., 2011). To close this gap, health care professionals must think differently about their practice. Just as Hamlet was conveying to Horatio, there are solutions to close these gaps; they just require new ways of thinking.

Two philosophical movements relevant to thinking differently about the quality and safety concerns in health care are logical positivism and postmodernism. Logical positivism is a philosophical movement started in the 1920s. Core tenets of the movement are based on the belief that only quantifiable and objective facts are relevant in our pursuit of understanding (Rodgers, 2018). This is in contrast with postmodernism, which was developed in the later part of the 20th century. The core tenets of postmodernism are based on the belief that truth is gained by understanding the individual viewpoint or experience (Rodgers, 2018).

These two movements are evident in efforts to transform health care, such as the Centers for Medicare & Medicaid Services (CMS) Hospital Compare website (www.medicare.gov/hospitalcompare/search.html?). Specifically, objective clinical outcomes and patient experience data collected via the Hospital Consumer Assessment of Healthcare Providers and Systems surveys are publicly reported for CMS participating hospitals. Similar examples are also provided by CMS for home care, skilled nursing facilities, and physician practices.

Considering these two philosophical movements, health care professionals are challenged to evaluate their practice using both quantifiable metrics and the experiences of patients, families, and colleagues. This careful analysis will undoubtedly reveal opportunities to change current practice. When evaluating these potential changes, it is important to remember that although all improvement is change, not all change is improvement (Institute of Healthcare Improvement [IHI], 2020). Health care professionals can use the tools, strategies, and insights from improvement science to discern which changes will be an improvement. In addition, tools and strategies from improvement science, such as the Plan-Do-Study-Act (PDSA) model and process flow mapping, can help health care professionals implement and sustain changes in their practice.

ENTER SCIENCE OF IMPROVEMENT: IMPLEMENTING AND SUSTAINING CHANGE IN HEALTH CARE

Granger (2018) noted the term *science of improvement* is often considered to be synonymous with quality improvement (QI). Although the science of improvement does encompass what has traditionally been thought of as QI (i.e., the use of data to drive process changes that add value [Perla et al., 2013]), the science of improvement encompasses a broader framework that consistently addresses three components. The three foundational questions that science of improvement seeks to address are (a) What is the goal? (b) Is the change an actual improvement? and (c) What can we change to see an improvement (Granger, 2018)? To help health care professionals address these questions, various theories, models, and frameworks have been developed, including the IHI model for improvement, the lean six sigma model, and Shewhart's theory of variation.

Grant and Osanloo (2014) described the use of models, theories, and frameworks as blueprints used to guide a research project. Although there are delineating features of models, theories, and frameworks, the definition, use, and application are often contraindicated in the literature. Nilsen (2015) noted theories encompass both descriptions and explanations of phenomenon. In contrast, Nilsen (2015) noted models and frameworks lack an explanation of phenomenon and provide only descriptions, often in the form of checklists related to aspects of proposed implementation. Despite the ambiguity and variation in the application of definitions, the blueprint analogy is consistent. Models, frameworks, and theories provide a blueprint for how health care professionals can design and create changes in their practice (Grant & Osanloo, 2014). They are essential to any improvement effort because they provide the foundation for identifying the clinical issue of focus and the methods for addressing the gap.

Irrespective of the model or framework used to implement change, all share similar underlying assumptions and common principles. For example, all leverage learning from small tests of change, require operational definitions, and focus on interprofessional collaboration. Learning from small tests of change is rooted in logical positivism because it requires data to draw conclusions (Rodgers, 2018).

Although common small test of change models such as PDSA cycles may lack the rigor of randomized controlled trials, they generate testable assertions and illuminate causal mechanisms in the system (Langley et al., 2009; Perla et al., 2013). From these assertions, health care professionals can determine if change is an improvement and if the goal was met (Granger, 2018; Perla et al., 2013).

Along with small tests of change, science of improvement work requires operational definitions. Operational definitions ensure health care professionals can communicate a shared understanding of their work (Perla et al., 2013). They are essential to establishing clear goals for improvement work. For example, concepts and adjectives such as "safe," "timely," and "good" generate misunderstandings between disciplines because each professional discipline defines these words with similar and different attributes. This impedes a team from working toward shared goals (Perla et al., 2013). By clearly articulating operational definitions, health care workers elevate discussions beyond opinions toward facts (Longest & Darr, 2019). For example, the establishment of an operational definition for safety being zero wrong-site surgeries makes it a fact that patients with wrong-site surgery are safety concerns.

The shared characteristic that science of improvement models rely on is interprofessional collaboration rooted in the concept of psychologism, which highlights the tendency to interpret events subjectively or exaggerate psychological factors (dictionary.com). Psychologism addresses an important gap in science of improvement work (Perla et al., 2013). Although formal ways of knowledge such as logic and philosophy can clearly describe objective standards, they do not provide insights into the often irrational human behaviors observed (Perla et al., 2013). For example, ethical standards and evidence-based guidelines support a best practice, but clinicians may not adopt the practice based on their rationalization that a practice does not fit in their unit, practice, or organizational culture. Science of improvement models and frameworks seek to address this paradox by implying both logic (what people should do) and psychology (what people do). This correlates with the common thread of interprofessional collaboration found across science of improvement models because innovation and learning are often facilitated by such collaborations (Perla et al., 2013).

THEORIES SUPPORTING SCIENCE OF IMPROVEMENT WORK

No discussion of the science of improvement would be complete without referencing the foundational work of W. Edward Deming. He, along with fellow science of improvement pioneers Kauro Ishikawa and Joseph Juran, developed fundamental frameworks in the automotive and manufacturing industries in the 1950s. These frameworks continue to guide health care improvement efforts today (Langley et al., 2009). Specifically, Deming's theory of profound knowledge provides the description and explanation needed to drive improvements within the health care system. The four key tenets are (a) an appreciation for the system, (b) understanding of variation, (c) theory of knowledge, and (d) psychology of change (Deming, 2000a).

The first tenet of Deming's theory of profound knowledge is systems thinking, which is rooted in the philosophical movement of logical positivism in that system thinking requires objective facts and data (Rodgers, 2018). As described by Senge (1990), systems thinking is the ability to understand the nonlinear connection of actions and reactions within a whole. This is contrasted by the linear mindset that "A" leads directly to "B" (Senge, 1990). Such linear thinking prevents health care professionals from realizing the delayed and sometimes detrimental impact of their interventions (Perla et al., 2013), and it is perpetuated by the unending use of numbered checklists. When considering these delayed impacts within health care systems, health care professionals must remember health care systems are open systems. As open systems, they can exchange information, products, and people within their environment and other systems (Perla et al., 2013).

The second tenet of Deming's theory of profound knowledge is understanding variation. This second tenet is also aligned with the philosophical movement of logical positivism because it seeks quantifiable data to draw understanding by applying Shewhart's theory of variation (Rodgers, 2018). One of the basic assumptions of Shewhart's theory of variation is that all systems produce variation (Nolan et al., 2016). Therefore, the challenge for health care professionals is to determine special cause from common cause variation (Nolan et al., 2016; Perla et al., 2013). Common cause variation is variation inherent in the system and is to be expected as a normal function of the inputs for the system. For example, because of traffic, it might take between 10 and 15 minutes to get to work each morning. A travel time of 11 minutes one day and 14 minutes the next day is to be expected. The common cause variation implies the system is stable and outcomes from the system are predictable. Although predictable, the outcomes may not meet the desired expectations (Nolan et al., 2016) and therefore warrant change.

Special cause variation is related to specific circumstances that are not part of the system's normal function (Nolan et al., 2016). Building on our commute time example, special cause variation could be road construction or a snowstorm. Either of these could extend the commute time beyond the 15-minute upper limit of the system. By identifying and addressing special cause variation, health care professionals can focus their efforts on circumstances influencing system performance (Nolan et al., 2016). The measurement of data over time in the form of run charts and/or control charts allows health care professionals to identify and address special cause variation and evaluate the impact of interventions (PDSA cycles) on system performance. For example, in our example of commute time, we could implement a new route or transportation mode. After several days of data collection, we could determine if the system had improved or not by evaluating the average commute time after our route change.

The third tenet of Deming's theory of profound knowledge is theory of knowledge. This tenet can be thought of as the following question: How do we know what we know? As with the previous tenets of Deming's theory, this one is aligned with logical positivism and the need for objective facts. Objective facts help avoid confirmation bias, which is a major barrier to improvement work. Confirmation bias is exemplified in the inclination to seek out information that validates preconceptions (Hunter, 2011).

Several QI tools are available to help health care professionals avoid confirmation bias. For example, process flow mapping allows health care professionals to compare the actual workflow with the ideal or assumed workflow (Roehrs, 2018). Along with process flow maps, the use of small test of change, such as the PDSA cycle, is a powerful tool that provides objective data and tests theory (Roehrs, 2018). The PDSA cycle provides a structured format to predict how a change might impact the system, make a change within a system, and monitor the outcomes (Roehrs, 2018). Deming argued that improvement required the ability to predict outcomes, and theory was prerequisite for any predictions. Therefore, these iterative PDSA cycles are the foundation of Deming's theory of knowledge (Roehrs, 2018).

The fourth and final tenet of Deming's theory of profound knowledge is the psychology of change. Unlike the previous tenets, the psychology of change tenet draws from the postmodernism movement in that change is an individualized experience that sometimes does not follow logical or data-driven algorithms (Kotter, 1995). To facilitate change within the system, Deming advocated for the development of leaders (Deming, 2000a). Leadership is essential to improvement work as leaders focus on quality by "remove[ing] the causes of failure: to help people to do a better job with less effort" (Deming, 2000b). By focusing on quality, leaders create a space where workers discover the pride of their chosen craft (Bowen & Neuhauser, 2013).

Although little is written to distinguish change management from change leadership, the differences are profound. Change management focuses on the tools and structures in the process of change and incorporates the steps and actions found in a project plan or protocol. Contrast this with change leadership that centers on the people side of change and the ability to influence, inspire, and accelerate change based on a keen awareness of the change schemas in an organization and how leaders demonstrate commitment, a compelling vision, and reinforcement of their belief in the work through their actions. Change leaders acknowledge the impact and importance of relationships and are aware of strengths and performance gaps that may exist (Hechanova et al., 2018). Deming

(2000b) was cognizant of the role of leaders in developing the culture and work environments and promoted this as a strategic lever to promulgate successful change. Although steps in a process may delineate how to accomplish work, it is the change leader that conveys confidence in team members through information, engagement, and support to design, implement, evaluate, and sustain change (Holten et al., 2020).

EXPLORING VARIOUS SCIENCE OF IMPROVEMENT MODELS AND FRAMEWORKS

With an understanding of some of the common principles and assumptions shared across the various improvement science models and frameworks, it is easier to analyze specific ones. Focusing on the application of the IHI model for improvement provides an in-depth discussion and exemplar. The IHI model for improvement, the Donabedian model, and a brief introduction to the lean six sigma model are provided. The chapter concludes with a discussion intended to differentiate implementation science (IS) from improvement science (Table 9-2).

Institute for Healthcare Improvement Model for Improvement

The IHI model is a framework for expediting improvement (IHI, 2020). Langley et al. (2009) described the model as a tool to address fundamental questions of improvement work that include addressing why a change is needed, obtaining feedback related to change, and knowing when to disseminate the change. The model incorporates three fundamental questions and the use of iterative PDSA cycles to gather information, evaluate the change intervention, and guide future interventions to accomplish improvement. A visual depiction of this model can be found at the IHI Open School (http://www.ihi.org/resources/Pages/HowtoImprove/ScienceofImprovementHowtoImprove.aspx; IHI, 2020). The three fundamental questions outlined by the model are (a) What are we trying to accomplish? (b) How will we know that change is an improvement? and (c) What change can we make that will result in improvement? (Langley et al., 2009, p. 24). To address these questions, the model uses iterative PDSA cycles as small tests of change (Table 9-3).

Plan-Do-Study-Act

Plan

The PDSA process begins with planning. Planning should include clear objectives (Langley et al., 2009; Moen & Norman, 2010). Both internal data and external data should be used to frame the objectives and make the case for why a change is needed (Kotter, 1995). Internal data might include unit performance metrics or observations made during process flow mapping. External data may include external benchmarks or published best practices. After developing clear goals and objectives, an aim statement should be created to succinctly summarize the team purpose. Aim statements are time-bound explicit objective goals for the team. They include specific details such as what is being accomplished, stakeholders, and the time the goal is expected to be completed (National Institute for Children's Health Quality, n.d.). For example, a team tasked to reduce falls might have the following aim statement: Unit X will see a 30% reduction in patient falls/1000 patient days by June 30th.

In addition to clearly defined aim statements, the planning phase should include a detailed timeline with clearly delimited prescribed roles and responsibilities (Moen & Norman, 2010). Planning may include creating a formal team charter, identifying key stakeholders, and collecting

TABLE **9-2**

Common Tools for Quality Improvement Work

TOOL	APPLICATION	COMMENTS
Process flow maps	A graphic representation of actions that define a process	Use for identifying gaps between current state and future state Use to plan interventions
Control charts	Differentiation of common cause vs. special cause variation	Includes upper and lower control limits to identify special cause variation
Run charts	Differentiation of common cause vs. special cause variation	Use to monitor data over time
Failure mode and effect analysis	Standardized tool to identify and quantify the impact of potential problems within the system	Use proactively during design of new intervention or process
Fishbone diagram/ Ishikawa diagram/ cause and effect diagram	Assists with organizing knowledge related to current understanding of causes for variation within the system	Often organized as how people, equipment, procedures, measurements, and materials impact observed outcome

Adapted from Langley, G. L., Moen, R., Nolan, K. M., Nolan, T. W., Norman, C. L., & Provost, L. P. (2009). *The improvement guide: A practical approach to enhancing organizational performance* (2nd ed.). Jossey-Bass Publishers and Langley et al. 2009; and Provost, M., & Murray, S. R. (2011). *The healthcare data guide: Learning from data for improvement.* Jossey-Bass Publishers.

TABLE **9-3**

Plan-Do-Study-Act Questions and Action Items

Plan	Aim statement
	Literature review—How did literature review change your aim statement?
	Plan
	  • Target population/number of participants for first PDSA
	  • Metrics—what will you measure? How will you obtain the metrics?
	  • What are the sequential steps needed to reach goal?
	  • Barriers—how will they be addressed?
	  • Timeline for project with milestones

Do	What barriers/challenges were encountered? What successes need to be celebrated?
Study	Compare outcome metrics to prediction To whom and how are these results reported
Act	Adopt, adapt, abandon

relevant internal and external data. Along with these activities, the planning phase must address how the team will use data. Specifically, the team must have a clearly defined process for identifying, collecting, and analyzing data to determine if a change occurred and if the change is an improvement (Langley et al., 2009).

Do

The do phase is the execution of the plan. As a small test of change, the do phase provides the health care professionals with valuable data related to what worked well and what did not work as planned. This information adds to a deeper understanding of the system and the ability to make informed predictions for future PDSA cycles (Perla et al., 2013). Although the actual intervention of the do phase is based on knowledge of the respective system, Powell et al. (2015) published a compilation of implementation strategies geared to help health care professionals implement changes. Their compilation included 73 discreet strategies covering a wide variety of tactics ranging from education and funding to policy changes (Powell et al., 2015). This work highlights the need to use multiple implementation strategies to ensure a planned change is effective.

Study

The study phase is the crux of Deming's theory of knowledge—how do we know what we know. During this phase, the data collected are analyzed and compared with the predictions made in the planning phase. Here careful attention should be paid to avoid confirmation bias, noting common and special cause variation aid in the analysis to guide decision making. A summary of what is learned should be created and used to inform the next iteration of the PDSA cycles (Moen & Norman, 2010).

Act

The act phase provides an opportunity to make course corrections before implementing the next PDSA cycle. Based on the "study" of data collected, the improvement team can choose to adopt, adapt, or abandon their PDSA experiment (Deming, 2000a). Adoption of the change would occur if the results matched the prediction of the planning phase, whereas adaption would occur if changes were needed to the intervention to meet the stated goals and objectives of the change. Finally, a change might be abandoned if the outcomes were detrimental to the system. The key to the act phase is to ensure rational actions are based on what was learned from the PDSA cycle and the data that were gathered (Langley et al., 2009).

Donabedian Model

Although the IHI model for improvement is a robust model to aid in the acceleration of improvement work, other models such as the Donabedian quality model and the lean six sigma model provide additional insights and frames to help improve care. The Donabedian quality model is composed of three core components: structure, process, and outcomes. These components provide a framework for evaluating the quality of health care and planning improvement initiatives. Specifically, the framework lends to the development of robust project metrics. As discussed earlier, clearly defined operational definitions are a prerequisite for science of improvement work. Before implementing a QI project, careful consideration should be given to the outcome, process, and balancing metrics that will be used to determine if the change has occurred and if the change was an improvement (Donabedian, 2005).

For example, a QI project aimed to reduce falls might include the following metrics: an outcome metric of actual falls per 1000 patient days. As an outcome metric, this variable is mapped to the aim or purpose of the project—a process metric of the percentage of patients with documented fall risk assessments complete. As a process metric, this variable reflects the way the team provides care. Finally, a balancing metric of patient mobility would be collected. This balancing variable would ensure there were intended consequences of decreased mobility to decrease falls (National Health Services, n.d.).

The Donabedian model is found in nursing practice and recognition systems in the American Nurses Credentialing Center Magnet Designation and Baldrige Award (Schulingkamp & Latham, 2015). The process, structure, and outcomes guide the evaluation of practice and quality outcomes residing foundationally on the attributes of leaders, systems, empiric measurement of outcomes, innovation, and engagement of stakeholders.

Lean Six Sigma

Although often referenced together, lean and six sigma represent two distinct approaches to improving quality. Lean is focused on the reduction of waste from the system, whereas six sigma focuses on the reduction of defects (IHI, 2020; Omachonu, 2019; Van den Heuvel et al., 2006). The eight distinct categories of waste targeted by lean are defects, excessive processing, overproduction, transportation, waiting, inventory, motion, and underutilization of personnel skill (Quality One International, 2020). The driving force for any waste reduction efforts is the customer or "voice of the customer" because they determine the value of the services and products being offered. Therefore, the purpose of lean is to maximize "value added time" (the need to include a form or feature needed for the customer to be satisfied) within the system. Examples of the application of lean in health care include just-in-time inventory and streamlining of workflows to gain efficiency.

In contrast to focusing on the elimination of waste, six sigma seeks to eliminate defects within the system. By focusing on the elimination of variation, six sigma seeks to ensure the system consistently generates acceptable results (Van den Heuvel et al., 2006). Six sigma's naming conventions are taken from the Greek symbol sigma, which denotes spread or variation. From a normal distribution curve, six sigma (six standard deviations) would correspond to a 99.99966% yield that system outputs would be free of defects. To achieve six sigma performance, a five-phase approach is used. The five phases are define, measure, analyze, improve, and control and are referred to as the *DMAIC process* (Jones et al., 2010; Omachonu, 2019).

Lean and six sigma methodologies are often used in conjunction to maximize results. A review of the DMAIC model highlights how the model evolved from the PDSA cycles outlined in the IHI model for improvement. This evolution has created a model that tends to be more quantitative than the traditional PDSA model. However, the model remains true to the tenets of Deming's theory of profound knowledge.

IMPLEMENTATION SCIENCE

The preceding discussion focused on the science of improvement, specifically how processes of care can be improved to create safe, timely, effective, efficient, equitable, and patient-centered health care (Granger, 2018). As health care professionals work to change processes, they must also seek to understand methods that promote and sustain the integration of evidence-based practices. Granger (2018) defined the study of these methods as IS. IS seeks to expand our knowledge of how to address barriers by expanding our theories and models to better translate evidence into practice

(Granger, 2018). Areas of focus for IS include root cause analysis for the barriers associated with the implementation of best practices, multisite studies aimed at showing the effectiveness of specific implementation strategies, and the addition of qualitative research designs to add context to implementation initiatives (Granger, 2018).

Conclusion

The challenges of today's health care environment require system changes. The science of improvement provides insights and tools to help health care professionals redesign their work environments. By using a data-driven, systematic approach, health care professionals can maximize their efforts to implement change. This chapter provided a broad overview of various theories, models, and frameworks used to implement change in health care.

As lifelong learners, health care professionals must commit to continue their study and proficiency in these concepts. Recommendations for further study include the IHI Open School. The IHI Open School is a free online training platform designed to equip interprofessional teams with the knowledge, skills, and attitudes needed to improve health care (IHI, 2000). In addition to IHI, the QSEN initiative aims to prepare future nurses with the knowledge, skills, and attitudes needed to continuously improve the quality and safety in their practice setting. QSEN provides a wealth of resources and teaching strategies applicable across disciplines (www.qsen.org). Finally, the MoreSteam (n.d.) toolbox provides a comprehensive set of tools and resources for QI work (www.moresteam.com).

Reflective Questions

1. Describe two improvement models, comparing their major constructs and how each model is applicable to change management.
2. Outline the principal tenets of lean six sigma, identifying implications for QI and waste reduction.
3. Compare improvement and implementation sciences and how they complement each other.

References

Agency for Healthcare Research and Quality. (2018). Six domains of health care quality. https://www.ahrq.gov/talkingquality/measures/six-domains.html

Bauer, M., Damschroder, L., Hagedorn, H., Smith, J., & Kilbourne, A. (2015). An introduction to implementation science for the non-specialist. *BMC Psychology, 3*, 32. https://doi.org/10.1186/s40359-015-0089-9

Bowen, M. E., & Neuhauser, D. (2013). Understanding and managing variation: Three different perspectives. *Implementation Science, 8*, S1. https://doi.org/10.1186/1748-5908-8-S1-S1

Centers for Medicare & Medicaid Services. (2020). Hospital compare. https://www.medicare.gov/hospitalcompare/About/What-Is-HOS.html

Dictionary.com (2021). Philosophy. https://www.dictionary.com/browse/philosophy

Dictionary.com (2021). Psychologism. https://www.dictionary.com/browse/psychologism

Deming, W. E. (2000a). *The new economics for industry, government edition* (2nd ed.). The MIT Press.

Deming, W. E. (2000b). *Out of the crisis* (1st ed.). The MIT Press.

Donabedian, A. (2005). Evaluating the quality of medical care. *The Milbank Quarterly, 83*(4), 691-729. https://doi.org/10.1111/j.1468-0009.2005.00397.x

Granger, B. B. (2018). Science of improvement versus science of implementation: Integrating both into clinical inquiry. *AACN Advanced Critical Care, 29*(2), 208-212. https://doi.org/10.4037/aacnacc2018757

Grant, C., & Osanloo, A. (2014). Conducting, selecting and integrating a theoretical framework in dissertation research: Creating the blueprint for your "house". *Administrative Issues Journal: Connecting Education. Practice and Research, 4*(2), 12-26.

Hechanova, M., Caringal-Go, J., Felice, J., & Magsaysay, J. (2018). Implicit change leadership, change management, and affective commitment to change comparing academic institutions vs business enterprises. *Leadership & Organization Development Journal, 39*(7), 914-925. https:/doi.org/o.1108/LODJ-01-2018-0013

Holten, A., Hancock, G., & Bollingtoft, A. (2020). Studying the importance of change leadership and change management in layoffs, mergers, and closures. *Management Decision, 58*(3), 393-409. https:/doi.org/10.1108/MD-03-2017-0278

Hunter, J. (2011). How do we know what we know? Deming's SoPK part IV. https://www.processexcellencenetwork.com/lean-six-sigma-business-performance/columns/an-introduction-to-deming-s-theory-of-knowledge-on

Institute of Healthcare Improvement. (2020). Open School. http://www.ihi.org/education/IHIOpenSchool/Pages/default.aspx

Institute of Medicine. (2000). *To err is human: Building a safer health system.* National Academy Press.

Institute of Medicine. (2001). *Crossing the quality chasm: A new health system for the 21st century.* National Academy Press.

Institute of Medicine. (2003a). *Health professions education: A bridge to quality.* National Academies Press.

Institute of Medicine. (2003b). *Patient safety: Achieving a new standard for care.* National Academies Press.

Jones, E., Riley, M., & Battieste, T. (2010). The value of industrial engineers in lean six sigma organizations. IIE Annual Conference. https://pdfs.semanticscholar.org/e393/c86f5541a2e1177dd53be108a85cc6f63b9a.pdf

Kotter, J. (1995). Leading change: Why transformation efforts fail. *Harvard Business Review.* https://hbr.org/1995/05/leading-change-why-transformation-efforts-fail-2

Langley, G. L., Moen, R., Nolan, K. M., Nolan, T. W., Norman, C. L., & Provost, L. P. (2009). *The improvement guide: A practical approach to enhancing organizational performance* (2nd ed.). Jossey-Bass Publishers.

Longest, B., Darr, K. (2019). Managerial problem solving and decision making. *Managing health services organizations and systems* (pp. 293-324). Healthcare Professional Press.

Moen, R. D., & Norman, C. L. (2010). Circling back: Clearing up myths about the Deming cycle and seeing how it is evolving. http://www.apiweb.org/circling-back.pdf

MoreSteam. (n.d.). Process improvement & lean six sigma tools. https://www.moresteam.com/toolbox/

Morris, Z., Wooding, S., & Grant, J. (2011). The answer is 17 years, what is the question: Understanding time lags in translational research. *Journal of the Royal Society of Medicine, 104*(12), 510-520.

National Health Services. (n.d.). ACT Academy. Online library of quality, service improvement and redesign tools: A model for measuring quality care. https://improvement.nhs.uk/documents/2135/measuring-quality-care-model.pdf

National Institute for Children's Health Quality. (n.d.). QI tips: A formula for developing a great aim statement. https://www.nichq.org/insight/qi-tips-formula-developing-great-aim-statement

Nilsen, P. (2015). Making sense of implementation theories, models, and frameworks. *Implementation Science, 10,* 53. https://doi.org/10.1186/s13012-015-0242-0

Nolan, T., Perla, R. J., & Provost, L. (2016). Understanding variation. *Quality Progress, 49*(11), 28-37.

Omachonu, V. (2019). *Healthcare value proposition: Creating a culture of excellence in patient experience.* Routledge Productivity Press, Taylor & Francis Group.

Perla, R. J., Provost, L. P., & Parry, G. J. (2013). Seven propositions of the science of improvement: exploring foundations. *Quality Management in Healthcare, 22*(3), 170-186.

Powell, B. J., Waltz, T. J., Chinman, M. J., Damschroder, L. J., Smith, J. L., Matthieu, M. M., Proctor, E. K., & Kirchner, J. E. (2015). A refined compilation of implementation strategies: Results from the expert recommendations for implementing change (ERIC) project. *Implementation Science, 10,* 21. https://doi.org/10.1186/s13012-015-0209-1

Provost, M., & Murray, S. R. (2011). The healthcare data guide: Learning from data for improvement. Jossey-Bass Publishers.

Quality and Safety Education for Nurses. (2020). www.qsen.org

Quality One International. (2020). https://quality-one.com/lean/

Rodgers, B. L. (2018). The evolution of nursing science. In J. B. Butts & K. L. Rich (Eds.), *Philosophies and theories for advanced nursing practice* (3rd ed., pp. 19-53). Jones and Bartlett Learning.

Roehrs, S. (2018). Building of profound knowledge. *Current Problems in Pediatric Adolescent Health Care, 48*(8), 196-197. https://doi.org/10.1016/j.cppeds.2018.08.013

Schulingkamp, R., & Latham, J. (2015). Healthcare performance excellence: A comparison of Baldrige Award recipients and competitors. *The Quality Management Journal, 22*(3), 6-22.

Senge, P. (1990). *The fifth discipline: The age and practice of the learning organization.* Currency Doubleday.

Shakespeare, W. (1992). *Hamlet.* C. Watts & K. Carbine (Eds.). Wordsworth Editions. (Original work published 1599)

Van den Heuvel, J., Does, R. J. M. M, & de Koning, H. (2006). Lean six sigma in a hospital. *International Journal of Six Sigma and Competitive Advantage, 2*(4), 377-388.

Exemplar 9-1

APPLICATION OF RUN AND CONTROL CHARTS

David H. James, DNP, MSHQS, RN, CCNS, NPD-BC

Run charts and control charts are powerful data analysis tools commonly used in QI initiatives. Although there are a wealth of books and other resources dedicated to the understanding and application of the statistical rules governing these charts, the purpose of this exemplar is to provide a foundational/basic overview of application. This exemplar highlights how run and control charts can be used to determine special cause variation within a system. For this exemplar, a case study of 30 glucose measurements taken over the course of 2 weeks is discussed (Figure 9-1). For the purpose of this example, a normal blood glucose is between 70 and 130 mg/dL.

DATA OVER TIME

Data collected over time provide insights into how well the system is performing and allow for predictions of future performance. Often data are presented as a "snapshot" in time. For example, the average wait time in the clinic is 20 minutes today. Although this information is valuable, it lacks the context for designing any meaningful innovations. Is today "normal"? Are there variations in wait times during the day, week, or time of month? By collecting and analyzing data over time, additional context and insights can be gained. These allow for the development and evaluation of small tests of change that are the foundation of improvement work.

CHANCE: COIN-FLIPPING ANALOGY

The role of chance in determining a coin toss (heads vs. tails) is one analogy for understanding how to distinguish special cause from common cause variation. For the analysis of the run chart, you need to first establish the mean of the data set. With the mean of the data set marked, you next examine how the data are organized around the mean. How many data points fall above or below the mean? This is where the coin-tossing analogy can be helpful. The determination of heads or tails on a coin toss is purely by chance (i.e., random). Therefore, any patterns in the number of heads vs. tails are attributed to common cause variation. For example, if I flip a coin 30 consecutive times, it is possible to have two or three "heads" in a row followed by two or three "tails" in a row. However, flipping 12 consecutive "heads" would fall outside the probability of chance and would indicate special cause variation. For example, perhaps a double-sided heads coin was substituted during the coin toss.

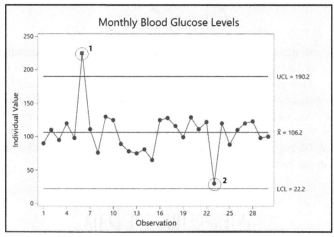

Figure 9-1. Blood glucose levels.

TABLE 9-4		

Tests Identifying Special Cause Variation

TEST	DESCRIPTION	NUMBER POINTS INDICATING SPECIAL CAUSE*
Nonrandom pattern	Too few or too many runs	< 11 runs > 21 runs
Shift	Too many points in a run on the same side of mean	> 8 data points
Trend	Too many points moving in the same direction (may cross the median)	> 5 data points
Astronomical data point	A data point strikingly above or below the median	Subjective assessment of data point
*Note the number of points indicating signals from the system is based on a data set of 30.		

RULES SIGNALING A POSSIBLE SPECIAL CAUSE VARIATION

Data plotted over time on a run chart will demonstrate similar patterns. There should be clear variation along the mean of the data set, with some data points falling above and some falling below the established mean. Just as with our coin toss example, a few consecutive data points above the mean and a few consecutive data points below the mean are to be expected. Therefore, the question becomes how to differentiate these expected common cause variations from special cause variation. There are four tests that are applied to run charts that indicate signals of possible special cause variation. Although more elaborate statistical analysis is needed to determine if the signals indicate special cause variation, they do provide insights into the system performance. Signals from the system can be interpreted using the four classic rules (Table 9-4). A minimum of 15 data points is needed to identify signals in the system. The more data the more reliable the determination is. Statisticians have developed tables describing a specific number of values needed to determine special cause variation based on the number of observed data points (Nolan et al., 2016; Provost & Murray, 2011).

Control Charts

Data with only common cause variation follow a normal bell curve distribution. Control charts add additional rigor to the analysis of data by providing upper and lower control limits based on the standard deviations of normally distributed data. By establishing the upper and lower control limits at ±3 standard deviations, any data points falling outside the control limits would most likely be due to special cause variation. Because 99.7% of observed data from a stable system should fall within ±3 standard deviations, there is only a 0.3% chance that the outside the limits is due to common cause variation (Provost & Murray, 2011). Figure 9-1 highlights special cause variation with data points falling outside the upper control limit.

Interpreting the Data

Two questions must be addressed when analyzing either a run or control chart. The first is to determine if the data are stable/predictable. If there is no special cause variation noted, then the system is deemed stable. Therefore, it can be assumed that unless changes are made, data from future observations will mirror the data observed. Special cause variation can negatively or positively affect the system. If special cause variation is evident, an investigation is warranted to determine the root cause(s) for the variation. The second question is to determine if the system is capable. Does the current performance as indicated by the observed data meet the customer's needs? If not, what changes need to be made to improve the process? These questions are driving forces for various science of improvement models, such as the lean six sigma or the IHI model for improvement.

Interpretation

Based on the data collected, we can expect future glucose levels to have an average measurement of 106.2 mg/dl. However, they will range between 22.2 and 190 mg/dl. This process does not meet customer needs because glucose levels below 60 mg/dl are dangerous. We note that one observation is above the upper control limit and indicates special cause variation. We also note that one observation is very low and clinically concerning even if it does not trigger special cause variation by falling below the lower control limit.

References

Nolan, T., Perla, R. J., & Provost, L. (2016). Understanding variation. *Quality Progress, 49*(11), 28-37.

Provost, M., & Murray, S. R. (2011). *The healthcare data guide: Learning from data for improvement.* Jossey-Bass.

Exemplar 9-2

APPLICATION OF QUALITY IMPROVEMENT CONCEPTS: COIN-SPINNING EXERCISE

David H. James, DNP, MSHQS, RN, CCNS, NPD-BC

Marti Rice, PhD, RN, FAAN

This chapter presented key concepts in the science of improvement, specifically the use of the IHI model for improvement. Although a review of concepts and definitions can be beneficial, the goal of this exemplar is to provide an example that explicates steps and processes for praxis. In alignment with this goal, what follows is an assignment to help students apply QI concepts to a "real-world" situation. This exercise was adapted from the IHI "QI Games: Learn How to Use PDSA Cycles by Spinning Coins" available at www.ihi.org (Lewis, n.d.). We encourage you to review the instructions and materials developed by the IHI along with the instructions and materials for this modified version.

THE SCENARIO

You are officers in the Tiddley Winks Coin Spinning Company and have been tasked to improve the coin-spinning time of the company's product tiddley wink coins. Currently, the coins spin for 2 to 3 seconds. Your task is to improve the coin-spinning time to at least 10 seconds so that the Tiddley Winks Coin Spinning Company can be competitive in the marketplace. You are required to test at least four PDSA cycles with a minimum of six spins each cycle and plot the data as a run chart(s). You are to record your work in a Microsoft PowerPoint slide presentation that will be shared with the board of the company.

STEPS TO COMPLETE THIS ASSIGNMENT

You will need to identify three to four friends or family members who can serve on your team. An alternative approach for the assignment is for faculty to place students in groups. Once your team has been identified, you will need to plan a team meeting to complete the activity. Team members should plan to spend 1 to 2 hours on the activity. At the meeting, choose a leader, designate responsibilities of the team members (timekeeper, spinner, etc.), and plan for at least four cycles (a minimum of four coins, three surfaces, a minimum of two spinners, and one other variable/condition of the team's choosing) and a minimum of six spins per cycle. For each cycle, you will need to include one variable and keep other areas the same. For example, you might start the first cycle with all the spinners, all spinners use a quarter, and all spinners spinning on a glass surface. The spinners are varied, the coin is a constant, and the surface is a constant. It is recommended that you do a "dry run" of the coin-spinning activity by yourself before engaging with your team. This will ensure you understand the process and have the necessary equipment.

TABLE 9-5

Outline for Coin-Spinning Presentation

FOCUS OF SLIDES	RECOMMENDED NUMBER OF SLIDES
Introduction • Aim statement, description of team	Two to three slides
Methods • Use of the Institute of Healthcare Improvement model for improvement • Plan-Do-Study-Act cycles • Application of midrange theory	Two to four slides
Results • Graphically display run chart from data collected during Plan-Do-Study-Act	One to two slides
Discussion • What do these results tell you? Was your aim met? • How did the application of the theory/model guide the project? (This may need to be in sentences vs. bullet points) • Limitations, lessons learned	Two to three slides
Conclusion • Abandon, adapt, or adopt • Based on results what will you do?	One to two slides

You will use the IHI model for improvement to complete this activity. In addition, the activity will require an analysis of data to determine the presence of signals (special cause variation). Your team will need to create a clear aim statement and address the three guiding questions from the IHI model for improvement: (a) What are we trying to accomplish? (b) How will we know a change is an improvement? and (c) What change can we make that will result in an improvement? (Langley et al., 2009).

After this discussion, you will need to define your data collection process. Once you complete your PDSA cycles, you will need to create a run chart or charts to analyze your data. Although control charts provide more robust analysis, run charts are easily made with the Microsoft Excel program and allow for the identification of signals in the data.

In addition to the IHI model for improvement, students are asked to apply a midrange theory to support their coin-spinning project. Such theories provide additional insights into how to implement and sustain improvement work. Although any number of theories can be applied, we recommend using a change theory or model. Such a model aligns well with Deming's theory of profound knowledge because it addresses the psychology of change tenet of Deming's theory (Deming, 2000).

The final step of the activity is to create a Microsoft PowerPoint presentation describing the QI process. Although you will not be formally submitting your presentation, creating a presentation to share with your team gives you an opportunity to practice your presentation skills and to organize the information. We recommend the following guidelines for the presentation. First, keep the presentation brief with approximately 12 to 15 slides. Ensure the presentation is well organized and uses appropriate font size and graphics (Table 9-5).

REFERENCES

Deming, W. E. (2000). *The new economics for industry, government edition* (2nd ed.). The MIT Press.

Langley, G. L., Moen, R., Nolan, K. M., Nolan, T. W., Norman, C. L., & Provost, L. P. (2009). *The improvement guide: A practical approach to enhancing organizational performance* (2nd ed.). Jossey-Bass Publishers.

Lewis, N. (n.d.). QI games: Learn how to use PDSA cycles by spinning coins. http://www.ihi.org/education/IHIOpenSchool/resources/Pages/AudioandVideo/QI-Games-Learn-How-to-Use-PDSA-Cycles-by-Spinning-Coins.aspx

INNOVATION AND TRANSLATION
Next Steps in Advancing Health Care
Through Implementation Science

Kristen Noles, DNP, RN, CNL, LSSGB
Rebekah Barber, BSN, MSN, DNP
Christina Fortugno, MSHA, MBA, BSN, RN, CCRN
Linda A. Roussel, PhD, RN, NEA-BC, CNL, FAAN
Patricia L. Thomas, PhD, RN, FAAN, FACHE, FNAP, NEA-BC, ACNS-BC, CNL

CHAPTER OBJECTIVES

- Outline the alignment of innovation and implementation science that brings health care to the next level of improvement
- Describe curiosity and inquiry and implication for state-of-the-art improvement
- Outline implementation and dissemination sciences and their impacts on population health and achieving the quadruple aim
- Describe innovation and the "next big idea" for improvement and sustainability through the exemplar models

Roussel, L. A., & Thomas, P. L. (Eds.). *Implementation Science in Nursing:*
A Framework for Education and Practice (pp. 163-176).
© 2022 Taylor & Francis Group.

KEY WORDS

- Accountable care
- Chronic care model
- Dissemination
- Frontline engagement

- Implementation science
- Innovation
- Inquiry

Innovation in health care is aimed to create or enhance existing resources that improve patient safety, timeliness of care, efficiency, and effectiveness with the patient always as the focal point (Institute for Healthcare Improvement [IHI], 2019). Innovation can be either disruptive, causing quick drastic changes, or iterative, progressing more gradually toward change. For decades, innovation has been the hallmark of American health care. Being curious and innovative must continue to be the driving forces of our country's health care system to enable us to conquer the unique and sustained challenges of achieving better patient outcomes, controlling costs, and coordinating and managing chronic diseases.

The science of improvement includes innovation, rapid cycle testing, and dissemination to generate an understanding about what changes produce improvements (IHI, 2019). The goal of improvement science is to ensure that improvement efforts are based on supportive evidence and best practices planned for implementation (Shojania & Grimshaw, 2005). Innovation and creativity greatly support enhanced nursing practice. Innovation is the essential component of nursing practice that permits response and adaptation to the variation presented in health care delivery (Rundio et al., 2016). To successfully implement changes at the point of care, a nurturing environment, the ability to function independently, and a willingness to take risks are all warranted (Fasnacht, 2003).

Frontline staff routinely identify needs for improvement and create "work-arounds" to complete physician orders, manage with less-than-optimal resources, and invent better ways to complete tasks needed for patient care. These work-arounds can be considered innovations, and, although clinicians' intentions are to do what is right, working around the current systems can put the patient at greater risk for an adverse event (Halbesleben et al., 2008). Some work-arounds prove to be better than current practice; however, the need for change is usually silenced, limiting diffusion. Rogers (2003) defined diffusion as the process in which innovation is communicated through certain channels by progression of the innovation among the members of a system. When there is a lack of communication about these work-arounds, health care leaders remain blinded to the reality of the challenges in current practice. Additionally, the underlying problems are not investigated; therefore, the underlying cause is never addressed. This creates an unsafe culture, putting the system at risk and increasing the chance for patient harm in an already risky setting. The message here is that innovation must be balanced with effective and safe care delivery. This is a challenge, particularly in fragmented and chaotic health care systems.

TRUST AND DIVERSITY: REQUISITES FOR FOSTERING INNOVATION

To foster innovation within organizations, health care leaders do not have to be innovators themselves; however, they need to create an innovative culture for frontline staff. One way to create this type of culture is by establishing trust with those working at the point of care. Cultivating a trusting relationship will facilitate the generation of new ideas, continual identification of problems, and engagement of the frontline staff to iteratively improve. In addition to a trust culture, it is also imperative to create a diverse team to enhance new patterns of thinking and decision making through the lens of multiple perspectives. Diversity coupled with the establishment of trust enhances overall innovation development, and fostering and supporting this type of culture aids in meeting the competing demands of regulatory, reimbursement, and safety requirements and everyone's care needs (Rundio et al., 2016).

Operationalizing innovations requires that efforts take place within a framework to closely evaluate outcomes and impact (Rundio et al., 2016). However, many existing care frameworks do not allow for the required level of engagement of frontline staff within their microsystems that is necessary to achieve innovative solutions to existing care delivery problems. Aligning existing care frameworks to focus efforts for rigorous improvement and implementation from the point of care will create a unified driving force to achieve optimal organizational outcomes.

Redesigning for Innovation

Redesigning health care to provide an infrastructure for innovation, rapid cycle improvement, and application of evidence-based implementation strategies is needed. Shifting from an individual focus to an environment of care focus where individuals develop relationships, both seek and openly provide feedback, and gain insight from experiences is imperative for survival in this chaotic health care environment (Malloch & Porter-O'Grady, 2010). This transforms individual inquiry to collective creativity and innovation. If value-added team innovation is to be realized to the fullest potential, the environment must be shaped for teamwork and supported by leadership. Two redesign models that demonstrate this are highlighted: the accountable care team (ACT) model and the clinical nurse leader (CNL) implementation model at the microsystem level.

Accountable Care Team Model: Implications for Implementation

The ACT model was started in 2012 when the Indiana University of Health Methodist Hospital leadership team redesigned care in the inpatient setting, centering care around ACTs (Kara et al., 2015). These teams are created at the microsystem level with a dedicated set of providers who take ownership for achieving outcomes for their respective inpatient unit (Kara et al., 2015). This model consists of three foundational domains: enhancing interprofessional collaboration, driving decision making with data, and providing leadership.

The enhancement of interprofessional collaboration is facilitated by dedicating providers to the same unit for an extended period. This allows for feelings of ownership, inclusion, and impact to have meaning, fostering a sense of purpose within the providers facilitating oversight of care delivery. The provider is considered qualified and capable and, in turn, is expected to round on all patients daily with the assigned bedside nurse, which minimizes the time wasted in seeking out information regarding the patient throughout other work demands of the day.

Rounding, as an evidence-based implementation strategy, is followed by a team huddle that consists of a brief discussion of all patients' needs for a safe transition out of the hospital (Kara et al., 2015). In these huddles, the expected day of discharge is discussed, and a time is provided; the day of discharge is the driver to execute purposeful action among the team. No health care provider would debate the importance of the timing of medication administration, and the knowledge of an expected discharge target is equally as important. The goal is set for at least 80% of discharged patients to be out of the hospital by 1,200 hours, creating a sense of urgency among all members of the team to make it happen and promoting a team striving to "win." This creates comradery, ownership, accountability, transparency, and celebration among the team, thus fostering a model that drives improvement. Additionally, gamification and competition to surpass previous milestones can be powerful motivators in driving continuous improvement. The 80% of patients discharged by 1,200 hours also facilitates consistent follow-up for leadership to review patient and staff outliers not achieving the expressed goal. This serves to provide new foci for improvement efforts.

Data driving the team's decision making enable unit leadership to maintain focus and receive ongoing feedback. At monthly interdisciplinary meetings, key metrics are monitored, trends discussed, and contributing factors identified (Kara et al., 2015). It is important that all the metrics are agreed on and clearly defined before the redesign begins and that all appropriate baseline data are gathered for accurate comparison and measurement during implementation. Evidence-based implementation such as rounding and team huddles are used. Data collection methods may need to be designed and implemented in the planning phase. The unit physician and nurse leader conduct weekly patient rounding. These rounds are not scripted but do include open-ended questions to seek both positive and negative feedback about the patient experience, providing qualitative data along with quantitative metrics.

In the ACT model, the commitment of the unit-level leadership is vital to ensure success. Because of changes in daily work and responsibilities, unit leadership must be supported, coached, and mentored as the culture is transformed. Using the ACT framework to purposefully redesign culture allows for education, alignment, and dedicated support for all staff to facilitate improvement and innovation.

Implementation of the Clinical Nurse Leader: Implications for Implementation

Another approach to health care redesign is the strategic implementation of the CNL at the microsystem level. The profession of nursing is well positioned to lead interprofessional improvement initiatives because nurses regularly interact with members of all patient care disciplines and have the most direct contact with their patients (Institute of Medicine, 2011). In 2007, the American Association of Colleges of Nursing (AACN) partnered with organizational nurse executives and outlined the CNL role to be the innovators and change agents at the point-of-care delivery (AACN, 2013). CNLs strengthen nursing leadership at the point of care to improve patient safety while strengthening the quality and outcomes of the care delivered. The CNL is trained to assess the microsystem, identifying gaps that need to be addressed to align improvement efforts within the organization. Once the gaps are identified, the CNL is also proficient in improvement science, applying evidence-based implementation strategies to conduct iterative cycles of testing, achieve sustainable positive patient outcomes, and diffuse new ideas into clinical practice.

The CNL embraces and uses the constructs of a high reliability organization, evidence-based practice (EBP), and process excellence (Harris et al., 2018). The essential aspects of CNL practice are a microsystem or point-of-care focus and include the role of clinician, outcomes manager, client advocate, educator, systems analyst/risk anticipator, information manager, team manager, member of a profession, and lifelong learner (AACN, 2013; Harris et al., 2018). The CNL leads the interprofessional teams that assume accountability for improving quality and safety outcomes for a specified group (Hatley et al., 2019). The CNL also serves as the facilitator to prioritize improvement, innovation, and change for positive health care outcomes.

CNLs have been implemented into nursing care models across the country and have shown measurable outcomes in many areas, including improving throughput and reducing length of stay (LOS). Wilson et al. (2012) embedded CNLs into their inpatient care units, working alongside bedside nursing staff to improve inefficient processes. After CNL implementation, they were able to reduce overall LOS by 39%, postprocedure LOS by 67%, and recovery unit LOS by 42%, for a total estimated cost savings of 1.5 million dollars (Wilson et al., 2012). Improved throughput has also been shown by CNLs in the operating room (OR). A CNL-led team using lean methods at one hospital was able to increase on-time OR case starts from 12% to 89% (Fairbanks, 2007). At a separate hospital, a CNL student in the OR facilitated an interdisciplinary team to examine turnaround time opportunities and implemented improvements leading to a 57% reduction in avoidable cancellations and a 22.25-hour increase in OR room usage (Wesolowski et al., 2014).

Bedside nurses need support to optimize creative problem solving to find better ways to provide safe, quality care in a timely manner. CNLs are prepared to be efficient in creating teams, assessing microsystems, mapping processes, recognizing patterns, and identifying areas to improve (Noles et al., 2019). In one study, the perception of innovation competence was compared between CNLs and other nurse leaders. CNLs rated their highest competency as interdisciplinary teamwork and collaboration followed by tenacity and resilience. Nurse leaders also rated their highest competency as interdisciplinary teamwork and collaboration but at a lower mean than CNLs (Noles et al., 2019). Implementing CNL practice with demonstrable positive outcomes is an excellent example of the application of translational science.

Chronic Care Model Framework: Implications for Implementation

Another common framework for making health care improvements is the chronic care model (CCM) developed by Dr. Ed Wagner and colleagues at the MacColl Institute for Healthcare Innovation (Improving Chronic Illness Care, 2016). One hundred eight million people in the United States suffer from a chronic condition (Cumbie et al., 2004). Almost half have multiple chronic conditions. There is a need to improve the current management of diseases such as diabetes, heart disease, depression, asthma, and others (Agency for Healthcare Research and Quality, 2016). The CCM identifies six fundamental aspects that encourage high-quality chronic disease management: self-management support; delivery system design; decision support; clinical information systems; organization of health care community; and creating health systems that provide safe, quality care (Improving Chronic Illness Care, 2019). Health care is constantly changing, with patients and communities becoming more diversified and complex.

Using the CCM as a framework to redesign heath care simplifies the focus of interventional improvement of health care outcomes. The management of the whole is more attainable when standardization of care for disease management is proven. This allows treatment of the disease but also more thought and focus on the individual differences by the care team. Members creating focus around diseases allows for defined, evidence-based interventions to occur, resulting in predefined expected outcomes. This focus allows the care team to include the patient and use human-centered design to first gain empathy for the population's current needs, barriers, and treatment. Gaining empathy allows the patient's voice to be heard and allows for compassionate problem solving to occur.

The CCM framework can better focus improvement efforts to other commonalities of specific populations. The number of adults older than 65 years of age is growing quickly (IHI, 2021). Older adults with multiple chronic conditions are the largest users of health care (Bynum et al., 2016; Parekh et al., 2011). Medicare beneficiaries with two or more chronic conditions account for 86% of Part A Medicare payments (Erdem et al., 2013). Care for these patients is fragmented because primary care clinicians work to coordinate care with multiple physicians that they may or may not know (Pham et al., 2009). To reduce fragmentation, it is ideal to have a smaller network of clinicians and for only one clinician to own the overall coordination of care to optimize the quality of life for the patient. The Age-Friendly Initiative follows an essential set of evidence-based practices related to the 4M framework of an Age-Friendly Health System (i.e., what matters, medication, mentation, and mobility; IHI, 2019). Like the CCM framework, these improvement efforts are focused around a certain population—adults older than 65 years of age.

Aligning Culture Change With Existing Frameworks

Institute for Healthcare Improvement's Quadruple Aim

One of the most used frameworks in health care is the IHI's Quadruple Aim, which originated as the Triple Aim. The Triple Aim was developed by the IHI and described an approach to optimize health system performance by improving the patient experience of populations, reducing costs, and maximizing efficiency and effectiveness (IHI, 2016). This framework was established as a compass to optimize health system performance (Bodenheimer & Sinsky, 2014).

Health care continues to evolve over time as a business model. This often results in clinician burnout, higher levels of stress, and a decrease in professional satisfaction in the work environment. As a result, a fourth aim was identified—improving the work life of clinicians and staff (Bodenheimer & Sinsky, 2014; Sikka, 2015). A fourth aim has been described as a meaningful addition to emphasize clinician well-being as a significant contributor to quality and safety. If healthcare professionals are exhausted or working in ineffective teams, the goals of the triple aim will not be attained or sustained.

Health care redesign aligning with this framework provides focus for improvement teams on the following four dimensions: improving the patient experience of care, improving the health of populations, reducing the cost of care per patient and/or population, and attaining joy at work through care team wellness (Bodenheimer & Sinsky, 2014). Several strategies can be harnessed to address each aim; however, it is imperative that the culture of the environment fosters trust, openness, and active problem identification and problem solving. These strategies are precursors to innovative implementation.

Facilitation Using New Agreement Tools (Three-Dimensional Approach): The Next Big Idea

David Dibble (2018) recently introduced a simple and efficient process for fostering a culture of innovation and ongoing improvement. His facilitation methods are generating a critical mass of leaders and managers to promote process improvement ownership within teams. His techniques use a "pull" strategy along with simple problem-solving methods to support teams to transform their culture to promote, sustain, and celebrate ongoing improvement. This simple problem-solving method focuses on facilitating teams to discover, distill and name, and identify the challenges to tackle first. The facilitator guides the team through this simple problem-solving process, known as *three-dimensional problem solving* and the *80/20 rule*, to help the team identify 20% of the problems causing 80% of the poor outcomes by leveraging emotional consensus (Dibble, 2018). The first step of the process, disruptive discovery, makes visible the individuals' challenges and stressors that can be mapped to system opportunities (Dibble, 2018). The facilitator simply asks the team, "What has been bothering you about work/unit/team?" The facilitator then allows the individuals to share their issues openly and honestly. The facilitator serves as the scribe and writes everything that is shared on a whiteboard. The discovery process does not stop until everyone has shared, and all issues are captured. Some refer to this as *brainstorming*; however, discovery is more specific to identifying the problems vs. jumping to solutions (Dibble, 2018).

Once the discovery phase has been completed, it is time to move on to the second phase, distillation and name. Part one of this second step is focused on distilling down the issues made visible through phase one (i.e., discovery; Dibble, 2018). The facilitator now asks the participants to group like items by using a different color for each group. The visual depiction that evolves from this process allows grouping of the frustrations into themes. As the momentum of the team slows, the facilitator will seek affirmation from the group to ensure shared ownership and agreement with the decisions before moving to a new color category (Dibble, 2018). After all items from the discovery phase are accounted for, the facilitator works with the team to name each color category. This is part two of the second phase (Dibble, 2018). All team members provide feedback in naming each group and build off one another's comments until the team has reached a consensus on each grouped category and name (Dibble, 2018). This exercise allows the team to add value and establish ownership for the collective voice of the feeling of frustration felt by everyone on the team.

The collective "blueprint" identified by the team through a ranking process, known as *80/20 ranking*, identifies the one thing that the team would want to improve (Dibble, 2018). The chaos of the team during this phase of the process is a palpable representation of the emotional frustrations felt by the team. It is critical that the facilitator capture this energy to establish emotional consensus (Dibble, 2018). The team must not be rushed during this phase. The emotional frustration of everyone will naturally expedite purposeful effort to improve the one thing that causes the most pain (Dibble, 2018). Once the top frustration category is identified, the facilitator moves to the second most important pain point (Dibble, 208). The number of categories identified depends on the size of the team, comfort with the process, and confidence in using improvement methods. It is more important to have success in removing a single frustration than having a magnitude of working groups addressing all the frustrations.

After selecting the one category to address, action items must be established. These actions are established, agreed on, and owned by the team to move the improvement forward (Dibble, 2018). This should be a simple, clear process identifying the action, the people accountable for completing the action, and a date of completion (Dibble, 2018). This process is primarily used to drive improvement, transform unit culture, and ultimately facilitate a mindset and an urge to own improvement that affects the team. In addition, these techniques facilitate the generation of innovative solutions once the work begins and the working groups work to come up with solutions for their "pain." Implementation strategies are aligned with owning the improvement. Processes to capture these innovative ideas and solutions must be documented and put in place so that all the effort from the frontline is captured. An established standardized process to capture the ideas of the frontlines is needed in every organization to redesign health care. This ensures the voice of those who interact with patients are heard and that active and focused work to continually improve care for patients, clinicians, families, and communities is the focal point.

Exemplars provide real-world experiences on how improvement, implementation, and innovation are interrelated and necessary to accomplish positive outcomes. Organizations exist that specifically focus on innovation and implementation science (IS). For example, the Center for Health Innovation and Implementation Science (CHIIS) is an organization centered on integrating innovation and IS through agile implementation (AI) methodology. CHIIS (2020) provides a website that describes AI as an evidence-based change methodology expressly created to improve health care. By leveraging AI, CHIIS is transforming care delivery systems into agile learning systems capable of addressing the quadruple aim for better care, improved outcomes, lower costs, and enhanced patient and clinician experiences. According to the website, CHIIS exists to create a network of change agents willing to advocate for improvement in the health care industry. CHIIS purports that through education and engagement, health care professionals learn the AI evidence-based change methodology designed specifically to improve health care.

Another example of innovation and implementation comes from the Institute of Public Health. Ramsey (2016) describes the importance of expanding the boundaries of IS within the translational science framework (T0-T4). Ramsey identifies three potential benefits to consider implementation issues before establishing innovation effectiveness. Specifically, benefits include accelerating the transfer of innovations into practice, improving the design and packaging of innovations, and refining organizational and system processes involved in implementation. Accelerating the transfer of innovations into practice involves collecting data on the perceptions of implementation (attitudes) and aligning effectiveness/utility testing. This process accelerates system-ready innovations by increasing effectiveness and implementation issues separately in a stepwise approach. Improving the design and packaging of innovations is accomplished through small-scale, early-stage implementation efforts that ensure more usable and useful innovations and inform ongoing and necessary adaptions with greater efficiency. Lastly, refining organizational system processes involved in implementation necessitates trialing implementation efforts, pilot testing implementation strategies, and modifying approaches as the evidence base for innovation. Doing this work will enhance preparation of the implementation setting and facilitate receptivity for timely uptake of the innovation.

Conclusion

Innovation requires a deep understanding of IS. Using evidence-based implementation strategies with fidelity and rigor can enhance creativity and sustained positive outcomes from the "next big ideas." IS considers the methodical approach to creating a culture of innovation through well-thought-out plans for improvement. Innovation cannot be advanced with a solid step and a clear path for sustainability and spread.

Reflective Questions

1. You are asked to lead a project to improve transitions of care within your acute health care system. You want to create a culture of innovation. Describe ways that you would apply innovation models and frameworks and strategies to sustain successful implementation.

2. Using the ACT model, describe an example from your practice illustrating the key components of the model through integration and application of innovation.

3. Apply the Dibble (2018) model in facilitating a team initiative (project). Describe this problem-solving process (three-dimensional problem solving and the 80/20 rule) as you work with your team through the various steps and phases of project planning and development.

References

Agency for Healthcare Research and Quality. (2016). Heath care/system redesign. http://www.ahrq.gov/professionals/prevention-chronic-care/improve/system/index.html

American Association of Colleges of Nursing. (2013). *Competencies and curricular expectations for clinical nurse leader education and practice.* https://www.aacnnursing.org/Portals/42/News/White-Papers/CNL-Competencies-October-2013.pdf

Bodenheimer, T., & Sinsky, C. (2014). From triple to quadruple aim: Care of the patient requires care of the provider. *Annals of Family Medicine, 12*(6), 573-576. https://doi.org/10.1370/afm.1713

Bynum, J. P. W., Meara, E., Chang, C. H., Rhoads, J. M., & Bronner, K. K. (2016). *Our parents, ourselves: Health care for an aging population: A report of the Dartmouth Atlas Project.* Dartmouth Institute for Health Policy and Clinical Practice.

Center for Health Innovation and Implementation Science. (2020, January 10). http://www.hii.iu.edu/about/

Cumbie, S., Conley, V., & Burman, M. (2004). Advanced practice nursing model for comprehensive care with chronic illness: Model for promoting process engagement. *Advances in Nursing Science, 27*(1), 70-80.

Dibble, D. (2018). *The new agreements for leaders: The 4 new agreements and 7 simple tools that develop emerging leaders and managers and grow excellent organizations.* David Dibble Publisher.

Erdem, E., Prada, S. I., & Haffer, S. C. (2013). Medicare payments: How much do chronic conditions matter? *Medicare & Medicaid Research Review, 3*(2), mmrr.003.02.b02. https://www.ncbi.nlm.nih.gov/pmc/articles/PMC3983726/

Fairbanks, C. B. (2007). Using six sigma and lean methodologies to improve OR throughput. *AORN Journal, 86*(1), 73-82.

Fasnacht, P. H. (2003). Creativity: A refinement of the concept for nursing practice. *Journal of Advanced Nursing, 41*(2), 195-202.

Halbesleben, J. R., Wakefield, D. S., & Wakefield, B. J. (2008). Work-arounds in health care settings: Literature review and research agenda. *Health Care Management Review, 33*(1), 2-12.

Harris, J., Roussel, L., & Thomas, P. (2018). *Initiating and sustaining the clinical nurse leader role: A practical guide.* (3rd ed.). Jones Bartlett Learning.

Hatley, A., Ralyea, T., Buttriss, G. O. C., & Rankin, V. L. (2019). Clarifying role expectations and practice standards sing a clinical nurse leader professional practice model illustration. *Journal of Nursing Care Quality, 34*(3), 269-272.

Improving Chronic Illness Care. (2016). The chronic care model. http://www.improvingchroniccare.org/index.php?p =Model_Elements&s=18

Improving Chronic Illness Care. (2019). Resource library. http://www.improvingchroniccare.org/index.php?p=1: _Models&s=363#targetText=The%20Chronic%20Care%20Model%20(CCM,a%20prepared%2C%20proactive%20 practice%20team

Institute for Healthcare Improvement. (2016). IHI Triple Aim Initiative. http://www.ihi.org/engage/initiatives/tripleaim /pages/default.aspx

Institute for Healthcare Improvement. (2019). Science of improvement. http://www.ihi.org/about/Pages/Scienceof Improvement.aspx

Institute for Healthcare Improvement (2021). What Is an Age-Friendly Health System? http://www.ihi.org/Engage/ Initiatives/Age-Friendly-Health-Systems/Pages/default.aspx

Institute of Medicine. (2011). *The future of nursing: Leading change, advancing health.* National Academies Press. https:// pubmed.ncbi.nlm.nih.gov/24983041/

Kara, A., Johnson, C. S., Nicley, A., Niemeier, M. R., & Hui, S. L. (2015). Redesigning inpatient care: Testing the effective-ness of an accountable care team model. *Journal of Hospital Medicine, 10*(12), 773-779.

Malloch, K., & Porter-O'Grady, T. P. (2010). *Introduction to evidence-based practice in nursing & healthcare* (2nd ed.). Jones & Bartlett Publishers.

Noles, K., Barber, R., James, D., & Wingo, N. (2019). Driving innovation in health care: Clinical nurse leader role. *Journal of Nursing Care Quality, 34*(4), 307-311.

Parekh, A., Goodman, R., Gordon, C., Koh, H., & HHS Interagency Workgroup on Multiple Chronic Conditions. (2011). Managing multiple chronic conditions: A strategic framework for improving health outcomes and quality of life. *Public Health Reports, 126*(4), 460-471.

Pham, H., O'Malley, A., Bach, P., Saiontz-Martinez, C., & Schrag, D. (2009). Primary care physicians' links to other physi-cians through Medicare patients: The scope of care coordination. *Annals of Internal Medicine, 150*(4), 236.

Ramsey, A. (2016). More than just the endgame: The role of implementation science for early stage innovations in be-havioral health. https://publichealth.wustl.edu/just-endgame-role-implementation-science-early-stage-innovations -behavioral-health-sciences/

Rogers, E. (2003). *Diffusion of innovations* (5th ed.). The Free Press.

Rundio, A., Wilson, V., & Meloy, F. A. (2016). *Nurse executive: Review and resource manual.* American Nurses Association.

Shojania, K. G., & Grimshaw, J. M. (2005). Evidence-based quality improvement: The state of the science. *Health Affairs, 24*(1), 138-150.

Sikka, R. (2015). The quadruple aim: Care, health, cost and meaning in work. *BMJ Quality & Safety, 24*(10), 608-610. https://doi.org/10.1136/bmjqs-2015-004160

Wesolowski, M., Casey, G., Berry, S., & Gannon, J. (2014). The clinical nurse leader in the perioperative setting: A precep-tor experience. *AORN Journal, 100*(1), 30-41.

Wilson, L., Orff, S., Gerry, T., Shirley, B., Tabor, D., Caiazzo, K., & Rouleau, D. (2012). Evolution of an innovative role: The clinical nurse leader. *Journal of Nursing Management, 21*, 175-181

Exemplar 10-1

HELP US SUPPORT HEALING: THE CREATION OF A SLEEP PROTOCOL TO LIMIT SLEEP INTERRUPTIONS ON A MEDICAL-SURGICAL UNIT

Shaun Lampron, DNP, MSN, BSN, RN

Donna Copeland, DNP, RN, NE-BC, CPN, CPON, AE-C

Hospitalized patients often experience poor sleep quality due to noise and sleep interruptions for clinical and nonclinical activities. The importance of sleep in maintaining physiological and psychological well-being is well documented (Gathecha et al., 2016; Vincensi et al., 2016). Sleep deprivation can also affect patients' perceptions of the overall hospital experience (Gathecha et al., 2016; Vincensi et al., 2016). However, by coordinating care among interprofessional health care providers, noise and sleep interruptions can be reduced to improve patients' perceptions of the hospital experience, as well as promote a healing environment.

Therefore, a quality improvement project was developed to reduce noise and sleep interruptions to improve patients' hospital experience by 5% in 16 weeks. An interprofessional project team developed a Help Us Support Healing (HUSH) protocol to coordinate patient care activities, allowing patients 6 or more hours of uninterrupted sleep. The inclusion criteria for the HUSH protocol were patients with a modified early warning score of ≤ 2 after at least 24 hours from the time of admission to the medical-surgical unit. This evidence-based implementation strategy was supported by the interdisciplinary team as they collaborated to provide patients with a more positive sleep experience (Cullen et al., 2017). The project team also wanted to facilitate a culture of innovation by engaging the team in simple problem-solving methods to transform their culture to promote, sustain, and celebrate ongoing improvement. This simple problem-solving method focuses on facilitating teams to discover, distill and name, and identify the challenges to tackle first. The facilitator guides the team through this simple problem-solving process, known as *three-dimensional problem solving* and the *80/20 rule*, to help the team identify 20% of the problems causing 80% of the poor outcomes by leveraging emotional consensus (Dibble, 2018).

Changes in patient perceptions of noise and number of hours of restful sleep were compared pre- and postimplementation of the HUSH protocol using the Hospital Consumer Assessment of Hospital Providers and Systems quiet domain scores and patient interviews during daily nurse leader rounding. After 16 weeks, there was a 9% improvement in the Hospital Consumer Assessment of Hospital Providers and Systems quiet domain scores. Patient interviews during nurse leader rounding indicated a positive response, with patients reporting more restful sleep with a reduction in unnecessary sleep interruptions during the night.

REFERENCES

Dibble, D. (2018). *The new agreements for leaders: The 4 new agreements and 7 simple tools that develop emerging leaders and managers and grow excellent organizations.* David Dibble Publisher.

Cullen L., Wagner, M., Matthews, G., & Farrington, M. (2017). Evidence into practice: Integration within an organizational infrastructure. *Journal of PeriAnesthesia Nursing, 32*(3), 247-256. https://doi.org/10.1016/j.jopan.2017.02.003

Gathecha, E., Rios, R., Buenaver, L. F., Landis, R., Howell, E., & Wright, S. (2016). Pilot study aiming to support sleep quality and duration during hospitalization. *Journal of Hospital Medicine, 11*(7), 467-472. https://doi.org/10.1002/jhm.2578

Vincensi, B., Pearce, K., Redding, J., Brandonisio, S., Tzou, S., & Meiusi, E. (2016). Sleep in the hospitalized patient: Nurse and patient perceptions. *Medsurg Nursing, 25*(5):351-356.

Exemplar 10-2

Using Design Thinking to Guide Innovation: Innovation in Action

Aakansha Gosain, BME

Zena Banker, BME

Innovative solutions are needed to address long-standing and frustrating problems. By using an innovation framework, different solutions emerge. This allows for innovative changes to be made to processes, protocols, and interventions often enabled by devices, software, and technologies.

Design thinking has been around as a term for decades. However, it became popularized in 2005 when Stanford University founded its d.school to teach design thinking as a generalizable approach to both social and technical innovation (Hasso Plattner Institute of Design at Stanford University, 2019). Design thinking is like rapid-cycle frameworks in that they are iterative steps that are moved through until an ideal solution is created. Design thinking, as taught by the Stanford University d.school, consists of five steps: empathize, define, ideate, prototype, and test (Hasso Plattner Institute of Design at Stanford University, 2010). Each of these steps is discussed in further detail.

Empathize

Empathy is understanding the thoughts, feelings, and conditions of another from their point of view (MastersInCommunication.org, 2019). It is the primary need to provide humane, compassionate care (Ameritech College of Healthcare, 2016). Gaining empathy is the crucial first step. Many innovators may not be the end user or customer of whatever problem they are trying to solve. Thus, it is imperative for the innovator to see the issue from the customer's perspective, learning what the current situation is, what the problems are, and why it is important to solve. Empathizing can happen through unobtrusive observations, watching and listening as people interact in the current environment or with the current product, as well as by interviewing customers with thoughtful open-ended questions to get to the heart of the issue (Hasso Plattner Institute of Design at Stanford University, 2010). In the context of health care innovations, a problem may be brought forth by a provider, but the patient may be an end user also, so it is important to understand the whole scope of the problem to gain empathy for all involved parties. After gaining empathy and before transitioning to the next step, innovators must thoughtfully consider all they have learned and "unpack" all the information by putting it into some type of visual form (Hasso Plattner Institute of Design at Stanford University, 2010).

DEFINE

After empathizing with all customers, the next step is definition. The end goal is to create an actionable and meaningful problem statement. By synthesizing all the separate bits of information gathered during the empathize phase by discerning patterns, an attempt to understand motivations, needs, and desires of the customers and innovators creates insights that focus the problem. It is important to be able to narrow the problem statement as much as possible in this phase because it will lead to better ideas and solutions in the next step. Having too broad of a focus in a problem statement can lead to solutions that may be acceptable to a greater number of people but may not be the best for the customers' issues that were the focus initially identified to be addressed (Hasso Plattner Institute of Design at Stanford University, 2010).

IDEATE

Once the problem is clearly defined, it is time to generate solution ideas. The goal of the ideation process is not to produce a single perfect solution but to generate as many ideas as possible, even those that may seem absurd or unachievable. Innovators need to expand their brain and move beyond the seemingly obvious and create a high volume of varied solution ideas (Hasso Plattner Institute of Design at Stanford University, 2010). It is important to establish with all the team members before ideating the necessity of not becoming emotionally attached to any single idea but rather remain open and objective throughout the entire process.

Brainstorming

One of the most popular ways to ideate is brainstorming. Each team member says ideas aloud while one person writes each idea on a separate sticky note. As members listen to the spoken ideas, it often generates new ideas as each person can build off the idea's others have offered. During brainstorming, it is important to not evaluate or judge feasibility yet because the goal of this process is to gather as many ideas as possible. Once the initial brainstorming is complete, ideas can be grouped or clustered into affinity or similarity groups to be evaluated.

Brainwriting

Brainwriting is like brainstorming. The difference is that ideas are written on slips of paper by individual team members. Although it is not possible to build off the ideas of others, it can be a useful strategy to get more participation in some teams if the members are soft spoken. Ideas can be shared and grouped, and multiple rounds of brainwriting can be facilitated.

There are other ideation techniques that may work better for different groups, such as mind mapping, sketching, building, or questioning (Hasso Plattner Institute of Design at Stanford University, 2010). The method chosen to generate ideas is secondary to the goal of getting everyone on the team to participate in generating diverse and voluminous ideas. After all ideas have been generated and discussed, voting criteria are established to narrow the selection of ideas down to two or three for the next phase of prototyping (Hasso Plattner Institute of Design at Stanford University, 2010).

Prototype

Prototyping the team's ideas serves several purposes including communicating ideas, starting conversations, testing possibilities, and problem solving. Because all ideas and prototypes will not lead to a feasible solution, the purpose of prototyping is to fail cheaply and quickly (Hasso Plattner Institute of Design at Stanford University, 2010). Better to find out in a few minutes of prototyping a cheap solution that it will not meet customer needs than to spend weeks or months creating an expensive version! Team members do not need to spend much time on any single prototype but do need to keep the customer in mind throughout the process and identify what facets they want to test with the customer (Hasso Plattner Institute of Design at Stanford University, 2010).

The aim of a prototype is to create a prototype the customer can interact or role-play with. This interaction typically brings out more meaningful responses than merely explaining or talking some-one through an idea. This phase, coupled with the testing phase, is iterative. Innovators are expected to continually refine the prototypes based on customer interactions (Hasso Plattner Institute of Design at Stanford University, 2010).

Test

The testing phase is when the team shows the prototypes to the customer and encourages them to interact with them. It is not merely finding out if the prototype is acceptable but rather a process of collecting feedback, asking why to refine and improve the prototypes to address the initial prob-lem definition. During the customer testing and interaction, it is important to step back initially and let the customers interact with the prototypes naturally before telling them how they were intended to function. This will bring insights that might otherwise be overlooked and allows the innovators to question their own assumptions about the prototypes (Hasso Plattner Institute of Design at Stanford University, 2010).

Design thinking is an iterative process and should not be expected to find the perfect solution in the first prototype. Perfect solutions are only found when the customer loves it, not when the innovation team does.

References

Ameritech College of Healthcare. (2016). *Tips for being empathetic when providing care.* https://www.ameritech.edu/blog/empathy-when-providing-care/

Hasso Plattner Institute of Design at Stanford University. (2010). *An introduction to design thinking: Process guide* [PDF document]. https://dschoolold.stanford.edu/sandbox/groups/designresources/wiki/36873/attachments/74b3d/ModeGuideBOOTCAMP2010L.pdf

Hasso Plattner Institute of Design at Stanford University. (2019). History & approach. https://web.stanford.edu/~mshanks/MichaelShanks/files/509554.pdf

MastersinCommunications.org. (2019). *Empathy: What it is, why it matters, and how you can improve.* https://www.mastersincommunications.org/empathy-what-why-how/

VOICES FROM HEALTH CARE AND NURSING CHAMPIONS
Implications for Implementation Science and Translational Nursing

Linda A. Roussel, PhD, RN, NEA-BC, CNL, FAAN
Carolynn Thomas Jones, DNP, MSPH, RN, FAAN
Patricia L. Thomas, PhD, RN, FAAN, FACHE, FNAP, NEA-BC, ACNS-BC, CNL

CHAPTER OBJECTIVES

- Describe the Implementation Science Research Development tool as a framework for implementation success that incorporates effective intervention strategies that contribute to spread and sustainability
- Outline a range of implementation factors that impact the positive outcomes of evidence-based practice interventions
- Provide exemplars from the field of nursing and health care that illustrate how implementation science and practice can be enhanced through the translation of research into practice

---

Roussel, L. A., & Thomas, P. L. (Eds.). *Implementation Science in Nursing: A Framework for Education and Practice* (pp. 177-225).
© 2022 Taylor & Francis Group.

KEY WORDS

- Evidence-based practice interventions
- Implementation science
- Implementation Science Research Development tool
- Translational nursing

Throughout the textbook, we have introduced a variety of concepts from translational science (TS) and practice. Specifically, we have presented theories, models, frameworks, evidence-based implementation strategies, outcomes, and exemplars to underscore the integration and application to translational nursing. According to Eccles and Mittman (2006), *implementation science* (IS) in health care has been defined as the scientific study of methods to promote the systematic uptake of clinical research findings and other evidence-based practices (EBPs) into routine practice and includes consideration of the influences of the organizational system and the impact on health care professional behaviors with the goal of improving the quality and effectiveness of health services. Implementation science reinforces innovative approaches to evidence-based interventions, tools, policies, protocols, and guidelines by understanding and overcoming barriers to adoption, adaptation, integration, scale-up, and sustainability (Fogarty International Center, n.d.). Specifically, TS and practice include developing valid and consistent tools and techniques for improving health-related processes and outcomes and to facilitate large-scale adoption of strategies. Additionally, IS also serves to develop insights and generalizable knowledge regarding the implementation process, barriers, facilitators, and strategies. A significant aspect of TS includes developing, testing, and refining implementation theories and hypotheses, methods, and measures (Mittman, 2015). The uptake of EBP continues to be a priority for health care providers. The World Health Organization has elucidated the implementation of EBP as one of the greatest challenges facing the global health community and has identified the importance of IS in scaling up evidence-based intervention (Peters et al., 2013).

In communication with doctor of nursing practice (DNP) program leaders and faculty, there were recurrent themes of concern regarding DNP projects specifically related to outcomes with implementation fidelity, impact, spread, and sustainment. Their voices resonated with the authors we discussed in our small group concerns about the DNP project. Our colleagues managing and teaching in DNP programs have incorporated EBP models and concepts with DNP students (i.e., DNP students are expected to implement EBP through searching for highest levels and most rigorous research evidence, including guidelines and protocols supported by systematic reviews, meta-analysis, and randomized controlled trials). DNP program leaders also described the importance of critical appraisal of evidence and putting together a well-written evidence synthesis. Our DNP colleagues shared that although their DNP program did have well-placed content on EBP, they described the need to have a stronger focus on TS and practice, specifically implementation and dissemination sciences. They voiced gaps noted in the fidelity and rigor of implementation and dissemination strategies. Despite including assignments and activities with a greater focus on contextual factors, such as organizational structure, culture, leadership, decision making, and access to resources, DNP projects often lacked the connection and alignment of the need (gap) and unique evidence-based intervention, evaluation, and dissemination strategies. Although there was grounding of the evidence throughout the DNP project, there was not always equal attention paid to the carrying out, "hardwiring," and sustainment factors necessary for long-term gains.

DNP leaders shared that DNP students' projects were stronger in improvement methodologies because the science had progressed through the impressive work of the Institute for Healthcare Improvement (IHI; i.e., the IHI offers several excellent resources including the IHI Open School, extensive on-demand videos on the model for improvement Plan-Do-Study-Act [PDSA], in-person trainings on improvement, worksheets, checklists, and a host of other resources to plan and develop project ideas and topics). Additionally, the IHI also has extensive content in patient safety, offering training and certification as a Certified Professional in Patient Safety. Although there is an emerging field of TS and practice, our DNP colleagues believe that more tools, strategies, and "how-tos" to develop tailored approaches to implementation and dissemination were important to incorporating didactic and experiential content into DNP programs. Our DNP colleagues expressed excitement about the new textbook that would provide a comprehensive perspective of all aspects of carrying out, implementing, disseminating, and sustaining projects with impact. This chapter serves to provide voices from the field to further incorporate this much-needed content into educational and practice programs.

What We Know

Proctor et al. (2011) proposed that successful implementation is a function of the effectiveness of the intervention being implemented and a range of implementation factors. As such, proven effectiveness of the intervention being implemented, although critical, is not enough to determine implementation success. A cadre of implementation factors affect the successful implementation of evidence-based interventions. Implementation scientists focus on studying these factors and their impact on implementation success. As a result, researchers striving to implement EBPs are tasked with identifying and synthesizing disparate literature to ensure that the key principles of IS are considered when designing an implementation project. This chapter provides examples through exemplars of real-world cases that can give us insight into how navigating organizational systems, collaborating with interprofessional partners, and building on success can enhance spread and sustainable outcomes.

To frame the chapter, the authors selected the Implementation Science Research Development (ImpRes) tool (King's Improvement Science, 2018), which was developed after a scoping review of the IS literature to delineate the core principles of IS. This work followed an iterative process including consultation with international experts in the field of IS. The model was created with the aim of addressing the challenge by providing researchers with a pragmatic and comprehensive resource. When planning and designing high-quality and rigorous implementation research and improvement projects, the ImpRes can serve as a foundational tool guiding the process. The ImpRes was selected because it illustrates a systematic step-by-step approach that assists in the selection of an appropriate theory, framework, or model that guides and evaluates implementation. Considering the barriers and facilitators to implementation, the tool can also help the research or project team to develop an implementation strategy that optimizes adoption, implementation, and sustainment through appropriate selection of implementation and health economic outcomes to measure. The tool also provides strategies that engage stakeholders, patients, and the public in the implementation project, as well as the consideration of unintended consequences of implementation efforts.

The ImpRes covers core principles and useful methods for implementation. These guidelines provide a mechanism for designing implementation research (King's Improvement Science, 2018). Figure 11-1 illustrates the ImpRes tool, showing 10 domains of implementation research development.

Domain 1: Implementation Research Characteristics

The ImpRes encourages research teams to design robust implementation research by clearly articulating the implementation aims that the research seeks to address, understanding the activities associated with each implementation stage, and selecting an appropriate study design. The

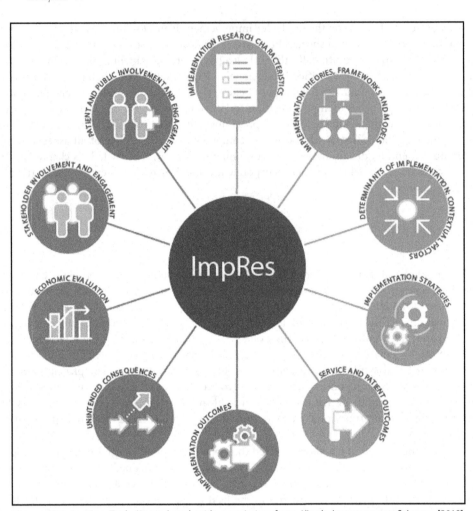

Figure 11-1. ImpRes Tool. (Reproduced with permission from King's Improvement Science. [2018]. Implementation science research development [ImpRes] Tool: A practical guide to using the ImpRes Tool [Version 1.0]. http://www.kingsimprovementscience.org/ImpRes King's Improvement Science, 2018, p.4.)

implementation team also considers the aim of the research, as well as the stages of implementation. The ImpRes tool cites Fixen et al.'s (2011) stages of implementation as part of their discussion on research characteristics. For example, the stages include exploration, installation, initial implementation, and full implementation. With each stage, activities are outlined. For example, during the exploration stage, activities such as assessing needs, examining intervention components, assessing capacity to implement, and determining barriers and facilitators are taken into account. Installation involves securing resources and preparing for organizational demands including implementation drivers and staff development. Initial implementation requires deployment of data systems as well as adjusting implementation facilitators and instituting improvement cycles. During full implementation, researchers and practitioners want to sustain improvement, monitor and manage implementation drivers, and achieve fidelity and outcome benchmarks. The ImpRes provides examples of study designs appropriate for implementation with excellent links to websites that can further advance users' understanding (King's Improvement Science, 2018). Chapter 2 of this textbook describes various research designs that align with this domain, specifically related to methods and measurement.

Domain 2: Implementation Theories, Frameworks, and Models

In this domain, theories, frameworks, and models are defined to provide the user the opportunity to understand how the implementation research and practice may be underpinned by each of these. *Theories* are a set of analytical principles created to structure observation, provide understanding and explanation of the world, and define variables. Also included is a set of relationships between the variables and specific predictions (Nilsen, 2015). Moving from theory, the ImpRes model describes a *framework* as a structure, overview, outline, system, or plan made up of various descriptive categories, such as concepts, constructs, or variables. Additionally, the relations between these categories that are presumed to account for a phenomenon are also included in the definition. Specifically, frameworks are not explanations; they only describe empirical phenomena by delineating them into a set of categories. Lastly, a *model* simplifies a phenomenon or a specific aspect of a phenomenon. According to Nilsen (2015), models do not need to be complete and accurate representations of reality to have value. The ImpRes model identifies several theories, models, and frameworks frequently cited in the literature including the normalization process theory, the Consolidated Framework for Implementation Research (CFIR), the theoretical domains framework, and the RE-AIM (Reach, Effectiveness, Adoption, Implementation, Maintenance) framework (Nilsen, 2015). The importance of selecting a theory, framework, and model is underscored as important to having a reference point (a priori vs. trial and error) and is significant in terms of replication. Citing Nilsen (2015), categories are suggested including process models that describe and guide the process of translating research into practice, understanding and explaining relationships and implementation outcomes (determinant frameworks, classic, and implementation theories), and evaluating implementation (evaluation frameworks). In selecting an appropriate theory, framework, and model, the research and project team considers the overall purpose, aims, and what the team would like to accomplish. Tabak et al. (2012) provided a cadre of theories, models, and frameworks cited in the literature and gave descriptions that the teams can use to determine the best fit based on features such as flexibility, sociocultural, and activities to be accomplished (implementation vs. dissemination). Birken et al. (2017) posited criteria for selecting implementation theories and framework based on their work from an international survey. The National Implementation Research Network is an excellent website that contains an interactive function to help the team select the best fit for a dissemination and implementation model based on the research question (population, purpose, aim, and the like). The website can be accessed through the following link: https://nirn.fpg.unc.edu/. Chapter 3 of this textbook also provides an excellent review of the various types of implementation and dissemination theories, models, and frameworks for greater detail and application.

Domain 3: Determinants of Implementation—Contextual Factors

Context is critical to successful TS and practice. In considering context, research and project teams want to identify barriers and facilitators to enhance successful implementation. Context can be described as the set of circumstances or situations that can impact implementation efforts and can be external to the intervention, which can block or strengthen its effects (Craig et al., 2008; Damschroder et al., 2009). The CFIR is an excellent example of a framework that considers inner and outer settings and process (Damschroder et al., 2009). The CFIR is one of the most widely used frameworks when considering context. The CFIR dimensions include the following: characteristics of the interventions, individuals involved, inner setting, outer setting, and process (Damschroder et al., 2009). Drilling down on the dimensions, the interventions' characteristics such as the trialability, design, complexity, and relative advantage are important to consider. Individuals involved in performing the intervention are essential to understanding their skills, competencies, work within the organization, and stage of change. The inner setting is concerned with the internal dimensions of the organization and system, such as the structure, culture, networks, resources available, strategic initiatives, leadership, and how communication and decision making "happen." The outer setting refers to what is external to the organizational systems, such as accreditation and regulatory requirements. It is important not to underestimate the processes involved in any implementation undertaken and include the planning, engagement of key stakeholders, execution, and evaluation. Chapter 8 describes organizational systems and leadership and the impact on translational nursing. Furthermore, Chapter 8 delineates change management responses on a continuum and the effectiveness of using a framework to enhance successful implementation. Chapters 6 and 7 focus on contextual factors as they relate to entry-level and graduate nursing education.

Domain 4: Implementation Strategies

Proctor et al. (2013) described implementation strategies as methods or techniques used to enhance the adoption, implementation, and sustainment of a guideline, protocol, or program. They further described implementation strategies as the active ingredient of the implementation process and the "how-to" component of changing health care practice (Proctor et al., 2013). To increase the utility of implementation strategies, the ImpRes model categorizes implementation strategies, and, within each category, examples of discrete strategies are identified. This is based on the work of Waltz et al. (2014). For example, within the category of develop stakeholder interrelationships, discrete strategies include identifying and preparing champions, informing local opinion leaders, and recognizing early adopters. Train and educate stakeholders as a category includes conducting ongoing training, distributing educational materials, and creating a learning collaborative. Another category, engage patient/service users, considers involving patients, family, and community members; preparing patient/service users to be participants; and increasing demand. Utilize financial incentives as a category can include altering incentive/allowance structure, using other payment schemes, and developing disincentives. The ImpRes model describes an impressive number of implementation strategies that can be used to tailor an improvement in practice underpinned by IS. The ImpRes model outlines the following guiding principles:

1. Select strategies to address the context and setting of a change effort to overcome barriers to implementation and/or harness facilitators to implementation.
2. Select strategies that have an adequate and relevant evidence base.
3. Engage stakeholders (i.e., health care professionals and patient and the public) in the selection and tailoring of strategies.
4. Select strategies based on expert ratings of importance and feasibility (i.e., most important strategy: assessing readiness and identify barriers and facilitators, least important strategy: changing liability laws, most feasible strategy: developing educational materials, and least feasible strategy: changing liability laws [King's Improvement Science, 2018, p. 25]).

When considering implementation strategies, how the team selects and develops an appropriate overall implementation strategy is dependent on the context of any given implementation effort and the systematic identification of implementation determinants such as facilitators and barriers. When selecting implementation strategies, the research and project team focuses on the implementation outcomes (e.g., informing local opinion leaders may increase the speed of implementation and improve fidelity; King's Improvement Science, 2018). Chapter 1 provides a framework to guide the selection of implementation strategies. We refer the reader to this chapter to further inform the development of evidence-based implementation strategies.

Domain 5: Service and Patient Outcomes

Proctor et al. (2011) described three types of outcomes in implementation research: service, patient, and implementation. Service outcomes include the consideration of efficiency, safety, effectiveness, equity, patient centeredness, and timeliness (Institute of Medicine's aims for quality). Patient (client) outcomes may include satisfaction, function, quality of life, and symptom management. Implementation outcomes entail consideration of acceptability, adoption, appropriateness, costs, feasibility, fidelity, penetration, and sustainability. We can all agree that paying attention to patient (client) and service outcomes is critical to meaningful work; however, we may miss important outcomes if we do not consider the actual process of implementation. It is important to consider the implementation research characteristics when outlining overall outcomes strategies inclusive of service and patient outcomes (King's Improvement Science, 2018). Service and patient outcomes are threaded throughout several chapters; see Chapters 8, 9, and 10 for additional examples and exemplars.

Domain 6: Implementation Outcomes

Measuring service and patient outcomes is essential in the overall context and direct services needed to impact outcomes. Table 5 in the ImpRes model document (https://www.effectiveservices.org/resources/implementation-science-research-development-impres-tool-a-practical-guide-to-using-the-impres-tool) provides implementation outcomes, definitions, and commonly used terms to describe the specific outcome. For example, the implementation outcome *appropriateness* is defined as "the perceived fit, relevance, or compatibility of the innovation or EBP for a given practice setting, provider, or consumer; and/or perceived fit of the innovation to address a particular issue or problem" (King's Improvement Science, 2018, p. 30). Commonly used terms to describe appropriateness include the following: perceived fit, relevance, compatibility, suitability, usefulness, and practicability (p. 30). Another example, fidelity, is described as "the degree to which an intervention was implemented as it was prescribed in the original protocol or as it was intended by the program developers" (King's Improvement Science, 2018, p. 30). Terms that are used to identify fidelity include delivered as intended, adherence, integrity, and quality of program delivery (King's Improvement Science, 2018, p. 31). Citing Proctor et al. (2011), the ImpRes outlines three functions that implementation outcomes address: serving as indicators of implementation success, proximal indicators of implementation processes, and key intermediate outcomes in relation to service or clinical outcomes in treatment effectiveness and quality of care research. If an intervention or treatment is poorly implemented, this impacts the overall effectiveness of the implementation plan and "serve[s] as necessary preconditions for attaining subsequent desired and/or hypothesized changes in clinical or service outcomes" (King's Improvement Science, 2018, p. 31). Included in the domain of implementation outcomes are measurement methodologies that can be qualitative or quantitative in nature. For example, qualitative methods could be interviews, focus groups, and observations. Quantitative methods identified may be data collected from surveys, audits, and administrative reports (i.e., quality indicators and benchmarks). Stakeholder group engagement and stages of implementation are also important considerations when evaluating implementation outcomes. Implementation outcomes are addressed in most of the chapters with a greater focus in Chapters 1, 4, and 5.

Domain 7: Unintended Consequences

Unintended consequences may occur when conducting implementation research or when implementing rigorous improvement projects. Researchers and practitioners are asked to be mindful and intentional when considering risk factors (the positive and negative consequences) of engaging in implementation efforts. Noted in the ImpRes model are three types of unintended consequences:

1. Unexpected benefit: a positive, unexpected benefit
2. Unexpected drawback: a negative, unexpected detriment occurring in addition to the desired effect
3. Perverse result: a perverse effect contrary to what was originally intended (King's Improvement Science, 2018, p. 34)

Domain 8: Economic Evaluations

The ImpRes illuminates the essential need to include an economic evaluation in the implementation process because it provides insight as to the specificity of implementation efforts being cost effective and how limited health care resources are used. Without considering costs, decision makers and key stakeholders are less likely to have successful widespread implementation and scale-up and spread of evidence-based treatment and practices. Table 6 of the ImpRes (https://www.effectiveservices.org/resources/implementation-science-research-development-impres-tool-a-practical-guide-to-using-the-impres-tool) provides an excellent listing of implementation costs and definitions to consider in the implementation process (King's Improvement Science, 2018, p. 37). For example, implementation project costs consider resources required for developing and delivering the implementation project and include factors that include setup costs for the implementation and fixed costs. Moreover, sustainability and long-term outcome tracking have associated costs as well.

Another example, *implementation cost-effectiveness*, is defined as the net implementation health benefit minus the net implementation cost. Return on investment, incremental cost-effectiveness ratio, policy cost-effectiveness, and cost-benefit ratio are also terms that can be used to describe and measure implementation cost-effectiveness (King's Improvement Science, 2018).

According to the ImpRes (King's Improvement Science, 2018), implementation research and practice need to consider the measurement requirements "to support a robust economic evaluation are considered at the early design phase of a project. Failure to do so will risk compromising the quality and value of research outputs for decisions makers" (p. 40). Specifically, consideration needs to be on the importance of deciding which implementation measures of outcomes and effectiveness will be translated into measures of impact of economic relevance (i.e., the implementation scientists will need to determine such outcomes; e.g., as improved health outcomes for patients as well as the resources needed [and costs] that accurately capture resource use and costs to reflect accepted methodological standards for economic analysis [King's Improvement Science, 2018, p. 40]). A conceptual framework for economic evaluation in a health service implementation context is illustrated in the ImpRes in Table 11-1 (King's Improvement Science, 2018, p. 41). Considering costs and the economic perspectives is important to implementation research and projects. Chapters 8, 9, and 10 provide additional examples that the reader can refer to for further detail.

Domain 9: Stakeholder Involvement and Engagement

The ImpRes underscores the importance of engaging stakeholders and getting them involved early in the process. Specifically, stakeholder engagement can be described as the active involvement by the research team with those implementing the strategies (frontline providers), who are more than participants in research. Early involvement, ongoing communication, and dissemination are ways to continually engage those who are critical to successful implementation efforts. Identifying champions, early adopters, and opinion leaders is an implementation strategy for early planning, intervention, and eventual sustainability. Providing incentives through education, recognition on publications, press releases, and other ways to build collaborative partnerships is essential to lasting relationships and improvement efforts. Stakeholder involvement and engagement are integral to successful implementation work, and as such most of the chapters include some aspect of this domain. For example, Chapters 5, 6, and 7 provide reinforcement of this domain from an academic nursing, including entry and graduate nursing, education.

Domain 10: Patient and Public Involvement and Engagement

The ImpRes underscores the importance of encouraging research teams to consider implementation research and practice as a true collaboration between research teams and patients and

TABLE 11-1

Knowledge to Action Framework Compared With Common Evidence-Based Practice Models

KNOWLEDGE TO ACTION FRAMEWORK (GRAHAM ET AL., 2006)	SEVEN STEPS OF EBP (MELNYK ET AL., 2018)	IOWA MODEL (IOWA MODEL COLLABORATIVE, 2017)
Identify problem; review and select knowledge	1. Problem inquiry 2. Ask the question 3. Search the evidence 4. Appraise the evidence	• Identify triggering issues • State the question or purpose • Form a team • Assemble, appraise, and synthesize the evidence
Adapt knowledge to local context	5. Integrate evidence with clinical expertise and patient preferences	• Design and pilot the practice change
Assess barriers to knowledge use		• Integrate and sustain practice change
Select, tailor, implement interventions		
Monitor knowledge use	6. Evaluate the outcomes	
Evaluate outcomes		
Sustain knowledge use	7. Disseminate findings	• Disseminate findings

Adapted from King's Improvement Science. (2018). Implementation science research development (ImpRes) tool: A practical guide to using the ImpRes Tool (Version 1.0). http://www.kingsimprovementscience.org/ImpRes.

the public. Patient and public engagement and involvement are part of a larger view of stakeholder involvement. The ImpRes supports research teams' efforts to delineate patient and public involvement in isolation to other stakeholder involvement because of its critical importance in facilitating the implementation of research evidence into clinical practice. This is essential to maximizing patient benefit and reducing health inequalities (Burton & Rycroft-Malone, 2015; Callard et al., 2012; King's Improvement Science, 2018; Ocloo & Matthews, 2016).

The ImpRes provides a way to consider IS and practice through systematic consideration of 10 domains: implementation research characteristics; implementation theories, frameworks, and models; determinants of implementation—contextual factors; implementation strategies; service and patient outcomes; implementation outcomes; unintended consequences; economic evaluations; stakeholder involvement and engagement; and patient and public involvement and engagement. As a critical domain, all chapters address this in some form through content, examples, and exemplars.

CONCLUSION

This chapter provided an overview of what to consider when applying concepts and principles to implementation research and practice that inform translational nursing. The 10 domains of the ImpRes were described as a road map that acknowledges the various steps, phases, and aspects of implementation to facilitate a successful update of EBP. Exemplars were provided to illustrate how the domains can be applied to a variety of clinical and educational settings. Using the ImpRes, researchers and practitioners are better equipped to comprehensively approach best practices in implementation and dissemination sciences.

REFERENCES

Birken, S. A., Powell, B. J., Shea, C. M., Haines, E. R., Kirk, M. A., Leeman, J., Rohweder, C., Damschroder, L., & Presseau, J. (2017). Criteria for selecting implementation science theories and frameworks: Results from an international survey. *Implementation Science, 12*, 124. https://doi.org/10.1186/s13012-017-0656-y

Burton, C., & Rycroft-Malone, J. (2015). An untapped resource: patient and public involvement in implementation. *International Journal of Health Policy Management, 4*(12), 845-847.

Callard, F., Rose, D., & Wykes, T. (2012). Close to the bench as well as at the bedside: Involving service users in all phases of translational research. *Health Expectations, 15*(4), 389-400.

Craig, P., Dieppe, P., Macintyre, S., Nazareth, M. S., & Petticrew, M. (2008). Developing and evaluating complex interventions: the new Medical Research Council guidance. *British Medical Journal, 337*, 11655.

Damschroder, L. J., Aron, D. C., Keith, R. E., Kirsh, S. R., Alexander, J. A., & Lowery, J. C. (2009). Fostering implementation of health services research findings into practice: A consolidated framework for advancing implementation science. *Implementation Science, 4*, 50. https://doi.org/10.1186/1748-5908-4-50

Eccles, M. P., & Mittman, B. S. (2006). Welcome to implementation science. *Implementation Science, 1*, 1. https://doi.org/10.1186/1748-5908-1-1

Fixen, D., Scott, V., Blasé, K., Naoom, S., & Wagar, L. (2011). When evidence is not enough: The challenge of implementing fall prevention strategies. *Journal of Safety Research, 42*(6), 419-422. https://doi.org/10.1016/j.jsr.2011.10.002

Fogarty International Center. (n.d.) Implementation Science Information and Resources. http://www.fic.nih.gov/research-topics/pages/implementationscience.aspx

Graham, I. D., Logan, J., Harrison, M. B., Straus, S. E., Tetroe, J., Caswell, W., & Robinson, N. (2006). Lost in knowledge translation: Time for a map? *Journal of Continuing Education in the Health Professions, 26*(1), 13-24. https://doi.org/10.1002/chp.47

Iowa Model Collaborative. (2017). Iowa model of evidence-based practice: Revisions and validation. *Worldviews on Evidence-Based Nursing, 14*(3), 175-182. https://doi.org/10.1111/wvn.12223

King's Improvement Science. (2018). Implementation science research development (ImpRes) tool: A practical guide to using the ImpRes Tool (Version 1.0). http://www.kingsimprovementscience.org/ImpRes

Melnyk, B. M., & Fineout-Overholt, E. (2018). *Evidence-based practice in nursing & healthcare: A guide to best practice* (4th ed.). Wolters Kluwer/Lippincott Williams & Wilkins.

Mittman, B.S., Weiner, B.J., Proctor, E.K. et al (2015). Expanding D&I science capacity and activity within NIH Clinical and Translational Science Award (CTSA) Programs: Guidance and successful models from national leaders. *Implementation Science, 10*, A38. https://doi.org/10.1186/1748-5908-10-S1-A38

Nilsen, P. (2015) Making sense of implementation theories, models and frameworks. *Implementation Science, 10*, 53. https://doi.org/10.1186/s13012-015-0242-0

Ocloo, J., & Matthews, R. (2016). From tokenism to empowerment: Progressing patient and public involvement in healthcare improvement. *BMJ Quality and Safety, 25*(8), 626-632.

Peters, D. H., Adam, T., Alonge, O., Agyepong, I. A., & Tran, N. (2013). Implementation research: What it is and how to do it. *BMJ, 347*, f6753. https://doi.org/10.1136/bmj.f6753

Proctor, E., Silmere, H., Raghavan, R., Hovmand, P., Aarons, G., Bunger, A., Griffey, R., & Hensley, M. (2011). Outcomes for implementation research: Conceptual distinctions, measurement challenges, and research agenda. *Administration and Policy in Mental Health, 38*(2), 65-76.

Proctor, E. K., Powell, B. J., & McMillen, J. C. (2013). Implementation strategies: Recommendations for specifying and reporting. *Implementation Science, 8*, 139. https://doi.org/10.1186/1748-5908-8-139

Tabak, R. G., Khoong, E. C., Chambers, D. A., & Brownson, R. C. (2012). Bridging research and practice: Models for dissemination and implementation research. *American Journal of Preventive Medicine, 43*(3), 337-350.

Waltz, T. J., Powell, B. J., Chinman, M. J., Smith, J. L., Matthieu, M. M., Proctor, E. K., Damschroder, L. J., & Kirchner, J. E. (2014). Expert Recommendations for Implementing Change (ERIC): Protocol for a mixed methods study. *Implementation Science, 9*, 39. https://doi.org/10.1186/1748-5908-9-39

Exemplar 11-1

IMPARTING KNOWLEDGE AND SUPPORTING EVIDENCE-BASED ACTION: THE ADULT NONALCOHOLIC FATTY LIVER DISEASE TOOLKIT

Kelly Casler, DNP, APRN-CNP, EBP-C, CHSE

Domains: theories, models, and frameworks; determinants of implementation—contextual factors; implementation strategies; implementation outcomes; service and patient outcomes

Nonalcoholic fatty liver disease (NAFLD) is rapidly increasing in prevalence and is poised to surpass hepatitis C and alcoholic liver disease as the leading cause of liver transplant (Fuch, 2019; Zezos & Renner, 2014). Despite NAFLD prevalence reaching epidemic levels, primary care providers struggle with diagnosing and managing NAFLD, especially knowing when to refer NAFLD patients for specialty care (Polanco-Briceno et al., 2016). These primary care provider knowledge gaps are impactful given that they can adversely affect patients because earlier identification and management of NAFLD have been associated with better patient outcomes (Dokmak et al., 2020; Fuch, 2019; Stål, 2015).

At a Midwestern primary care practice, my colleagues and I encountered multiple patients with NAFLD. There was a lack of clarity on how to best manage them, especially how to determine when they should be referred to a hepatologist for care. Other patients in the practice had "silent" NAFLD without any clinical signs or symptoms, and NAFLD was not identified until it resulted in a severe exacerbation that necessitated hospitalization.

After recognizing this problem, I consulted with colleagues in a state professional nurse practitioner (NP) program and performed a literature review to determine the extent of the problem outside just our clinic. The literature demonstrated that primary care provider knowledge gaps regarding NAFLD occurred not only nationally but also globally. Collaboration with colleagues in the state professional NP organization identified knowledge gaps and missed opportunities in care that matched the descriptions in the retrieved research literature. Moreover, colleagues at the clinical practice site and state NP organization agreed that there was a need for an EBP change project focused on NAFLD.

The Knowledge to Action (KTA) framework was selected as the guiding framework for the practice change. The KTA framework focuses on the process of knowledge translation and, like EBP models, approaches implementation using a systems and collaboration lens (Graham & Tetroe, 2010). It emphasizes the collaboration between knowledge producers (researchers) and knowledge users (clinicians) as well as the dynamic and fluid process that occurs when knowledge is translated into meaningful action. Additionally, emphasis is placed on the influence of the local culture when moving from a "knowing" mindset to a "doing" mindset (i.e., action). There are two cycles in the KTA framework (Graham et al., 2006). The first cycle, knowledge creation, begins when knowledge is produced, usually by researchers. As individuals or organizations look to solve clinical practice problems, they query the knowledge that has been produced (knowledge inquiry). Next, knowledge is synthesized and then transformed into tools and products that can be used at the site of patient care. Practice guidelines, clinical decision aids, and algorithms are examples of tools and products

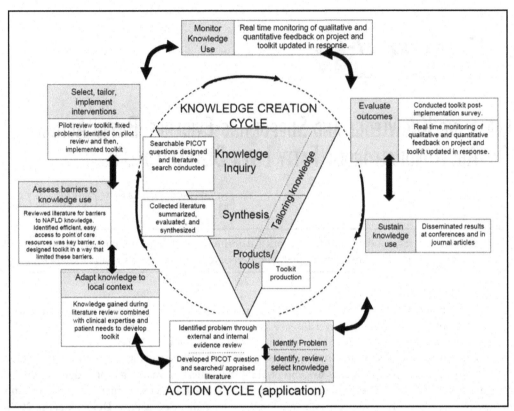

Figure 11-2. Knowledge to Action framework. Gray boxes/triangles identify steps in Knowledge to Action cycles. White boxes identify corresponding action for the Non-Alcoholic Fatty Liver Disease Toolkit. (Adapted with permission from Graham, I. D., Logan, J., Harrison, M. B., Straus, S. E., Tetroe, J., Caswell, W., & Robinson, N. [2006]. Lost in knowledge translation: Time for a map? *Journal of Continuing Education in the Health Professions, 26*(1), 13-24. https://doi.org/10.1002/ch.47.)

that are created in this cycle. The second cycle, or action cycle, focuses on the "what" and "how" of putting knowledge into practice as well as the anticipation of and planning for barriers to knowledge use. There are seven steps in the action cycle that are usually completed simultaneously, although they can also occur in a sequential manner. Figure 11-2 illustrates the steps. A strength of the KTA framework is that the steps were developed after careful analysis of shared attributes between 31 different planned action theories (Graham & Tetroe, 2010). The KTA framework shares many similarities with other frequently used EBP models, and a comparison with two of the most common is provided in Table 11-1. Like other models, the KTA framework notes interdisciplinary teamwork and collaboration as imperative to success (Graham et al., 2006).

After identifying the knowledge gap problem, searchable clinical questions were drafted in the PICOT (Population, Intervention, Comparison, Outcome, Time) format, and a literature search was completed to query the knowledge base and further clarify the scope of the problem and its solution. The evidence was compiled, evaluated, and synthesized using tables to compare the retrieved information. Initial inquiry questions explored not only appropriate approaches to NAFLD diagnosis, management, and referral but also to best practices in translating knowledge into practice. A brief clinical immersion was completed with experts in NAFLD to create a robust clinical expertise to supplement the knowledge gained during the literature inquiry. Common patient concerns and challenges were noted and later used to create knowledge tools that could be used to educate patients.

When exploring the evidence for methods to deliver the new knowledge successfully and with the best chance for it to be put into practice, electronic tool kits delivered online were identified as the most efficient and effective solutions (Barac et al., 2014). Therefore, the Adult NAFLD Toolkit was designed using free, online web design software and was hosted on a free web hosting platform. The tool kit was purposely designed to be easy to navigate and access through either handheld or personal computer devices.

The tool kit allowed clinicians to select resources based on their areas of knowledge needs. The available options included pathophysiology and epidemiology, diagnosis, management, and patient education. Without any treatments for severe NAFLD at the time of the project, management primarily focused on early identification and management and referral when severe disease was identified. Therefore, one important aspect of the tool kit was a diagnosis algorithm, which also guided clinicians on when to refer patients. Guidance on completing nutrition and exercise coaching, the mainstay of NAFLD treatment, was also provided as a tool. Additionally, the patient education module provided clinicians with modifiable patient education materials as a tool. All tools were developed during the knowledge creation cycle. After the tool kit was finalized, a pilot review was conducted, and necessary modifications were made.

Implementation of the tool kit was completed with the primary care clinic and the statewide NP organization described earlier. Before accessing the tool kit, clinicians were asked to complete a presurvey to assess baseline knowledge and approaches to NAFLD management. The presurvey helped in evaluating the impact of the tool kit; after using the tool kit, clinicians were asked to complete a postsurvey that asked the same questions as the presurvey. The postsurvey also allowed for narrative feedback on the tool kit. Evaluation of the survey responses and changes from before and after tool kit use showed that the tool kit significantly improved primary care NPs' knowledge regarding NAFLD, at least in the short term. Clinicians also felt more prepared to care for NAFLD patients, and their self-reported approach to patient care (application of knowledge) more closely aligned with recommended practices (Casler et al., 2020). Several narrative comments reported that the tool kit was valuable and useful, especially the algorithms and patient education components.

The Adult NAFLD Toolkit was able to address clinician knowledge gaps and speed the translation of research regarding the disease into clinical practice. The KTA framework proved to be a useful guide for conceptualization and implementation of this evidence-based intervention. Its applicability to the dynamic and continuous nature of most practice change projects was another beneficial aspect of this implementation framework.

Author's Commentary: In the future, the researchers may want to consider the work of Brownson et al. (2012) specific to the taxonomy of dissemination and implementation outcomes. Reviewing the outcomes (i.e., acceptability, reach, feasibility) could provide additional dimensions for successful sustainment of the use of the tool kit. Consideration of the state of implementation and specific evidence-based implementation strategies could also have enhanced the work of the researchers (Cullen et al., 2018).

REFERENCES

Barac, R., Stein, S., Bruce, B., & Barwick, M. (2014). Scoping review of toolkits as a knowledge translation strategy in health. *BMC Medical Informatics and Decision Making, 14*, 1. https://doi.org/10.1186/s12911-014-0121-7

Brownson, R. C., Colditz, G. A., & Proctor, E. K. (Eds.). (2012). *Dissemination and implementation research in health: Translating science to practice.* Oxford University Press.

Casler, K., Trees, K., & Bosak, K. (2020). Readiness for the epidemic: The adult non-alcoholic fatty liver disease toolkit for primary care nurse practitioners. *Journal of the American Association of Nurse Practitioners, 32*, 323-331. https://doi.org/10.1097/JXX.0000000000000223

Cullen, L., Hanrahan, K., Farrington, M., DeBerg, J., Tucker, S., & Kleiber, C. (2018). *Evidence-based practice in action: Comprehensive strategies, tools, and tips from the University of Iowa Hospitals and Clinics.* Sigma Theta Tau International.

Dokmak, A., Lizaola-Mayo, B., & Trivedi, H. D. (2020). The impact of Non-alcoholic Fatty Liver Disease in primary care: A population health perspective. *The American Journal of Medicine.* Advance online publication. https://doi.org/10.1016/j.amjmed.2020.08.010

Fuch, M. (2019). Managing the silent epidemic of nonalcoholic fatty liver disease. *Federal Practitioner, 36*(1), 12-13.

Graham, I. D., Logan, J., Harrison, M. B., Straus, S. E., Tetroe, J., Caswell, W., & Robinson, N. (2006). Lost in knowledge translation: Time for a map? *Journal of Continuing Education in the Health Professions, 26*(1), 13-24. https://doi.org/10.1002/chp.47

Graham, I. D., & Tetroe, J. M. (2010). The knowledge to action framework. In J. Rycroft-Malone & T. Bucknall (Eds.), Models and frameworks for implementing evidence-based practice: Linking evidence to action (pp. 207-219). Wiley Blackwell.

Polanco-Briceno, S., Glass, D., Stuntz, M., & Caze, A. (2016). Awareness of non-alcoholic steatohepatitis and associated practice patterns of primary care physicians and specialists. *BMC Research Notes, 9*, 157-169. https://doi.org/10.1186/s13104-016-1946-1

Stål, P. (2015). Liver fibrosis in non-alcoholic fatty liver disease - Diagnostic challenge with prognostic significance. *World Journal of Gastroenterology, 21*(39), 11077. https://doi.org/10.3748/wjg.v21.i39.11077

Zezos, P., & Renner, E. (2014). Liver transplantation and non-alcoholic fatty liver disease. *World Journal of Gastroenterology, 20*(42), 15532-15338. https://doi.org/10.3748/wjg.v20.i42.15532

Exemplar 11-2

NURSING LEADERSHIP AND EVIDENCE-BASED PRACTICE AMIDST THE PANDEMIC

Kelli Chovanec, DNP, RN, NE-BC

Domains: determinants of implementation—contextual factors; implementation strategies; implementation outcomes

Nurse leaders are on the forefront of driving the changes in the rapidly changing and fast-paced health care landscape, and it is more critical now than ever to integrate the current best available evidence into nursing practice. The current coronavirus disease 2019 (COVID-19) pandemic has increased the demand for health care systems leaders to develop, implement, and evaluate rapid change cycle projects across all care settings. The limiting factors for IS can be moderated through an effective nursing leadership approach, the application of a change management model, and the dissemination of outcomes. Competency and political acumen in networking, interpersonal skills, and emotional intelligence are essential to leverage for the informing of strategic decisions and the change management process.

Supporting or limiting factors can influence the adoption and effectiveness of approaches to TS and evidence-based nursing practice. Nurses' knowledge and attitudes are significantly associated with the implementation of EBPs (Algahtani et al., 2019). Nurses' viewpoints about EBP can be adverse, with some favoring customary approaches compared with incorporating new methods into practice (Farokhzadian et al., 2015). The barriers to evidence-based nursing practice include nurses' lack of confidence and skill in deducing and understanding the outcomes of the studies and discerning the relative applicability of evidence to practice (Farokhzadian et al., 2015). The most impactful supporting factors for the adoption of TS are effective nursing leadership and mentorship (Farokhzadian et al., 2015). It is the role of the nurse leader to address and overcome the barriers to the translation of evidence into practice, including supporting a culture that optimizes the knowledge, skill, and attitudes of the nurses within the practice setting.

The nurse leader serves as a catalyst for driving and fostering changes in the health care organization, with a focus on addressing the health of the populations served. Clinical expertise and relationship building skills are applied to influence collaborative efforts to improve the quality of care delivery and patient outcomes (Stanley & Stanley, 2018). These ambitious aims can be achieved through the process of translating the best available evidence into practice, and the subsequent dissemination of outcomes ensures the sustainability of the changes. The sharing of timely and relevant findings about nursing practice and EBP changes elevates the nursing profession and drives quality improvement (Oermann et al., 2018). Nursing leaders contribute to the general body of nursing knowledge through the sharing of EBP projects, results, and implications for practice.

The PDSA cycle change management model provides a framework to support the process of implementing a practice change. The model can be applied to guide the change management and quality improvement progression, allowing for testing of the practice change and continuous revisions to processes that are based on implications from the measurement and analysis of outcomes (Berwick, 1996). The study component of the PDSA model refers to the analysis of the data resulting from the rapid cycle change (Leis & Shojania, 2017). Outcomes are collected, and the analysis leads to revisions to the plan and further action (Leis & Shojania, 2017). It is important for the nurse leader to perform ongoing formative evaluation of the implementation process, making changes to the project as necessary.

The demand for effective health care systems leaders is great during the COVID-19 pandemic. The leaders and teams are driven to develop, implement, and evaluate rapid change cycle projects under extremely stressful circumstances. Leaders are compelled to support ongoing clinical inquiry and inform decisions based on the evolving, emerging evidence. The pandemic experience reinforces the importance of remaining agile, flexible, and open to modifying plans if there is a need for a change. Even with the comprehensive and thoughtful development of implementation plans, the strategy to successfully implement the project can change rapidly because of the context of the health care environment. Changes to the implementation strategy can cause stress, which is associated with adverse psychological effects and can be surmounted through resilience (Li & Hasson, 2020). Effective nurse leaders demonstrate resiliency and other key competencies to influence EBP and IS in the health care setting.

An example of a rapid cycle change project during the pandemic involves the management of transitions of care for emergency room and hospital-discharged patients who have a COVID-19 diagnosis. A team of interdisciplinary leaders collaboratively developed an algorithm and process for the telephonic nursing outreach based on the best available evidence. The initial outreach is the day after discharge, and subsequent calls are daily between days of illness 8 through 14 when the patient is at high risk for adverse outcomes. All nursing outreach calls include a review of symptoms, especially worsening shortness of breath, confusion, and a review of oxygen saturation readings for patients on oxygen. A technology platform has been leveraged to support the nurse telephone triage using COVID-19 protocols. The guidelines are updated regularly in alignment with the emerging and changing evidence and Centers for Disease Control and Prevention guidance, and the nurses apply the adult and pediatric protocols to assess symptoms and provide care advice for patients diagnosed with COVID-19. The implementation of this practice change to support transitions of care for this population requires dedicated nursing leadership and ongoing collaboration with interprofessional team members.

A leadership style that involves political acumen and interprofessional skills, leveraging the relationships with other leaders and team members, enables a leader to effectively drive the necessary practice change. Serving as a health care system leader amidst the COVID-19 pandemic presents challenges, including the need to take decisive action in a timely manner. There is a risk to assertive leadership qualities, and they must be present in balance with emotional intelligence to serve as a driving force for the overall leadership approach. The emotionally intelligent nurse leader remains self-reflective to understand and manage central emotions, demonstrating an appreciation of the emotions of others through empathetic expression of respect, awareness, and accountability (Yekta & Abdolrahimi, 2016). Leaders proficient in these areas consider the impact a decision will make to the health care organization, weighing the benefits and necessity of the decision against the potential impact and advocating for what is right.

The current health care context presents an unprecedented opportunity for nurses to leverage competencies in EBP and leadership to influence, drive, and manage nursing practice changes. Nurse leaders are challenged to apply TS and change management strategies in an approach that fosters a culture that conveys the values of inquiry and aims to continuously improve and elevate the profession of nursing. This is an exciting time to serve as a nurse leader, translating the implications derived from the best available evidence into nursing practice.

Author's Commentary: This well-designed quality improvement project could be enhanced by the application of an implementation theory, model, or framework that would specifically guide the researchers' work in conceptualizing the implementation phase of the project. Guided by phases of the PDSA, the researchers may want to consider the evidence-based implementation strategies as described by Cullen et al. (2018) in their work on evidence-based implementation strategies for sustainability, which captures specific interventions during the various phases of implementation (i.e., create awareness and interest, build knowledge and commitment, promote action and adoption, and pursue integration and sustained use).

REFERENCES

Algahtani, N., Oh, K., Kitsantas, P., & Rodan, M. (2019). Nurses' evidence-based practice knowledge, attitudes, and implementation: A cross-sectional study. *Journal of Clinical Nursing, 29*(1), 274-283.

Berwick, D. (1996). A primer on leading the improvement of systems. *British Medical Journal, 312*(7031), 619-622.

Cullen, L., Hanrahan, K., Farrington, M., DeBerg, J., Tucker, S., & Kleiber, C. (2018). *Evidence-based practice in action: Comprehensive strategies, tools, and tips from the University of Iowa Hospitals and Clinics.* Sigma Theta Tau International.

Farokhzadian, J., Khajouei, R., & Ahmadian, L. (2015). Evaluating factors associated with implementing evidence-based practice in nursing. *Journal of Evaluation in Clinical Practice, 21*(6), 1107-1113.

Leis, J., & Shojania, K. (2017). A primer on PDSA: executing plan-do-study-act cycles in practice, not just in name. *BMJ Quality and Safety, 26*(7), 572.

Li, Z., & Hasson, F. (2020). Resilience, stress, and psychological well-being in nursing students: a systematic review. *Nursing Education Today.* Advance online publication. https://doi.org/10.1016/j.nedt.2020.104440.

Oermann, M., Christenbery, T., & Turner, K. (2018). Writing publishable review, research, quality improvement, and evidence-based practice manuscripts. *Nursing Economics, 36*(6), 268-275.

Stanley, D., & Stanley, K. (2018). Clinical leadership and nursing explored: A literature search. *Journal of Clinical Nursing, 27*(9), 1730-1745.

Yekta, Z., & Abdolrahimi, M. (2016). Concept analysis of emotional intelligence in nursing. *Nursing Practice Today, 3*(4), 158-163.

Exemplar 11-3

BUILDING A PEER SUPPORT SYSTEM TO MITIGATE PSYCHOLOGICAL TRAUMA IN HEALTH CARE WORKERS

Donna Copeland, DNP, RN, NE-BC, CPN, CPON, AE-C

Domains: determinants of implementation—contextual factors; stakeholder involvement and engagement

Secondary victimization as a topic of interest was presented to the hospital's Interprofessional Evidence-Based Practice Council (IEBPC). Further discussion among the council members indicated personal encounters of and an interest in exploring psychological trauma and its effects on health care workers and the hospital system. A literature review was performed by the IEBPC to establish the prevalence, contributing factors, and consequences of psychological trauma of health care workers.

Results of the literature review indicate that health care is stressful due to high workloads, lack of social support, exposure to suffering and dying patients, and unintended adverse events (Portoghese et al., 2014). Repeated exposures to high levels of stress lead to burnout, an occupational hazard that is experienced by over one half of physicians and one third of nurses (Reith, 2018). Other effects of psychological trauma include depression, feelings of inadequacy, exhaustion, shame, distraction, low morale, cynicism, substance abuse, and suicide (Duffy et al., 2015; Joint Commission, 2018; Sirriyeh et al., 2010; Yung et al., 2012). Furthermore, negative consequences on the health care system include high rates of turnover, chronic absenteeism, increased medical errors, lower patient satisfaction, longer wait and patient recovery times, and increased overall costs (West et al., 2018).

Recommendations of the IEBPC include a system-wide, organized approach to addressing psychological trauma in health care workers. Health care organizations that implement interventions to address psychological trauma can reduce staff turnover and burnout, improve employee retention, decrease costs, and increase patient satisfaction. Leadership and stakeholder buy-in has been established. The next steps of the IEBPC include raising organizational awareness and developing an advisory committee to develop a peer support program to mitigate the negative effects of psychological trauma of health care workers.

Author's Commentary: Because the researchers are beginning their work on incorporating a system-wide approach to addressing psychological trauma in health care workers, this is an excellent opportunity for the team to consider the application of an implementation theory, model, or framework that would specifically guide the researchers' work in conceptualizing the implementation phase of the project. The researchers may want to consider the evidence-based implementation strategies as described by Cullen et al. (2018) in their work on evidence-based implementation strategies for sustainability, which captures specific interventions during the various phases of implementation (i.e., create awareness and interest, build knowledge and commitment, promote action and adoption, and pursue integration and sustained use).

References

Cullen, L., Hanrahan, K., Farrington, M., DeBerg, J., Tucker, S., & Kleiber, C. (2018). *Evidence-based practice in action: Comprehensive strategies, tools, and tips from the University of Iowa Hospitals and Clinics.* Sigma Theta Tau International.

Duffy, E., Avalos, G., & Dowling, M. (2015). Secondary traumatic stress among emergency nurses: A cross-sectional study. *International Emergency Nursing*, 23, 53-58. https://doi.org.10.1016/j.ienj.2014.05.001

Joint Commission. (2018). Supporting second victims. jointcommission.org

Portoghese, I., Galletta, M., Coppola, R., & Finco, G. (2014). Burnout and workload among health care workers: The moderating role for job control. *Safety and Health at Work*, 5, 152-157. https://doi.org/10.1016/j.shaw.2014.05.004

Reith, T. (2018). Burnout in United States healthcare professionals: a narrative review. *Cureus*, *10*(12), e3681. https://doi.org/10.7759/cureus.3681

Sirriyeh, R., Lawton, R., Gardner, P., & Armitage, G. (2010). Coping with medical error: A systematic review of papers to assess the effects of involvement in medical errors on healthcare professionals' psychological well-being. *Quality Safety in Healthcare*, 19(6), e43. https://doi.org/10.1136/qahc.2009.035253

West, C., Dyrbye, L., & Shanafelt, T. (2018). Physician burnout: Contributors, consequences, and solutions. *Journal of Internal Medicine*, 281, 516-529. https://doi.org/10.1111/joim.12752

Yung, Y., Fix, M., Hevelone, N., Lipsitz, S., Greenberg, C., & Weissman, J. (2012). Physicians' needs in coping with emotional stressors. *JAMA Surgery*, 147(3), 212-217 https://doi.org/10.1001/archsurg.2011.312

Exemplar 11-4

Implementing New Informed Consent Practices for Pediatric Coronavirus Disease 2019 Clinical Trials: Innovations, Collaborations, Resilience, and Team Science During a Pandemic

Carolynn Thomas Jones, DNP, MSPH, RN, FAAN

Mallory E. Rowell, MS, BSN, RN

> **Domains:** implementation research characteristics; theories, models, and frameworks; determinants of implementation—contextual factors; implementation strategies; implementation outcomes; service and patient outcomes

When the disease severe acute respiratory syndrome coronavirus 2, also known as *COVID-19*, emerged in January 2020, health care systems and clinical research departments were challenged on multiple fronts. Patient care and operational and clinical research expectations were initially based on reports from China and Europe. It was difficult to imagine that this pandemic would land in the United States at such a rapid and intense force. In response, U.S. researchers quickly launched COVID-19–related preclinical and clinical trials for both adult and pediatric populations. The clinical research challenges were to rapidly diagnose cases (requiring studies on diagnostic test assays); test the population at large; perform contact tracing; find best treatments to mitigate disease impact; and collect specimens to learn about the biology and genetics of the virus itself, the effectiveness of immune response and antibodies, postinfection, convalescent plasma, and new clinical trials for antivirals and vaccines. Before COVID-19, clinical trials were conducted within a strict set of regulations for institutional review board (IRB) approval, informed consenting, and risk-based monitoring. Participants (whether adult or children) were seen in person (in the hospital room or clinic) during specified study visits, and data were obtained through testing, observations of signs and symptoms, and other study-required methods. Protocols remained relatively static, although sometimes amendments were required when new information came about.

Between January and July 2020, more than 548 COVID-19 studies have been registered in clinicaltrials.gov. With COVID-19, everyone in the health care, regulatory, and clinical trial enterprise was jettisoned onto the "COVID fast train" to innovation, communication, and team science while also ensuring participant safety and study integrity in clinical trials. Mitigating patient infection was paramount, and many treatments, tests, and surgeries were canceled and put on hold. At a Children's Hospital, during the local arrival of COVID-19, there was initial reluctance to further disrupt the already stressed hospital floors with COVID-19 clinical trials. Nurse managers were appreciably concerned about personal protective equipment (PPE), staffing, infection control, shutdowns, and multiple meetings. Yet, clinical trials in COVID-19 were essential and especially affected emergency departments (EDs), hospital floors, and intensive care units (ICUs). Moreover, IRBs were tasked

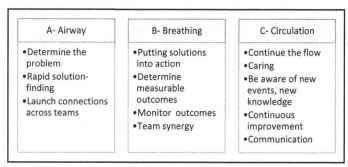

A- Airway	B- Breathing	C- Circulation
•Determine the problem •Rapid solution-finding •Launch connections across teams	•Putting solutions into action •Determine measurable outcomes •Monitor outcomes •Team synergy	•Continue the flow •Caring •Be aware of new events, new knowledge •Continuous improvement •Communication

Figure 11-3.

with unique problem solving, being given new "daily" regulatory challenges. Study coordinators and clinical research nurses were obtaining informed consent and assessing COVID-19 patients for study eligibility; yet, they were often having to rely on hospital staff to conduct study tasks because at first research staff were initially not allowed access to the patient rooms. Moreover, research staff, being from a different department, lacked PPE supplies. Learning the effective use of PPE and to manage a new supply chain for PPE acquisition was required to operationalize research activities safely and inserted unexpected clinical research department costs. Patient family members and caregivers were segregated from the patient and were not allowed in the building. The COVID-19 virus itself was a moving target. Because it was a novel virus, little was known about it. As new information about this RNA virus and its effect on patients emerged, protocols changed rapidly, with at least one protocol change per week per study. For example, knowledge of influenza and respiratory syncytial virus gave investigators a starting point for targeting assessments of signs and symptoms; however, new information on the negative effects of the virus on sensory taste and smell required adjustments to assessments and case report forms. Moreover, study visit schedules required flexibility, and IRBs became amenable to risk-based approaches to handling protocol deviations and new approvals. To keep up with the response pace, real-time approvals were needed.

Proper informed consent and pediatric assent are key requirements in protecting human participants in clinical research. Required social distancing led to restrictions whereby hospitalized pediatric patients were often segregated from their family members, necessitating alternative consenting measures. Verbal telephone consents and the use of DocuSign for consent signatures were implemented, also requiring rapid regulatory approval and special consent witnessing. This was a new process that heretofore had been against policy. At the center of the pandemic, the adoption of team science approaches and strong communication planning were essential, especially with the numerous policy and process changes that were occurring. As the number of COVID-19 trials increased, an institutional plan to consolidate studies was implemented so that patients and their family members were not approached by multiple study team members at one time seeking informed consent. Emerging pediatric issues related to organ damage, neurologic manifestations, and cardiovascular and circulatory complications began to be noticed. What was initially thought to be best practice was replaced with new evidence-based approaches from research that was being disseminated in real time.

To assist researchers and sponsors to manage clinical trials during COVID-19, guidance documents emerged from the U.S. Food and Drug Administration, Centers for Disease Control and Prevention, and other clinical trial experts and IRBs. One article suggested that the COVID-19 response to clinical trial management was like a code blue and developed an "A-B-C" algorithm to keep moving forward effectively (Lee et al., 2020; Figure 11-3).

Using the University of Iowa implementation strategy methods (Cullen & Adams, 2012), the complexities of evolving new practices for informed consent during a pandemic are illustrated (Figure 11-4). These strategies have been reported as future innovative practices before COVID-19

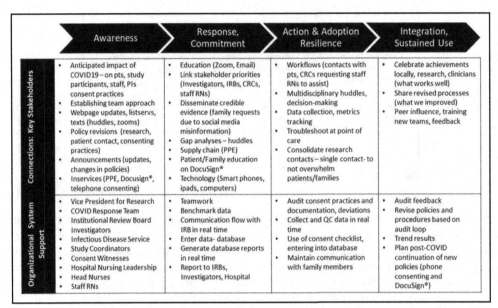

	Awareness	Response, Commitment	Action & Adoption Resilience	Integration, Sustained Use
Connections: Key Stakeholders	• Anticipated impact of COVID19 – on pts, study participants, staff, PIs consent practices • Establishing team approach • Webpage updates, listservs, texts (huddles, zooms) • Policy revisions (research, patient contact, consenting practices) • Announcements (updates, changes in policies) • Inservices (PPE, Docusign®, telephone consenting)	• Education (Zoom, Email) • Link stakeholder priorities (Investigators, IRBs, CRCs, staff RNs) • Disseminate credible evidence (family requests due to social media misinformation) • Gap analyses – huddles • Supply chain (PPE) • Patient/Family education on DocuSign® • Technology (Smart phones, ipads, computers)	• Workflows (contacts with pts, CRCs requesting staff RNs to assist) • Multidisciplinary huddles, decision-making • Data collection, metrics tracking • Troubleshoot at point of care • Consolidate research contacts – single contact- to not overwhelm patients/families	• Celebrate achievements locally, research, clinicians (what works well) • Share revised processes (what we improved) • Peer influence, training new teams, feedback
Organizational System Support	• Vice President for Research • COVID Response Team • Institutional Review Board • Investigators • Infectious Disease Service • Study Coordinators • Consent Witnesses • Hospital Nursing Leadership • Head Nurses • Staff RNs	• Teamwork • Benchmark data • Communication flow with IRB in real time • Enter data- database • Generate database reports in real time • Report to IRBs, Investigators, Hospital	• Audit consent practices and documentation, deviations • Collect and QC data in real time • Use of consent checklist, entering into database • Maintain communication with family members	• Audit feedback • Revise policies and procedures based on audit loop • Trend results • Plan post-COVID continuation of new policies (phone consenting and DocuSign®)

Figure 11-4. The implementation strategy for revised consent practices during coronavirus disease 2019. (Adapted with permission from Cullen, L. & Adams, S. [2012]. Planning for Implementation of Evidence-Based Practice. *Journal of Nursing Administration, 42*(4), 222-230.)

but had not gained traction with academic medical center IRBs or the FDA until the pandemic struck.

The FDA published a guidance document with newly approved allowances for protocol deviations, new informed consent processes using technology, and telemedicine study visits. The new consent innovations arising out of the COVID-19 clinical trials resulted in disruptive but long-awaited changes for current and upcoming trials (Ross, 2020). As COVID-19 clinical trials continued to increase, other academic medical centers began to report evolving approvals for the use of remote consenting (Rai & Frei, 2020). The University of Minnesota Clinical and Translational Science Institute published their use of a remote signature for consenting using REDcap (Reseach Electronic Data Capture), achieving an unprecedented 10-day approval by their IRB (University of Minnesota Clinical and Translational Science Institute, n.d.). The use of remote consenting and DocuSign at this institution paves the way for other types of innovations and pragmatic clinical trial methods. The connections between teams and effective communication planning have set the stage for future collaborations and confidence to continue conducting effective studies in COVID-19 within the ever-changing pandemic landscape. Continuous improvement assessments included conversations concerning the following: "What did we do?" "What went well?" "What bioethical issues are arising?" "What can we do better?" and "What do we know today that we did not know yesterday?" These remain agenda items for the frequent Zoom meetings and huddles associated with the COVID-19 response. Implementing new informed consent practices is just one of the rapid innovations required for clinical research and clinical care in pediatric COVID-19 patients. Key words for implementing new clinical research practices during a pandemic include knowledge, flexibility, resilience, creativity, communication, team science, accountability, caring, safety, and documentation.

Authors' Commentary: The researchers did excellent work in identifying an evidence-based model (University of Iowa) as well as incorporating implementation strategies from the phases of implementation proposed by Cullen et al. (2018). In the future, the researchers may want to consider the work of Brownson et al. (2012) specific to the taxonomy of dissemination and implementation outcomes. Reviewing the outcomes (i.e., acceptability, reach, feasibility) could provide additional dimensions for successful sustainment of the use of their informed consent practices.

References

Brownson, R. C., Colditz, G. A., & Proctor, E. K. (Eds.). (2012). *Dissemination and implementation research in health: Translating science to practice.* Oxford University Press.

Cullen, L., & Adams, S. L. (2012). Planning for implementation of evidence-based practice. *The Journal of Nursing Administration, 42*(4), 222–230. https://doi.org/10.1097/NNA.0b013e31824ccd0a

Cullen, L., Hanrahan, K., Farrington, M., DeBerg, J., Tucker, S., & Kleiber, C. (2018). *Evidence-based practice in action: Comprehensive strategies, tools, and tips from the University of Iowa Hospitals and Clinics.* Sigma Theta Tau International.

Lee, J. Y., Hong, J. H., & Park, E. Y. (2020). Beyond the fear: Nurses' experiences caring for patients with Middle East respiratory syndrome: A phenomenological study. *Journal of Clinical Nursing, 29*(17-18), 3349–3362. https://doi.org/10.1111/jocn.15366

Rai, A.T., & Frei, D. J. (2020). A rationale and framework for seeking remote electronic or phone consent approval in endovascular stroke trials – special relevance in the COVID-19 environment and beyond. *J NeuroIntervent Surg, 12*(7), 654-657. https://doi.org10.1136/neurintsurg-2020-016221

Ross, J. (2020). The exacerbation of burnout during COVID-19: A major concern for nurse safety. *Journal of PeriAnesthesia Nursing, 35*(4), 439–440. https://doi.org/10.1016/j.jopan.2020.04.001

University of Minnesota Clinical and Translational Science Institute. (n.d.). https://ctsi.umn.edu/

Exemplar 11-5

BEST PRACTICES FOR EMBEDDING IMPLEMENTATION SCIENCE IN DOCTOR OF NURSING PRACTICE PROJECTS

Linda A. Roussel, PhD, RN, NEA-BC, CNL, FAAN

Jeannie Scruggs Corey, DNP, RN, NEA-BC

Domains: theories, models, and frameworks; implementation strategies; implementation outcomes

BACKGROUND

Bauer et al. (2015) described IS as the scientific study of methods to facilitate the systematic uptake of research findings and other EBPs into routine practice with the purpose to improve the quality and effectiveness of patient care and health system's services. Quality improvement and dissemination methods share common elements with IS, but there are differences. Specifically, implementation studies use a mix of methods that include both quantitative-qualitative designs and identify factors that impact uptake across multiple levels, including patient, provider, clinic, facility, organization, and often the broader community and policy environment. A solid grounding in theory and the involvement of transdisciplinary research teams are essential to IS. DNP project outcomes are expected to create impact and be sustainable over time. DNP project outcomes focus on improving patient safety, quality of care, and organizational systems. EBP practice and quality improvement methodological frameworks are the underpinning of DNP projects. It is imperative to incorporate IS frameworks into DNP projects to provide a principled approach when executing evidence-based implementation strategies.

When IS is not a key component of the DNP project, DNP projects may not be sustainable. Two faculty from two different schools retrospectively reviewed a sampling of DNP projects with the intent of determining the use of theories, frameworks, and models from the field of IS. Additionally, faculty were concerned about the rigor and fidelity of implementation strategies described in DNP projects and the research evidence and methods selected. Faculty developed an audit tool for the retrospective review. The conclusion at both universities was that there was a lack of use of clearly documented IS concepts in most DNP projects that were reviewed. There is a need for intentional use of IS strategies in DNP projects to create rigor, impact, sustainability, and the potential for replication of work.

Purpose

The overall goal for the quality improvement project was to determine the degree to which DNP projects in two universities embedded theories, models, and frameworks from IS and used evidence-based implementation strategies.

Methods

A PDSA methodological framework was used in conducting this project to determine the use of theories, models, and frameworks from IS as well as identifying evidence-based implementation strategies in DNP projects at two university DNP programs. A faculty-developed audit tool was used to retrospectively review a sampling of DNP projects using descriptive statistics to determine the degree to which IS is a part of DNP project development and evaluation.

Findings/Results

The results revealed a lack of consistency in the use of theories, models, and frameworks from IS from both universities. Although students outlined their implementation plan for their DNP projects, there was limited attention to the "why" and "how" of the students' decision-making process in selecting specific implementation strategies. There was a lack of alignment of theoretical underpinning of identified strategies for implementing DNP projects.

Implications for Practice

Implications for practice and education are described as important to fidelity in replicating EBP guidelines and protocols. This is critical to creating sustainable and scalable DNP projects.

> *Authors' Commentary:* The faculty identify their quality improvement project and use an implementation framework to integrate their intervention strategies. Should the faculty continue their work (additional PDSA cycles), they may want to consider the evidence-based implementation strategies as described by Cullen et al. (2018) in their work on evidence-based implementation strategies for sustainability, which captures specific interventions during the various phases of implementation (i.e., create awareness and interest, build knowledge and commitment, promote action and adoption, and pursue integration and sustained use).

References

Bauer, M. S., Damschroder, L., Hagedorn, H., Smith, J., & Kilbourne, A. M. (2015). An introduction to implementation science for the nonspecialist. *BMC Psychology, 16*, 3-32. https://doi.org/10.1186/s40359-015-0089-9

Cullen, L., Hanrahan, K., Farrington, M., DeBerg, J., Tucker, S., & Kleiber, C. (2018). *Evidence-based practice in action: Comprehensive strategies, tools, and tips from the University of Iowa Hospitals and Clinics.* Sigma Theta Tau International.

Exemplar 11-6

Evidence-Based Best Practice for Decreasing Inappropriate Referrals to a Comprehensive Vascular Access Team

Somali Nguyen, DNP, CRNP, AGACNP-BC
April Garrigan, DNP, APRN, FNP-BC
Shea Polancich, PhD, RN, FAAN

Domains: implementation strategies; implementation outcomes; service and patient outcomes

Background

At ACME University Hospital, a comprehensive vascular access team (CVAT) was created in 2017 to reduce delays in medical therapy, specifically therapy involving fluid management and medication administration. The CVAT serves as a specialty consult team for intravascular (IV) access and other more advanced vascular access procedures, such as peripheral IV accesses, ultrasound-guided peripheral IV (USGPIV) catheters, modified Seldinger technique midlines, peripherally inserted central catheters, and central venous lines as appropriate for patients' treatment plans.

The Problem

In 2018, the CVAT received more than 2,200 consults for peripheral IV access from hospital staff. This figure represented approximately 25% percentage of all consults to the CVAT. During this time period, RN/staff nurses in the ED were requesting a higher volume of CVAT consultations, not only for peripheral IV accesses but also for laboratory work, on patients who were not considered difficult IV access opportunities, in turn increasing the CVAT volume. The ED nursing staff would most often avoid attempts at peripheral IV placement in three specific patient populations: adults with a history of chronic kidney disease, patients with end-stage renal failure, and patients with morbid obesity. This pattern of consults resulted in a higher volume of inappropriate consults and an inefficient use of CVAT resources.

Evidence-Based Application

Provider attempts at establishing vascular access using superficially visible veins, palpation of deeper veins, and the identification of landmarks while blindly inserting an IV device with a goal of successful cannulation of the appropriate vascular structure have been the norm (Bahl et al., 2016). This blind technique often renders multiple unsuccessful attempts at establishing vascular access, which may result in delayed medication administration, dissatisfied patients, and physician intervention, likely ending with unnecessary central venous line insertions for difficult-to-access patients (Bahl et al., 2016).

Recent studies have shown that USGPIV accesses are equally as dependable and as safe as, if not superior to, the IV lines inserted using the blind technique (Saltarelli et al., 2015; Warrington et al., 2012; Witting et al., 2017).

IMPROVEMENT INTERVENTION

Using the PDSA (Institute for Healthcare Improvement, n.d.; Langley et al., 2009) small test of change improvement model as the methodological framework for the improvement, two APRNs with ED and CVAT experience developed an improvement intervention to target staff nurse training and competency assessment for using USGPIV placement. Participants were provided training sessions within the organization's simulation laboratory. The project team APRNs led the sessions, which included a review on IV insertion skills, an overview of basic ultrasound functions, and a combination of implementing the two skills simultaneously. A 25% decrease in total CVAT consultation and placement volume for peripheral IV access indicated a successful improvement project. Percentage measurement was derived before the project implementation and at the end of a 6-week observation period after training and competency assessment of the ED nursing staff.

DATA COLLECTION AND FINDINGS

Descriptive statistics (frequency and percentage) were used to analyze the project results. Using April and May 2019 as a baseline, the CVAT inserted 438 USGPIV accesses during the 2-month time period, which averaged approximately 219 peripheral IV placements per month. During the intervention time period between June 1, 2019, and July 15, 2019, the CVAT and the ED RNs placed a total of 430 USGPIV lines. The CVAT placed 341 of the 430, 79% of the USGPIV lines. Of the total 430 USGPIV lines placed during the intervention time frame, the ED RNs placed a total of 89 peripheral IV catheters, resulting in a 21% decrease in CVAT consults and placements.

CONCLUSION

Using an evidence-based approach for improvement is an effective method to decrease the number of inappropriate referrals to a CVAT. The project team found that because of the simulation training and competency validation, ED RNs using the USGPIV technique decreased the total volume of CVAT consults for peripheral IV insertion. Although the project goal of a 25% reduction in the referrals and use of the CVAT for peripheral IV placement was not met, the team did observe a 21% decrease in CVAT referrals and placement for peripheral IV lines over 6 weeks. The improvement team believed that although the 21% decrease in consults and placement of peripheral IV lines by the CVAT failed to be statistically significant, the outcome was clinically significant.

> ***Authors' Commentary:*** This well-designed quality improvement project could be further informed by the application of an implementation theory, model, or framework that would specifically guide the researchers' work in conceptualizing the implementation phase of the project. Guided by phases of the PDSA, the researchers may want to consider the evidence-based implementation strategies as described by Cullen et al. (2018) in their work on evidence-based implementation strategies for sustainability, which captures specific interventions during the various phases of implementation (i.e., create awareness and interest, build knowledge and commitment, promote action and adoption, and pursue integration and sustained use).

REFERENCES

Bahl, A., Pandurangadu, A. V., Tucker, J., & Bagan, M. (2016). A randomized controlled trial assessing the use of ultrasound for nurse performed IV placement in difficult access ED patients. *American Journal of Emergency Medicine, 34*(10), 1950-1954. https://doi.org/o.1016/j.ajem.2016.06.098

Cullen, L., Hanrahan, K., Farrington, M., DeBerg, J., Tucker, S., & Kleiber, C. (2018). *Evidence-based practice in action: Comprehensive strategies, tools, and tips from the University of Iowa Hospitals and Clinics.* Sigma Theta Tau International.

Institute for Healthcare Improvement. (n.d.). http://www.ihi.org/resources/Pages/Tools/PlanDoStudyActWorksheet.aspx

Langley, G., Moen, R., Nolan, K., Nolan, T., Norman, C., & Provost, L. (2009). The improvement guide: A practical approach to enhancing organizational performance (2nd ed.). Jossey-Bass.

Saltarelli, N. A., VanHouten, J., Boyd, J., Rupp, J., & Ferre, R. M. (2015). Infiltration rates are similar in ultrasound-guided and traditionally placed peripheral IVs in admitted emergency department patients with difficult IV access. *Annals of Emergency Medicine, 66*, S137.

Warrington, W. G., Aragon Penoyer, D., Kamps, T. A., & Van Hoeck, E. H. (2012). Outcomes of using a modified Seldinger technique for long term intravenous therapy in hospitalized patients with difficult venous access. *Journal of the Association for Vascular Access, 17*(1), 24-30.

Witting, M. D., Moayedi, S., Dunning, K., Babin, L. S., & Cogan, B. M. (2017). Power injection through ultrasound-guided intravenous lines: Safety and efficacy under an institutional protocol. *Journal of Emergency Medicine, 52*(1), 16-22.

Exemplar 11-7

PATIENT SAFETY IMPLEMENTATION

Jaclyn Castano, MSN, RN, CPPS

Domains: theories, models, and frameworks; determinants of implementation—contextual factors; implementation strategies; implementation outcomes

Adverse events are unanticipated events that affect a patient leading to the categorizations of no harm, mild harm, moderate harm, severe harm, permanent harm, or death (Williams et al., 2015). The patient safety role is an integral part of learning from these errors. This is done through a systematic approach instead of an individual approach to find process variation and search for a sustainable mitigation. Patient safety works to identify opportunities to mitigate harm to a patient and continuously reviews actions taken to protect patients. This is a step toward the journey of prevention along with becoming a high reliability organization (HRO). An HRO is preoccupied with failure, is reluctant to simplify, is sensitive to operations, practices deference to expertise, and is committed to resiliency (Agency for Healthcare Research and Quality, 2019).

PATIENT SAFETY AND THE SWISS CHEESE THEORY

Along with HRO principles, the organization has chosen to use the Swiss cheese theory to assist in understanding why errors occur and develop or adjust system processes that take as much of the human factor out of the decision making as possible. The theory behind the Swiss cheese process is that active failures, which have immediate effects and latent conditions, can influence the situation (Larouzee & Guarnieri, 2015). In this theory, errors can be prevented through defense layers implemented throughout the system. These defense layers provide a barrier until a variation in process or change in conditions allows for a vulnerability in the defense (Neuhaus et al., 2018). The Swiss cheese theory lends itself to the thought that if defenses are implemented and staff and leadership are involved, then fewer errors should occur. Leadership support or lack of support can create an environment where trust is built or damaged, which can lead to other errors occurring.

PATIENT SAFETY REPORTING

An organization creates an environment focused on patient safety when combining the two concepts of HRO and the Swiss cheese theory. A way to apply these concepts in a proactive light is through the Patient Safety Reporting (PSR) system. The PSR system is a reactive form of annotation offering the staff an opportunity to anonymously report a patient safety concern, whether it reached the patient or was a near-miss report. In an HRO setting, reporting is encouraged to learn about

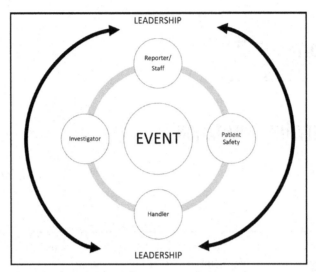

Figure 11-5. The Patient Safety Reporting cycle.

organization failures and the reluctance to simplify. The PSR also encourages transparency and creates a standardized process to decrease variability throughout the organization. When a report is submitted, it allows both the frontline staff and the leadership to be involved in finding a sustainable solution for the organization.

PATIENT SAFETY REPORTING LEADERSHIP CONCEPT

The question that has been discussed is how to create an environment where preventable harm is emphasized in the hospital setting. The current concept behind the PSR system is linear, which does not allow for the continuous review. In the process improvement initiative, the PSR Leadership Concept, the flow is in a circular direction, which encourages continuous reviewing of the process (Figure 11-5). When applying the PSR Leadership Concept to the current PSR process, leadership organization failures and the reluctance to simplify. The PSR also encourages transparency and creates a standardized process to decrease variability throughout the organization. When a report is submitted, it allows both the frontline staff and the leadership to be involved in finding a sustainable solution for the organization.

PATIENT SAFETY REPORTING LEADERSHIP CONCEPT

The question that has been discussed is how to create an environment where preventable harm is emphasized in the hospital setting. The current concept behind the PSR system is linear, which does not allow for the continuous review. In the process improvement initiative, the PSR Leadership Concept, the flow is in a circular direction, which encourages continuous reviewing of the process (Figure 11-5). When applying the PSR Leadership Concept to the current PSR process, leadership is involved earlier in the process. This encourages full support and resources in implementing any changes that may need to be applied to the process and distributing information throughout the enterprise. Adding leaders to this process encourages a full understanding of the root cause of the adverse event and provides the support to create and sustain implementations of changes. Ultimately, with the use of the PSR Leadership Concept, preventable harm is continuously brought to the forefront of all employees, handlers, investigators, and leadership.

IMPLEMENTATION

The implementation process occurred over 1 year. It specifically focused on decreasing the number of patient safety reports, which were overdue. The initial step in the implementation plan was to share with hospital leaders what the current data showed for overdue patient safety reports and overall open patient safety reports. This was completed through the performance improvement update brief. From there, a strategy was put in place to provide a monthly PSR 101 training to facilitate learning how to thoroughly investigate a report. Approximately 75 staff members have been trained. The patient safety team reviewed and updated the PSR contact handler and investigator list to ensure contacts were available to complete the PSR. To ensure leadership understood their role and the importance of the PSR process, the chief of patient safety presented this information at the three main patient care hospital sections' monthly meetings. The leaders were requested to begin asking for PSR data and trends from their junior leaders to assist in focusing their process improvement planning. An avenue to reach junior leaders was through the patient safety functional management team. During this monthly meeting, PSR data and trends were discussed, along with the importance of completing a thorough investigation in a timely manner. Finally, to specifically focus on the overdue patient safety reports, the list was sent to the executive level leaders on a weekly basis, with the overall open PSR list being sent to the handlers and investigators. The overdue patient safety report numbers went from 305 in June 2019 to 11 PSRs in September 2020, and the total open patient safety reports went from 255 in July 2019 to 59 in September 2020.

This author can attribute the success of this process improvement implementation to several things. First was the continuous application of the HRO principles—reporting to learn and increase transparency. These two principles allow the entire organization to learn from an error that may have occurred in one location, minimizing the silo affect that has occurred in the past. Second was the increased leadership dedication to learning from the reports. This shows the organization that each report is taken seriously and can be applied to create further improvement in the organization. Third, an increased focus on education and facilitating accountability throughout the organization was accomplished with assistance from the patient safety team. Focusing efforts on the "why" and the "how" behind the PSR process further aids in the staff's understanding and desire to continue to report to learn.

Author's Commentary: In the future, the researcher may want to consider the work of Brownson et al. (2012) specific to the taxonomy of dissemination and implementation outcomes. Reviewing the outcomes (i.e., acceptability, reach, feasibility) could provide additional dimensions for successful sustainment of the use of the patient safety team. The researcher may want to consider the evidence-based implementation strategies as described by Cullen et al. (2018) in their work on evidence-based implementation strategies for sustainability, which captures specific interventions during the various phases of implementation (i.e., create awareness and interest, build knowledge and commitment, promote action and adoption, and pursue integration and sustained use). It may also be useful for the team to consider the application of an implementation theory, model, or framework that would specifically guide the researcher's work in furthering this work.

REFERENCES

Agency for Healthcare Research and Quality. (2019). Patient safety network: High reliability. https://psnet.ahrq.gov/primer/high-reliability

Brownson, R. C., Colditz, G. A., & Proctor, E. K. (Eds.). (2012). *Dissemination and implementation research in health: Translating science to practice*. Oxford University Press.

Cullen, L., Hanrahan, K., Farrington, M., DeBerg, J., Tucker, S., & Kleiber, C. (2018). *Evidence-based practice in action: Comprehensive strategies, tools, and tips from the University of Iowa Hospitals and Clinics*. Sigma Theta Tau International.

Larouzee, J., & Guarnieri, F. (2015). From theory to practice: Itinerary of Reason's Swiss cheese model. Centre of Research on Risks and Crises (MINES Paristech).

Neuhaus, C., Huck, M., Hofmann, G., Pierre, M. S., Weigand, M. A., & Lichtenstern, C. (2018). Applying the human factors analysis and classification system to critical incident reports in anesthesiology. *Acta Anaesthesiologica Scandinavica, 62*(10), 1403-1411. https://doi.org/10.1111/aas.13213

Williams, T., Szekendi, M., Pavkovic, S., Clevenger, W., & Cerese, J. (2015). The reliability of AHRQ common format harm scales in rating patient safety events. *Journal of Patient Safety, 11*(1), 52-59.

Exemplar 11-8

INTERPROFESSIONAL EVIDENCE-BASED PRACTICE COUNCIL FOR COLLABORATIVE PRACTICE

Donna Copeland, DNP, RN, NE-BC, CPN, CPON, AE-C

Domains: determinants of implementation—contextual factors; implementation strategies

To foster the principles of both interprofessional collaboration and EBP in a hospital setting, there must be shared leadership, collective decision making, and effective communication and teamwork (Quality and Safety Education for Nurses, 2018). Thus, an academic–practice partnership was formed to develop and implement an IEBPC. The goal of the council was to engage and empower an interprofessional team of frontline staff in the translation of best available evidence to foster a healthy work environment. The creation of an interprofessional EBP council is unique in that many shared governance councils are nurse driven; however, few have taken an interprofessional approach (Harper et al., 2017).

Hospital administrative support for the project was established, and preliminary data were collected to understand the current beliefs, knowledge, and organizational readiness for change. Data revealed that both frontline staff and leadership regarded EBP as essential; however, EBP competencies and implementation were incongruent between frontline staff and leadership. Furthermore, both the staff and leadership described the culture as needing improvements in the widespread efforts for implementing EBP. Thus, a steering committee was formed to develop the structure of the IEBPC including (a) the mission, purpose, goals, and bylaws; (b) a leadership and reporting structure; (c) an orientation manual for IEBPC members; (d) an organizational EBP appraisal tool; and (e) a curriculum for training staff and leadership on EBP and interprofessional collaboration. Staff input and feedback were critical to creating an environment of shared leadership, and an interprofessional structure allows for ownership of all disciplines in achieving a healthy work environment.

Author's Commentary: The researcher may want to consider the evidence-based implementation strategies as described by Cullen et al. (2018) in their work on evidence-based implementation strategies for sustainability, which captures specific interventions during the various phases of implementation (i.e., create awareness and interest, build knowledge and commitment, promote action and adoption, and pursue integration and sustained use). It may also be useful for the researcher to consider the application of an implementation theory, model, or framework that would specifically guide the researcher's work in furthering this work. In the future, the researcher may want to consider the work of Brownson et al. (2012) specific to the taxonomy of dissemination and implementation outcomes. Reviewing the outcomes (i.e., acceptability, reach, feasibility) could provide additional dimensions for the research.

References

Brownson, R. C., Colditz, G. A., & Proctor, E. K. (Eds.). (2012). *Dissemination and implementation research in health: Translating science to practice*. Oxford University Press.

Cullen, L., Hanrahan, K., Farrington, M., DeBerg, J., Tucker, S., & Kleiber, C. (2018). *Evidence-based practice in action: Comprehensive strategies, tools, and tips from the University of Iowa Hospitals and Clinics*. Sigma Theta Tau International.

Harper, M., Gallagher-Ford, L., Warren, J., Troseth, M., Sinnot, L., & Thomas, B. K. (2017) Evidence-based practice and U.S. healthcare outcomes: Findings from a national survery with nursing professional development practicioners. Journal for Nurses in Professional Development, 33, 170-179. https://doi.org/10.1097/nnd.0000000000000360

Quality and Saftey Education for Nurses. (2018). QSEN competencies: Overview. http://qsen.org/competencies/pre-licensure-ksas/

Exemplar 11-9

Implementing P6 Acupressure in Conjunction With Pharmacotherapy to Decrease Chemotherapy-Induced Nausea and Vomiting: A Nurse-Led Evidence-Based Practice Initiative to Improve Care and Quality of Life

Megan Maloney, RN, BSN, DNC
Mary L. Schumann, RN, MA, AOCN, OCN
Heather Ugolini, BSN, RN

Domains: implementation strategies; service and patient outcomes; implementation outcomes; stakeholder involvement and engagement

A nursing team came together with the goal of improving the care of patients with chemotherapy-induced nausea and vomiting (CINV) using an EBP approach. At one large National Cancer Institute–designated cancer center, data from the first two quarters of 2018 showed that 58% of patients seen in the ED for nausea and/or vomiting required admission, and the primary method of management was pharmacologic interventions. Using these data, the following PICOT (Population, Intervention, Comparison, Outcome, Time) question was formulated: In patients with CINV, how do pharmacotherapy interventions compared with pharmacotherapy with acupressure affect nausea and/or vomiting?

A literature search was conducted using PubMed, CINAHL, and Cochrane over a 5-year period (2012-2017). The key word search included the following terms: chemotherapy-induced nausea and vomiting, nonpharmacologic interventions, patient satisfaction, length of stay, alternative therapies, complementary therapies, complementary and alternative method, cost, nurse, patient, acupressure, and side effects. The search identified 39 articles, and after the initial screening, three were eliminated because of a lack of relevance to the topic of acupressure and CINV. Four additional articles were identified from references and added for a total of 41 "keeper" articles. Critical appraisal of the articles demonstrated a high level of evidence; 22% were Level 1 systematic reviews, 39% were Level 2 randomized controlled trials, and the remaining 39% were between Level 3 and Level 7.

A review of the literature revealed that nonpharmacologic interventions showed varied results. Most studies compared various types of complementary therapies while using standard antiemetic medications. Interventions included acupuncture, P6 acupressure (digital/wristbands), auricular acupressure, aromatherapy, inhaled ginger, and ingested ginger. Of these interventions, P6 acupressure, when added to standard antiemetics, emerged as an effective intervention for CINV. Twenty-one studies found P6 acupressure to decrease both acute and delayed CINV. Four of the reviewed articles demonstrated no statistical significance of a decrease in CINV; however, subjectively, patients reported a decrease in symptoms. Using acupressure to the P6 point was noninvasive, safe, effective, low cost, and without undesirable side effects.

As part of the external evidence search, seven comparable cancer centers were contacted, and responses were received from five. None of the responding centers were offering acupressure as a nonpharmacologic treatment for the control of CINV. Internal evidence identified different methods of complementary therapies being offered through the integrative medicine department. Services included acupuncture, massage, touch, and music therapies. Although acupressure was available, it was only used by patients who specifically requested it. Patient education on acupressure (both a written pamphlet and a video) was already available to staff and patients and was consistent with the evidence but was woefully underused. Providing multiple methods to teach this to patients (video, written, and demonstration) ensures patients with different learning styles could reduce CINV using P6 acupressure when used in conjunction with pharmacotherapy.

To ensure successful implementation, institution-wide involvement was essential. The team created a standard of care, which was presented to the shared governance councils. This provided an opportunity to expose nurses in these venues to the evidence and get their feedback on the implementation plan. Once approved, it was shared with the nursing staff institution wide via email. Acupressure education was then incorporated into the department of nursing orientation for new employees as well as the chemotherapy/biotherapy course. For sustainability, content was included in the annual required education program. Five different nursing documentation forms were updated to incorporate P6 acupressure in the electronic health record so that education and utilization of acupressure can be documented.

As frontline care providers, nurses are in a unique position to identify problems and offer solutions. The evidence-based approach offers the profession an opportunity to positively impact patient care. Our team was empowered by our organization, which led to this nurse-driven initiative being incorporated into the institution's standard of care for CINV.

ACKNOWLEDGMENTS

We would like to acknowledge the hard work of our colleagues Robell Calucag, BSN, RN, CPAN; Stephanie McEneaney, RN, MSN, OCN; and Natasha Ramrup, RN, MSN, AOCNS, OCN, who were instrumental in reviewing the evidence and implementing this change.

Authors' Commentary: In the future, the researchers may want to consider the evidence-based implementation strategies as described by Cullen et al. (2018) in their work on evidence-based implementation strategies for sustainability, which captures specific interventions during the various phases of implementation (i.e., create awareness and interest, build knowledge and commitment, promote action and adoption, and pursue integration and sustained use). The researchers may want to consider the work of Brownson et al. (2012) specific to the taxonomy of dissemination and implementation outcomes. Reviewing the outcomes (i.e., acceptability, reach, feasibility) could provide additional dimensions for successful sustainment of the use of a nurse-led EBP initiative. It may also be useful for the team to consider the application of an implementation theory, model, or framework that would specifically guide the researcher's work in furthering this work.

REFERENCES

Brownson, R. C., Colditz, G. A., & Proctor, E. K. (Eds.). (2012). *Dissemination and implementation research in health: Translating science to practice*. Oxford University Press.

Cullen, L., Hanrahan, K., Farrington, M., DeBerg, J., Tucker, S., & Kleiber, C. (2018). *Evidence-based practice in action: Comprehensive strategies, tools, and tips from the University of Iowa Hospitals and Clinics*. Sigma Theta Tau International.

Exemplar 11-10

DIVERSITY AND INCLUSION: BIAS IN PERIOPERATIVE CARE

Mercedes Weir, PhD, APRN, CRNA

Domains: determinants of implementation—contextual factors; implementation strategies

A patient is vulnerable once they enter the health care system (Medicine & Committee on Quality of Health Care in America, n.d.; Pelligrini, 2020). They are especially so in the perioperative area. The patient must trust that team to provide the best care, especially because at some point they may be rendered unconscious. Not only must the patient navigate myriad known and documented institutionally generated obstacles to safely exit the hospital or outpatient center, but also there are provider-influenced patient safety dangers largely unknown to the providers themselves.

Bias can be defined as a disproportionate preference for or prejudice against one thing, person, group, or idea, usually resulting in a judgment that is close minded or unfair (Stevenson & Lindberg, 2010). Explicit or conscious bias is described as attitudes or beliefs we hold on a conscious level and with sufficient belief in its accuracy to act on that judgment, whereas implicit or unconscious bias refers to the attitudes or stereotypes that unconsciously affect our understanding, actions, and decisions (Ruhl, 2020). Unconscious bias is insidious because it operates outside the full awareness of the provider. Although it is not easy to pinpoint, measure, or fix, there is sufficient evidence to suggest that implicit bias among health care professionals is a clear and present danger to patient safety and significantly affects patient care outcomes (FitzGerald & Hurst, 2017; Hall et al., 2015).

According to the *National Healthcare Disparities Report* (Agency for Healthcare Research and Quality, 2019a), in these United States, people of color continue to disproportionately face disparities in access to health care, quality of care, and health outcomes compared with White patients who receive better quality of care than Black, Hispanic, American Indian, and Asian patients. Addressing health disparities is increasingly important because the population is becoming more diverse. Projections are that people of color will comprise 52% of the population in 30 years, with the largest growth being among Hispanic individuals (Agency for Healthcare Research and Quality, 2019a).

I consented an older Mexican woman for a same-day surgical procedure at a hospital in Orlando, Florida. We used a certified translator via video as provided by the hospital. The patient was able to communicate in English but not sufficiently for complete understanding of the surgical and anesthesia consent. Her daughter was present and fluent in English but was not permitted to be used for the consent purposes. I speak rudimentary Spanish picked up from my Central American mother, high school and college courses, and providing health care services to a largely Cuban population in Miami for 20 years. The surgical technologist in the operating room (OR) happened to be fluent in Spanish and assisted with communication once we arrived in the room. We all had a very pleasant interaction, and the patient was anesthetized and awakened without incident. The OR RN and I took the patient to the recovery room and began with identification of the patient. Hearing the very Hispanic–sounding name, the postanesthesia care unit (PACU) RN interrupted the report, sighed aloud, and said, "I hope she speaks English." The patient, circulator, and I all looked at each other, and I saw the engaging pleasant patient retreat into a blank shell. I told the nurse that yes, the patient understands and speaks English, but it is not her preferred language. The PACU RN was visibly relieved upon hearing this information, received the rest of the information, and proceeded to assess the patient. As the OR RN and I left the patient, we could see that the patient fully understood that brief statement and that it had altered how the interaction with her nurse would proceed. When we left, she was responding with head movements only and avoiding eye contact or using words. The PACU RN stating her explicit bias aloud may have caused both the patient and the nurse to lean into their respective explicit and implicit biases about each other.

Before becoming a certified registered nurse anesthetist, I was a critical care RN at a Level 1 trauma center in Tennessee. During the holidays on the night shift, we would be ready, almost predictably at around 1 to 3 a.m., for the intoxication-related accidents. These could be botched suicide attempts, rattlesnake bites, shooting mishaps, or motor vehicle accidents. Nurses often remark on the likelihood of survival directly related to the number of tattoos (implicit bias?). Early on one such morning, we had a horrific incident. An imminently pregnant mother was traveling through with her husband after Thanksgiving dinner and got hit by a drunk driver headed the wrong direction on the interstate. The airbags deployed in her vehicle and ruptured her uterus; the 38-week baby (first) died, and the mother had her uterus removed. Her husband fractured his femur. The drunk driver had a concussion and was in a separate ICU in the same hospital, but they had him transferred to another hospital because of a visiting room altercation between families. I remember when they brought her beautiful baby girl, who had just passed away, to hold in her arms. I was her nurse; it was early in my career but unforgettable. I know that there may remain some implicit bias I hold toward drunk drivers to this day.

I am not alone in this. Everyone has explicitly or implicitly held biases. Most educational interventions rely on providers' awareness of the bias to address it, and although this may be effective for explicit bias, it is less so for implicit bias. Implicit bias begins to be ingrained from early ages and can possibly take years and a determined effort to ameliorate its effects. Factor in production pressures, an overburdened ineffective health care system, and cognitively overloaded providers in a pressured same-day surgery center, ED, or ICU and the likelihood of patients receiving biased and selective attention because of mental shortcuts and stereotyping increases.

Implementation Strategies

So, how do we combat an unseen enemy? First, be aware that it indeed exists. All health care providers presumably enter the profession vowing to treat "all patients equally" regardless of race or creed, but is this truly so? Implicit bias is an unseen, ubiquitous deterrent to patient safety. The Implicit Association Test is the most widely used and frequently cited of several measures used to assess implicit bias. Although this test has strengths and limitations, it, along with education, is a first step to awareness. Burgess et al. (2007; Figure 11-6) introduced a conceptual framework based on social cognitive psychology that may be helpful in attenuating bias.

Based on this framework, the following are some strategies and recommendations to help providers, particularly in the perioperative setting.

1. Acknowledge that bias is ever present in the human psyche, but we can work toward modulating our unconsciousness.
2. Take steps to understand your own implicit bias. Try taking the Implicit Association Test (https://implicit.harvard.edu/implicit/) and reading books (e.g., Banaji & Greenwald, 2016).
3. When interacting with patients who are different from you, strive to seek common ground.
4. Be especially conscious to exercise patience when caring for incapacitated patients.
5. Have concerted efforts to encourage hiring practices that will build a diverse, culturally competent team.

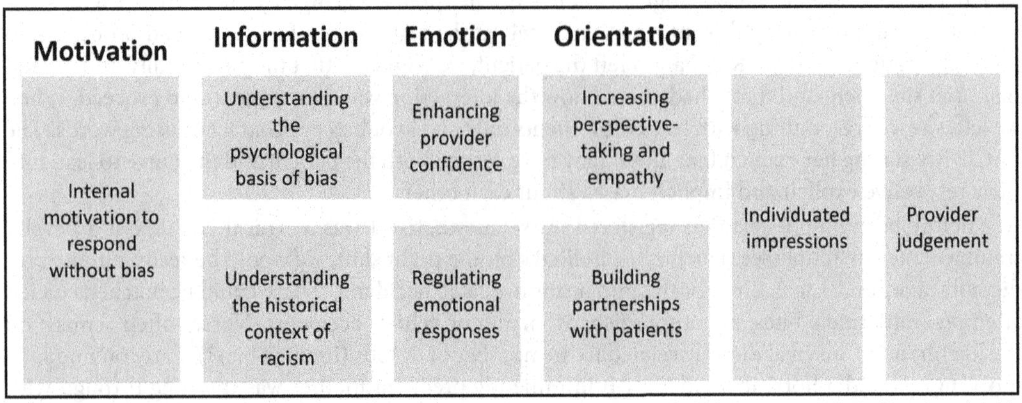

Figure 11-6. The conceptual framework for reducing racial bias among health care providers. (Reprinted with permission from Burgess, D., van Ryn, M., Dovidio, J., & Saha, S. [2007]. Reducing racial bias among health care providers: Lessons from social-cognitive psychology. *Journal of General Internal Medicine, 22*(6), 882-887. https://doi.org/10.1007/s11606-007-0160-1.)

6. Self-care is important. Be aware that our emotional state affects our ability to be empathetic to our patients.

7. Commit to using evidence-based protocols so that every patient who walks in with chest pain, for instance, is cared for the same.

8. Decide to grow and no longer be complicit due to a lack of self-awareness. Our patients deserve no less.

Author's Commentary: Because the researcher is beginning her work in diversity and inclusion in perioperative care, this is an excellent opportunity for her team to consider the application of an implementation theory, model, or framework that would specifically guide the researcher's work in conceptualizing the implementation phase of the project. The researcher may want to recognize the evidence-based implementation strategies as described by Cullen et al. (2018) in their work on evidence-based implementation strategies for sustainability, which captures specific interventions during the various phases of implementation (i.e., create awareness and interest, build knowledge and commitment, promote action and adoption, and pursue integration and sustained use). The researcher may also want to integrate the work of Brownson et. al (2012) specific to the taxonomy of dissemination and implementation outcomes. Reviewing the outcomes (i.e., acceptability, reach, feasibility) could provide additional dimensions for successful sustainment of the use of a nurse-led EBP initiative.

REFERENCES

Agency for Healthcare Research and Quality. (2019a). 2018 national healthcare disparities report. US Department of Health and Human Services.

Banaji, M. R., & Greenwald, A. G. (2016). Blindspot: Hidden biases of good people. Random House.

Brownson, R. C., Colditz, G. A., & Proctor, E. K. (Eds.). (2012). *Dissemination and implementation research in health: Translating science to practice*. Oxford University Press.

Burgess, D., van Ryn, M., Dovidio, J., & Saha, S. (2007). Reducing racial bias among health care providers: Lessons from social-cognitive psychology. *Journal of General Internal Medicine, 22*(6), 882-887. https://doi.org/10.1007/s11606-007-0160-1

Cullen, L., Hanrahan, K., Farrington, M., DeBerg, J., Tucker, S., & Kleiber, C. (2018). *Evidence-based practice in action: Comprehensive strategies, tools, and tips from the University of Iowa Hospitals and Clinics.* Sigma Theta Tau International.

FitzGerald, C., & Hurst, S. (2017). Implicit bias in healthcare professionals: A systematic review. *BMC Medical Ethics, 18,* 1. https://doi.org/10.1186/s12910-017-0179-8

Hall, W. J., Chapman, M. V., Lee, K. M., Merino, Y. M., Thomas, T. W., Payne, B., Eng, E., Day, S. H., & Coyne-Beasley, T. (2015). Implicit racial/ethnic bias among health care professionals and its influence on health care outcomes: A systematic review. *American Journal of Public Health, 105*(12), e60-e76. https://doi.org/10.2105/ajph.2015.302903

Medicine & Committee on Quality of Health Care in America. (n.d.). https://www.nationalacademies.org/our-work/the-quality-of-health-care-in-america

Pelligrini, C. A. (2020, February 1). Revisiting to err is human 20 years later. Bulletin of the American College of Surgeons. https://bulletin.facs.org/2020/02/revisiting-to-err-is-human-20-years-later/

Ruhl, C. (2020, July 1). Implicit or unconscious bias. Simply Psychology. https://doi.org/www.simplypsychology.org/implicit-bias.html

Stevenson, A., & Lindberg, C. A. (Eds.). (2010). New Oxford American Dictionary. Oxford University Press. https://doi.org/10.1093/acref/9780195392883.001.0001

Exemplar 11-11

EVIDENCE-BASED PRACTICE ADVOCATE PROGRAM FOR DIRECT CARE NURSES

Paula E. Dunham, DNP, ND, MSA, NPD-BC, EBP-C
Debi Sampsel, DNP, RN

Domains: determinants of implementation—contextual factors; implementation strategies

BACKGROUND/SIGNIFICANCE

EBP has been shown in the literature to improve patient outcomes, contribute to high-quality patient care, and reduce hospital expenses (Kim et al., 2016; Melnyk et al., 2017; Pitkanen et al., 2015). Even though this is well known, most nurses do not routinely engage in EBP activities and, instead, rely on experience and advice from coworkers (Duncombe, 2017; Pitkanen et al., 2015; Saunders et al., 2016). Hospitals have struggled to promote a climate of EBP where direct care nurses use EBP in their daily practice (Sanares-Carreon et al., 2015). Barriers to EBP use include variable EBP education in nursing schools, lack of knowledge and skills, and lack of leadership support (Bovino et al., 2017; Christenbery et al., 2016; Melnyk et al., 2017).

PROBLEM

When a Midwestern medical center EBP committee was charged with increasing EBP use among direct care nursing staff, they went to the literature. The work group looked for interventions that improved EBP use, barriers and facilitators, and specific educational topics and techniques to produce optimal EBP utilization.

The PICOT question was as follows: In direct care staff RNs, how does a formal EBP educational program compared to no formal education affect EBP utilization over 12 months?

SEARCH STRATEGY

The team divided the search strategy and searched the CINAHL, PubMed, Joanna Briggs, and Cochrane databases using the following search terms: EBP, education, utilization, training, hospital, and related combinations and terms. The search was limited to the prior 5 years and excluded academic programs but did not exclude other disciplines.

Search Results

The search revealed 14 applicable articles that were appraised using the Johns Hopkins appraisal tools. The results were placed into three outcomes synthesis tables. The first table identified literature showing the benefits of EBP education on EBP use including improved beliefs correlated to implementation (Bovino et al., 2017; Kim et al., 2016; Melnyk et al., 2017); organizational readiness for EBP (Breckenridge-Sproat et al., 2015); increased knowledge, confidence, and ability (Crabtree et al., 2016); increased implementation (Pitkanen et al., 2015); and job satisfaction and empowerment (Christenbery et al., 2016; Kim et al., 2016; Sanares-Carreon et al., 2015).

The second table identified known facilitators and barriers to EBP use. Facilitators included mentors (Bovino et al., 2017; Christenbery et al., 2016; Connor et al., 2016; Duncombe, 2017; Farokhzadian et al., 2015; Kim et al., 2016; Melnyk et al., 2017; Pitkanen et al., 2015; Sanares-Carreon et al., 2015; Saunders et al., 2016; Spiva et al., 2017), knowledge and classes (Bovino et al., 2017; Christenbery et al., 2016; Duncombe, 2017; Farokhzadian et al., 2015; Pitkanen et al., 2015; Saunders et al., 2016; Spiva et al., 2017), leadership support (Breckenridge-Sproat et al., 2015; Christenbery et al., 2016; Connor et al., 2016; Duncombe, 2017; Farokhzadian et al., 2015; Pitkanen et al., 2015; Saunders et al., 2016; Spiva et al., 2017), librarian support (Breckenridge-Sproat et al., 2015; Connor et al., 2016; Farokhzadian et al., 2015; Spiva et al., 2016), and dedicated time (Connor et al., 2016; Duncombe, 2017; Farokhzadian et al., 2015; Pitkanen et al., 2015; Sanares-Carreon et al., 2015).

The third table identified specific educational topics, time frames, and techniques used in successful educational programs. Topics deemed crucial to include were the steps of EBP (Melnyk et al., 2017), asking questions and PICOT (Breckenridge-Sproat et al., 2015; Connor et al., 2016; Melnyk et al., 2017), searching and appraising the literature (Breckenridge-Sproat et al., 2015; Connor et al., 2016; Melnyk et al., 2017); and types of research and literature (Connor et al., 2016; Melnyk et al., 2017; Sanares-Carreon et al., 2015). The course structure very strongly recommended a project-based program (Breckenridge-Sproat et al., 2015; Pitkanen et al., 2015). Time frames varied widely from 1 day, 1 full week, or sessions spaced throughout 1 year.

Implementation

Based on the appraised literature, an educational program was developed and termed the *EBP Advocate Program*. The program consisted of one 8-hour session monthly for 6 months (a total of 48 hours). The first 3 days consisted of general EBP education, including the steps of EBP, a session on library searching, practice using appraisal tools, and developing synthesis tables. The last 3 days of the program were devoted to each participant's unit-based project with a mentor. The program was limited to 10 participants because each was assigned a mentor. RN applicants could be associate degree or bachelor of science in nursing prepared and were limited to direct care staff.

Admission to the program was competitive based on the applicant's project topic and limited to one nurse per unit. The nurse managers agreed to allow their participants to attend each of the six sessions, and some allowed additional time as needed. The program ended with a graduation ceremony/poster presentation where hospital and nursing leadership were able to see progress toward outcomes. The EBP committee chair and cochair oversaw the program, provided lectures, and acted as mentors when needed.

Results

The 10 participants developed 10 separate EBP projects and had a 100% program completion rate. Two years after the program completion, 80% practice changes have been completed or are planned. The program received 100% positive feedback, and one unit-based project has spread hospital wide and has been presented at several national venues. One participant has been involved in additional EBP projects as the owner and mentor.

Lessons Learned

Through the program, although volunteer mentors were assigned to each participant, the mentor knowledge and availability were variable. Mentors need additional mentor-specific training to assure a minimum level of competency, and they should be granted the same protected time as participants. Even though all proposed projects were endorsed by the unit manager, several were not an actual problem in our facility. More attention should be paid to potential projects to ascertain the necessity and facility benefit. In a large medical center, it is unrealistic to expect projects to be completed within 3 months of practice recommendation. After completion of the 6-month program, the direct care staff and mentors did not have any additional protected time for implementation and data collection. Continued implementation has been slow, and the EBP committee chair and cochair have served as ongoing mentors.

Conclusion

The goal of this unique educational EBP initiative was to increase EBP use by direct care nurses. The work group used the EBP seven-step method for evidence translation and the KTA framework to facilitate implementation. Using established frameworks allowed the work group to systematically identify the problem, evaluate the literature, apply nursing expertise, consider learner preferences and values, and implement the practice recommendation in a manner that improves adoption, outcomes, and sustainment.

Authors' Commentary: This EBP project includes several improvement and implementation strategies, such as identifying barriers and facilitators, the use of advocates, and educational offerings. Should the project coordinators want to further their work, this is an excellent opportunity for the team to consider the application of an implementation theory, model, or framework that would specifically guide the researchers' work in conceptualizing the implementation phase of the project. The researcher may also want to recognize the evidence-based implementation strategies as described by Cullen et al. (2018) in their work on evidence-based implementation strategies for sustainability, which captures specific interventions during the various phases of implementation (i.e., create awareness and interest, build knowledge and commitment, promote action and adoption, and pursue integration and sustained use). The researchers may want to integrate the work of Brownson et. al (2012) specific to the taxonomy of dissemination and implementation outcomes. Reviewing the outcomes (i.e., acceptability, reach, feasibility) could provide additional dimensions for successful sustainment of the EBP Advocate Program for direct care nurses.

REFERENCES

Bovino, R., Aquila, A., Bartos, S., McCurry, T., Cunningham, C., Lane, T., Rogucki, N., DosSantos, J., Moody, D., Mealia-Ospina, K., Pust-Marconem, J., & Quiles, J. (2017). A cross-sectional study on evidence-based nursing practice in the contemporary hospital setting. *Journal for Nurses in Professional Development, 33*(2), 64-69. https://doi.org/10.1097/NND.0000000000000339

Breckenridge-Sproat, S., Throop, M., Raju, D., Murphy, D., Loan, L., & Patrician, P. (2015). Building a unit-level mentored program to sustain a culture of inquiry for EBP. *Clinical Nurse Specialist CNS, 29*(6), 329-37. https://doi.org/10.1097/NUR.0000000000000161

Brownson, R. C., Colditz, G. A., & Proctor, E. K. (Eds.). (2012). *Dissemination and implementation research in health: Translating science to practice.* Oxford University Press.

Christenbery, T., Williamson, A., Sandlin, V., & Wells, N. (2016). Immersion in EBP fellowship program. *Journal for Nurses in Professional Development, 32*(1), 15-20. https://doi.org/10.1097/NND.0000000000000197

Connor, L., Dwyer, P., & Oliveira, J. (2016). Nurses' use of EBP in clinical practice after attending a formal EBP course. *Journal for Nurses in Professional Development, 32*(1), E1-7. https://doi.org/10.1097/NND.0000000000000229

Crabtree, E., Brennan, E., Davis, A., & Coyle, A. (2016). Improving patient care through nursing engagement in EBP. *Worldviews in Evidence Based Nursing, 13*(2), 172-175. https://doi.org/10.1111/wvn.12126

Cullen, L., Hanrahan, K., Farrington, M., DeBerg, J., Tucker, S., & Kleiber, C. (2018). *Evidence-based practice in action: Comprehensive strategies, tools, and tips from the University of Iowa Hospitals and Clinics.* Sigma Theta Tau International.

Duncombe, D. (2017). A Multi-institutional study of the perceived barriers and facilitators to implementing EBP. *Journal of Clinical Nursing, 27*(5-6), 1216-1226. https://doi.org/10.1111/jocn.14168

Farokhzadian, J., Khajouei, R., & Ahmadian, L. (2015). Evaluating factors associated with implementing evidence-based practice in nursing. *Journal of Evaluation in Clinical Practice, 21*(6), 1107-1113.

Kim, S., Stichler, J., Ecoff, L., Brown, C., Gallo, A., & Davidson, J. (2016). Predictors of EBP implementation, job satisfaction, and group cohesion among regional fellowship participants. *Worldviews in Evidence Based Nursing, 13*(5), 340-348. https://doi.org//10.1111/wvn.12171

Melnyk, B. M., Fineout-Overholt, E., Giggleman, M., & Choy, K. (2017). A test of the ARCC model improves Implementation of EBP, healthcare culture & patient outcomes. *Worldviews in Evidence Based Nursing, 14*(1), 5-9. https://doi.org/10.1111/wvn.12188

Pitkanen, A., Alanen, S., Rantanen, A., Kaunonen, M., & Aalto, P. (2015). Enhancing nurses' participation in implementing EBP. *Journal for Nurses in Professional Development, 31*(2), E1-E5. https://doi.org/10.1097/nnd.0000000000000161

Sanares-Carreon, D., Comeau, O., Heliker, D., Marshall, D., Machner, C., Bell, L., Brumfield, V., Kwarciany, G., & Sandridge. J. (2015). An educational pathway to fast track EBP at the bedside. *Journal for Nurses in Professional Development, 31*(1), E1-E6. https://doi.org/10.1097/nnd.0000000000000113

Saunders, H., Vehvilainen-Julkunen, K., & Stevens, K. (2016). Effectiveness of an educational intervention to strengthen nurses' readiness for EBP: A single-blind RCT. *Applied Nursing Research, 31,* 175-185. https://doi.org/10.1016/japnr.2016.03.004

Spiva. L., Hart, P., Patrick, S., Waggoner, J., Jackson, C., & Threatt, J. (2017). Effectiveness of an EBP nurse mentor training program. *Worldviews on Evidence Based Nursing, 14*(3), 183-191. https://doi.org/10.1111/wvn.12219

Spiva, L., Hand, M., VanBrackle, L., & McVay, F. (2016). Validation of a predictive model to identify patients at high risk for hospital readmission. *Journal for Healthcare Quality, 38*(1), 34–41. https://doi.org/10.1111/jhq.12070

Exemplar 11-12

Nursing Academic–Practice Partnerships

Mary G. Carey, PhD, RN, FAHA, FAAN

> **Domains:** determinants of implementation—contextual factors; service and patient outcomes; implementation outcomes; stakeholder involvement and engagement; implementation strategies

Our Implementation Science Story

At the University of Rochester in New York, our nursing academic–practice partnership between the School of Nursing and the hospital has been in existence since the beginning of the medical campus. Both the flagship hospital, Strong Memorial Hospital, and the school were built at the same time. The School of Nursing was established in 1925 as a diploma program administered by Strong Memorial Hospital. The school's graduate programs were developed beginning in the 1950s, with the diploma program replaced with a baccalaureate degree program in 1960. In 1972, the School of Nursing became an independent school with the leadership of Dr. Lee Ford, the pioneer of the unification model and the NP role. The nursing PhD program was added in 1979 and has subsequently graduated 150 PhD students.

The activities of the dean of the School of Nursing and the University of Rochester Medical Center's chief nursing executive are those of academic and administrative leadership in the university and medical center and top-level policy formulation for the discipline of nursing. A unification model was established that assisted the School of Nursing in assuming accountability and responsibility in practice, education, and research. With an enrollment of nearly 900 students across its academic programs, the school is focused on developing exceptional team-oriented health care providers, researchers, educators, clinical leaders, and innovators, who continually strive to improve health care provision. The hospital has nearly 900 beds and employs over 4000 nurses; thus, our partnership provides extensive support to the nursing discipline (AACN-AONE Task Force on Academic-Practice Partnerships, 2012). To continue to benefit and optimize a collaborative and productive relationship between academia and practice, which includes fundamental mutual respect and trust between academia and practice; knowledge is gained and exchanged between academia and practice; the transition of students and new nurses is optimized using evidence-based programs; academia and practice are committed to maximizing the potential of every nurse to achieve their highest level of practice; organizational processes develop, implement, and evaluate academic and clinical accomplishments; better understand the nursing workforce, academia, and practice both systematically analyze data to anticipate the future needs of our discipline (Phillips et al., 2019). Nursing practice continues to serve as the primary site for all clinical training of nurses, and our School of Nursing continues to provide education to our diverse workforce.

The School of Nursing's Center for Research Support serves as the central resource for academic research; it is organized into three divisions: Pre- and Post-Award, Research Facilitation, and Training and Education. The center includes experienced, highly trained staff that provides accessible, consistent, high-quality services to nursing practice.

CENTER FOR RESEARCH SUPPORT

The center and its staff offer comprehensive support to School of Nursing faculty and students, including drafting proposals, identifying funding sources, designing experiments, gathering and analyzing data, and connecting with expert collaborators across the university. The Research Facilitation group provides key support services for research and scholarly activities. The group's goals include but are not limited to providing services for preliminary and pilot studies, providing orientation, and consulting in project oversight; structures exist to provide direct access to timely assistance with both developing and carrying out ongoing projects. In addition, hospital practice has the Clinical Nursing Research Center, which is directed by a nurse scientist and provides high-quality support to all nurses. The Edward G. Miner Library provides the University of Rochester Medical Center and the greater Rochester community with resources, expertise, and an inviting space to support health, discovery, teaching, and learning. Despite the unique research capacity of nursing, especially related to patient-, nurse-, and family-oriented outcomes (Shepard Battle, 2019), schools of nursing are only awarded 0.4% or $133 million of the National Institutes of Health research budget. Notably, the School of Nursing is ranked 21st nationally among all nursing schools with nearly 3 million dollars of grant funds.

The clinical institution continues to provide tuition support for all nursing programs. Also, the School of Nursing tuition grant, which was instituted at the end of 2018, offers scholarships to fill the gaps where tuition benefits fall short, giving University of Rochester nurses tuition-free access to the following programs:

- RN to bachelor of science (BS) program
- Clinical nurse leader (master of science [MS], post-MS)
- Nursing education (MS, post-MS, and RN to BS to MS entry points)
- Health care management organization and leadership (MS)

CURRENT MODEL

Our academic–practice partnership model is led by the chief nursing executive and dean, with 18 nursing directors, seven directors, three chief nursing officers who are clinical operations related (e.g., critical care), and eight nursing directors providing support services (e.g., Clinical Nursing Research Center). Among the nursing directors, more than half have a clinical appointment in the School of Nursing, and the director of the research center is a tenured nursing faculty.

For nearly 100 years, all the hospital chiefs of nursing and the schools' deans have provided leadership for our relationship in academia and practice. Plus, over the years, nurses in both academia and practice consistently contribute to the shared strategic plans. Being part of an academic medical center is a tremendous boost to the partnership. The School of Nursing not only falls within the greater University of Rochester academic community as one of six stand-alone schools, but it is also a component of the University of Rochester Medical Center, which allows for better integration of nursing research, education, and practice. In addition, the academic–practice partnership enjoys the benefit of six affiliate hospitals, including Strong Memorial, Highland, F.F. Thompson,

Noyes Memorial, Jones Memorial, and St. James Memorial Hospitals. Strong is the largest hospital with nearly 900 beds, and F.F. Thompson is the smallest with fewer than 100 beds. This provides the partnership with a wide variety of opportunities in large academic teaching hospitals or a small community setting.

IMPLEMENTATION STRATEGY

To continue to benefit and optimize collaborative and productive relationships between an academic practice, our vision includes the following (Beal, 2019):

- Fundamental mutual respect and trust between academia and practice
- Pursuit and exchange of knowledge shared between academia and practice
- Optimized transition of students and new nurses using evidence-based programs
- A commitment to maximizing the potential of every nurse to achieve their highest level of practice plus increase the diversity of the workforce
- Organizational processes developing, implementing, and evaluating academic and clinical accomplishments
- Practice's commitment to serving as the primary location for all the clinical training of our nurses
- A better understanding of the nursing workforce; academia and practice both systematically analyze data to anticipate the future needs of our discipline

Overall, through this academic–practice partnership, the school is a top-ranking educational institution recognized 3 years in a row for the Health Professions Higher Education Excellence in Diversity Award, and the hospital is a four-time Magnet-designated institution providing world-class nursing education and nursing care.

Author's Commentary: The author shares the work of her team in developing a strong academic–clinical partnership. This project includes several determinants of contextual implementation factors such as organizational processes, nursing workforce, academia, and practice. As the project continues to evolve, the author may want to integrate an implementation theory, model, or framework that would specifically guide the work in conceptualizing the implementation phase of their academic–clinical partnerships. Using additional evidence-based implementation strategies as described by Cullen et al. (2018) in their work on evidence-based implementation strategies for sustainability may also enhance the author's work. It may be helpful to integrate the work of Brownson et al. (2012) specific to the taxonomy of dissemination and implementation outcomes. Reviewing the outcomes (i.e., acceptability, reach, feasibility) could provide additional dimensions for successful sustainment of the academic–clinical partnership.

REFERENCES

AACN-AONE Task Force on Academic-Practice Partnerships. (2012). Guiding principles to academic-practice partnerships. https://www.aacnnursing.org/Academic-Practice-Partnerships/The-Guiding-Principles

Beal, J. A., & Zimmermann, D. (2019). Academic-practice partnerships: Update on the national initiative. *Journal of Nursing Administration, 49*(12), 577-579. https://doi.org/10.1097/NNA.0000000000000817

Brownson, R. C., Colditz, G. A., & Proctor, E. K. (Eds.). (2012). *Dissemination and implementation research in health: Translating science to practice.* Oxford University Press.

Cullen, L., Hanrahan, K., Farrington, M., DeBerg, J., Tucker, S., & Kleiber, C. (2018). *Evidence-based practice in action: Comprehensive strategies, tools, and tips from the University of Iowa Hospitals and Clinics.* Sigma Theta Tau International.

Phillips, J., Phillips, C., Kauffman, K., Gainey, M., & Schnur P. (2019). Academicpractice partnerships: A win-win. *Journal of Continuing Education in Nursing, 50*(6), 282-288. https://doi.org/10.3928/00220124-20190516-09

Shepard Battle, L. (2019). Academic-practice partnerships and patient outcomes. *Nursing Management, 49*(1), 34-40. https://doi.org/10.1097/01.NUMA.0000527717.13135.f4

FINANCIAL DISCLOSURES

Zena Banker has no financial or proprietary interest in the materials presented herein.

Dr. Rebekah Barber has no financial or proprietary interest in the materials presented herein.

Dr. Mary G. Carey has no financial or proprietary interest in the materials presented herein.

Dr. Kelly Casler has no financial or proprietary interest in the materials presented herein.

Jaclyn Castano has no financial or proprietary interest in the materials presented herein.

Dr. Kelli Chovanec has no financial or proprietary interest in the materials presented herein.

Clista Clanton has no financial or proprietary interest in the materials presented herein.

Dr. Donna Copeland has no financial or proprietary interest in the materials presented herein.

Dr. Paula E. Dunham has no financial or proprietary interest in the materials presented herein.

Christina Fortugno has no financial or proprietary interest in the materials presented herein.

Dr. April Garrigan has no financial or proprietary interest in the materials presented herein.

Aakansha Gosain has no financial or proprietary interest in the materials presented herein.

Dr. David H. James has no financial or proprietary interest in the materials presented herein.

Dr. Shaun Lampron has no financial or proprietary interest in the materials presented herein.

Andrew Loehr has no financial or proprietary interest in the materials presented herein.

Megan Maloney has no financial or proprietary interest in the materials presented herein.

Dr. Margaret Moore-Nadler has no financial or proprietary interest in the materials presented herein.

Dr. Somali Nguyen has no financial or proprietary interest in the materials presented herein.

Dr. Kristen Noles has no financial or proprietary interest in the materials presented herein.

Dr. Cynthia Peltier Coviak has no financial or proprietary interest in the materials presented herein.

Dr. Shea Polancich has no financial or proprietary interest in the materials presented herein.

Dr. Marti Rice has no financial or proprietary interest in the materials presented herein

Dr. Linda A. Roussel has no financial or proprietary interest in the materials presented herein.

Mallory E. Rowell has no financial or proprietary interest in the materials presented herein.

Dr. Debi Sampsel has no financial or proprietary interest in the materials presented herein.

Mary L. Schumann has no financial or proprietary interest in the materials presented herein.

Dr. Jeannie Scruggs Corey has no financial or proprietary interest in the materials presented herein.

Dr. Tedra S. Smith has no financial or proprietary interest in the materials presented herein.

Dr. Carolynn Thomas Jones has no financial or proprietary interest in the materials presented herein.

Dr. Patricia L. Thomas has no financial or proprietary interest in the materials presented herein

Dr. Tiffany Tscherne has no financial or proprietary interest in the materials presented herein.

Dr. Sharon Tucker has no financial or proprietary interest in the materials presented herein.

Heather Ugolini has no financial or proprietary interest in the materials presented herein.

Dr. Mercedes Weir has no financial or proprietary interest in the materials presented herein.

Dr. Janet E. Winter has no financial or proprietary interest in the materials presented herein.

Index

accelerated second-degree nursing program, 89, 91

accountable care team (ACT) model, 164, 165–166

accreditation, 89, 92–93

ACE Star Model of Knowledge Transformation, 23

ACT. *See* accountable care team model

adaptation, 2, 11–13, 31–32, 34

adoption, 2, 10

Adult Nonalcoholic Fatty Liver Disease (NAFLD) Toolkit, 187–190

advanced nursing practice roles, 73

Advancing Research and Clinical Practice Through Close Collaboration (ARCC), 23

application, 56, 57

appropriateness, 183

ARCC (Advancing Research and Clinical Practice Through Close Collaboration), 23

baccalaureate nursing program, 89, 90–92

bias in perioperative care (diversity and inclusion), 214–217

Braden Scale, implementation of, for predicting pressure injury risk in the emergency department, 144

Canadian Institutes of Health Research (CIHR), 41–42

Carper's way of knowing, 19, 20

CCM (chronic care model), 164, 167

CFIR (Consolidated Framework for Implementation Research), 43–45

change management, 134, 137, 145, 149–150

change responses, 134, 137

checklists and instruments associated with dissemination science and implementation science frameworks, 47–50

chemotherapy-induced nausea and vomiting, using evidence-based practice approach to improve care of patients with, 211–213

chronic care model (CCM), 164, 167

CIHR (Canadian Institutes of Health Research), 41–42

client and service outcomes, 182–183

clinical nurse leaders (CNLs), 109, 124–127, 166–167

clinical rotations, 92, 94

coin-spinning exercise (application of quality improvement concepts), 159–161

collaboration, 56, 59, 61, 106, 123–124, 138–139, 209–210, 222–225

community health promotion project implementation, 70–71

comprehensive vascular access team, using evidence-based approach for decreasing inappropriate referrals to, 202–204

consequences, unintended, 183

Consolidated Framework for Implementation Research (CFIR), 43–45

context, 25, 181–182

core value, vision, and mission congruence, 95
crisis prevention program for staff, development of, 143
curriculum, 92, 94–95, 124–127

definitions, 3–5
deimplementation, 2, 5, 13–15
design thinking as guide for innovation, 174–176
didactic learning, 73, 80–81
diffusion, 79
diffusion of innovations theory, 42–43
direct care nurses, evidence-based practice advocate program for, 218–221
discovery, 56, 57, 68–69
dissemination, 7, 164
dissemination and implementation outcomes, 9–11, 183
dissemination frameworks, 39, 42–43
dissemination practice, 4
dissemination research, 2, 5, 6, 30, 32–34
dissemination science, 2, 4, 19, 56, 89, 108
dissemination science vs. implementation science, 22
dissemination strategies, 19, 30, 32–33
diversity, 164–165
diversity and inclusion in perioperative care, 214–217
doctor of nursing practice, 108, 109–110
doctor of nursing practice projects, embedding implementation science in, 200–201
doctor of philosophy and doctor of nursing practice collaboration, 108, 123–124
Donabedian model, 152–153

economic evaluations, 184
effectiveness trials, 19, 27
efficacy trials, 19, 26–27
80/20 rule, 168–169
electronic data, knowledge discovery from, 68–69
entry level of practice, 89–106
    accreditation, role of, 92–93
    addressing barriers to ensure entry-level implementation science practices, 98–100
    baccalaureate nursing curriculum, 92, 94–95
    exemplars and assignments, 82–84, 106
    implementation practices in the clinical setting
        advancing the placement site's strategic plan, 96–97
        congruency in vision, mission, and core values, 95
        exercises, 95, 97
        indicator performance practices in the clinical experience, 96–97
    pathways to baccalaureate nursing, 90–92
    simulation-based experiences, 101–104
        aspects of fidelity, 102
        simulation methodologies, 103
evidence-based practice, 2, 4, 19, 22

Evidence-Based Practice Attitude Scale, 141

evidence-based practice, evolution of, 1–18

    evidence-based practice uptake, 2, 5–6

    and path to implementation and dissemination science, 6–9

evidence-based practice interventions, 178

exemplars

    Adult Nonalcoholic Fatty Liver Disease Toolkit, 187–190

    application of quality improvement concepts (coin-spinning exercise), 159–161

    application of run and control charts, 156–158

    building a peer support system to mitigate psychological trauma in health care workers, 194–195

    community health promotion project implementation, 70–71

    creation of sleep protocol to limit sleep interruptions on a medical-surgical unit, 172–173

    decreasing inappropriate referrals to a comprehensive vascular access team, 202–204

    design thinking as guide for innovation, 174–176

    diversity and inclusion (bias in perioperative care), 214–217

    embedding implementation science in doctor of nursing practice projects, 200–201

    enhancing staff confidence in de-escalating a crisis situation, 143

    evidence-based practice advocate program for direct care nurses, 218–221

    implementation of Braden Scale for predicting pressure injury risk in the emergency department, 144

    implementing new informed consent practices for pediatric coronavirus disease 2019 clinical trials, 196–199

    implementing P6 acupressure in conjunction with pharmacotherapy to decrease chemotherapy-induced nausea and vomiting, 211–213

    interprofessional collaboration, 106

    interprofessional evidence-based practice council for collaborative practice, 209–210

    knowledge discovery from electronic data, 68–69

    nursing academic-practice partnerships, 222–225

    nursing leadership and evidence-based practice amidst the pandemic, 191–193

    patient safety implementation, 205–208

    pediatric patient/family education in a cardiovascular intensive care setting, 130–131

experiential learning, 73, 81

fidelity, 2, 12–13, 19, 89, 96, 102, 183

framework, definition of, 40, 146

frameworks for nursing education, 75–82

frameworks, models, and theories for promoting evidence-based practice in nursing, 23–24

frameworks, models, and theories in implementation and decision science, 39–53

    dissemination frameworks, 42–43

    frameworks for either dissemination or implementation, 45–47

    implementation frameworks, 43–45

    Implementation Science Research Development tool and, 181

    instruments, checklists, and methods associated with frameworks, 47–50

    major theorists and scientists, 40–42

    resource websites for translational science concept measurement, 49

frontline engagement, 164–165

graduate nursing education, 73

graduate nursing education and advanced practice, 107–131

    exemplars and assignments, 84–85, 130–131

    nursing research, nursing practice, and translational science, 109–112

    translational science competencies in master's-level graduates, 116–117

    translational science competency development

        doctor of philosophy and doctor of nursing practice collaboration, 123–124

        doctoral nursing program clinical and simulation experiences, 121–122

        doctoral nursing program content, 112, 117–121

        experiences for developing evidence-based practice competencies in practice-focused doctoral programs, 119

        master of science in nursing student competencies and curriculum for evidence-based practice, 124–127

        recommended clinical nurse leader curriculum experiences, 126

    translational science competency differences in research-focused vs. practice-focused graduates, 113–115

health systems thinking, 134–136

historical perspective of translational science, 20–22

IHI (Institute for Healthcare Improvement) model for improvement, 150

IHI's (Institute for Healthcare Improvement) Quadruple Aim, 168

implementation and decision science history, context, and application, 19–37

    conducting investigations, 28

        dissemination strategies, 30, 32–33

        implementation strategies, 28–30, 182

        potential design applications and adaptations for research, 34

        potential participant differences from efficacy trial samples and potential design adaptations, 31–32

        tools for planning research, 33

    historical perspective of translational science, 20–22

    implementation science, dissemination science, and translational nursing science, 25–26

    testing interventions, 26–28

implementation and decision science theories, frameworks, and models, 39–53

    dissemination frameworks, 42–43

    frameworks for either dissemination or implementation, 45–47

    implementation frameworks, 43–45

    Implementation Science Research Development tool and, 181

    instruments, checklists, and methods associated with frameworks, 47–50

    major theorists and scientists, 40–42

    resource websites for translational science concept measurement, 49

implementation and dissemination outcomes, 9–11, 183

implementation checklist, 39, 47–50

Implementation Citizenship Behavior Scale, 140

Implementation Climate Scale, 140

implementation cost-effectiveness, 184

Implementation Leadership Scale, 140

implementation measurement, 39, 47–50, 183

implementation practice, 3, 73, 89
implementation research, 2, 5, 28–30, 34
implementation research characteristics, 179–180
implementation science, 2, 3, 5–6, 19, 56, 73, 89, 108, 145, 164, 178
implementation science frameworks, 39, 43–45
implementation science models, 39, 41
Implementation Science Research Development (ImpRes) tool, 178, 179–185
implementation science theories, 39, 40–41
implementation science vs. dissemination science, 22
implementation strategies, 19, 28–30, 83–84, 182
Implementation Strategies for Evidence-Based Practice, 75–78, 141
implementation tools, 39, 47–50
improvement and implementation sciences (student assignment), 84–85
improvement science, 4, 145, 146
improvement science, application of, 145–161
    exemplars
        application of quality improvement concepts (coin-spinning exercise), 159–161
        application of run and control charts, 156–158
    implementation science and, 153–154
    implementing and sustaining change in health care, 147–148
    models and frameworks
        common tools for quality improvement work, 151
        Donabedian model, 152–153
        Institute for Healthcare Improvement model for improvement, 150
        lean six sigma, 153
        Plan-Do-Study-Act, 150–152
    philosophical perspective on improving health care, 146–147
    theories supporting science of improvement work, 148–150
indicator performance practices in the clinical experience, 96–97
individual, organization, and policy outcomes, 10–11
influence, 134, 139
informed consent protocol innovations for pediatric coronavirus disease 2019 clinical trials, 196–199
innovation, 164
innovation and translation, 163–176
    aligning culture change with existing frameworks
        facilitation using new agreement tools (the next big idea), 168–170
        Institute for Healthcare Improvement's Quadruple Aim, 168
    exemplars
        creation of sleep protocol to limit sleep interruptions on a medical-surgical unit, 172–173
        using design thinking to guide innovation, 174–176
    redesigning for innovation, 165
        accountable care team (ACT) model, 165–166
        chronic care model (CCM) framework, 167
        clinical nurse leaders, 166–167
    trust and diversity, 164–165
inquiry, 56, 57–58, 164
Institute for Healthcare Improvement model for improvement, 150

Institute for Healthcare Improvement's Quadruple Aim, 168
instruments and checklists associated with dissemination science and implementation science frameworks, 47–50
Integrated Promoting Action on Research Implementation in Health Services (i-PARIHS), 43–45
integration, 2, 56, 57
interprofessional, 56, 57
interprofessional collaboration, exemplar for, 106
interprofessional evidence-based practice council for collaborative practice, 209–210
interventions, developing and testing, 26–28
Iowa Model of Evidence-Based Practice, 23
i-PARIHS (Integrated Promoting Action on Research Implementation in Health Services), 43–45

Johns Hopkins Nursing Evidence-Based Practice Model, 24

knowledge discovery from electronic data, 68–69
knowledge, skills, and attitudes (KSAs) for implementation science in nursing education, 113–117
Knowledge to Action framework compared with common evidence-based practice models, 185
Knowledge to Translation model, 78–79
knowledge translation, 2, 3, 39, 41–42
KSAs (knowledge, skills, and attitudes) for implementation science in nursing education, 113–117

leadership. *See* organizational systems and leadership
lean six sigma model, 153
master of nursing competencies, 108, 116–117, 124–127

measurement methods and issues, 9–11, 47–50, 183
message, 134, 139
mission, vision, and core value congruence, 95
model, definition of, 40, 146
models (frameworks) for nursing education, 75–82
models, frameworks, and theories for promoting evidence-based practice in nursing, 23–24
models, frameworks, and theories in implementation and decision science, 39–53
    dissemination frameworks, 42–43
    frameworks for either dissemination or implementation, 45–47
    implementation frameworks, 43–45
    Implementation Science Research Development tool and, 181
    instruments, checklists, and methods associated with frameworks, 47–50
    major theorists and scientists, 40–42
    resource websites for translational science concept measurement, 49

Nonalcoholic Fatty Liver Disease (NAFLD) Toolkit, 187–190
nurse scientist, 56
nursing education, 73–87
    evolution of implementation science and nursing, 74
    frameworks for
        implementation, 79
        Registered Nurses' Association of Ontario, 78–79
        teaching-learning strategies, 80–82

University of Iowa Hospitals and Clinics, 75–78

graduate nursing education and advanced practice, 107–131

doctor of philosophy and doctor of nursing practice collaboration, 123–124

doctoral nursing program clinical and simulation experiences, 121–122

doctoral nursing program content, 112, 117–121

exemplars and assignments, 84–85, 130–131

experiences for developing evidence-based practice competencies in practice-focused doctoral programs, 119

master of science in nursing student competencies and curriculum for evidence-based practice, 124–127

nursing research, nursing practice, and translational science, 109–112

recommended clinical nurse leader curriculum experiences, 126

translational science competencies in master's-level graduates, 116–117

translational science competency differences in research-focused vs. practice-focused graduates, 113–115

undergraduate nursing education, 89–106

accreditation, role of, 92–93

addressing barriers to ensure entry-level implementation science practices, 98–100

baccalaureate nursing curriculum, 92, 94–95

exemplars and assignments, 82–84, 106

implementation practices for optimizing learning in the clinical setting, 95–97

pathways to baccalaureate nursing, 90–92

simulation-based experiences, 101–104

nursing interventions, developing and testing, 26–28

nursing leadership amidst the pandemic, 191–193

nursing practice, 108, 109–112

nursing research, 108, 109–112

organization, individual, and policy outcomes, 10–11

organizational assessment tools, 134, 139–141

organizational systems, 134

organizational systems and leadership, 133–144

best practice assessment tools and strategies, 139–141

Evidence-Based Practice Attitude Scale, 141

Implementation Citizenship Behavior Scale, 140

Implementation Climate Scale, 140

Implementation Leadership Scale, 140

change management and change responses, 137

exemplars

development of crisis prevention program for staff, 143

implementation of Braden Scale for predicting pressure injury risk in the emergency department, 144

influence and messaging, 139

systems thinking, 134–136

team science, 138–139

organizational vision, mission, and core values, 95

organization's strategic plan, enhancing, 96–97

outcomes, dissemination and implementation, 9–11, 183

outcomes, patient and service, 182–183

PARIHS (Promoting Action on Research Implementation in Health Services), 43–45
patient and public involvement and engagement, 184–185
patient and service outcomes, 182–183
patient safety implementation, 205–208
patient safety, systems thinking perspective on, 135
patterns of knowing, 56, 57
PCT. *See* pragmatic clinical trial
pediatric patient/family education in a cardiovascular intensive care setting, evidence-based approach for, 130–131
peer support program development to mitigate psychological trauma in health care workers, 194–195
Plan-Do-Study-Act, 145, 150–152
policy, individual, and organization outcomes, 10–11
population health, 2, 8
practice immersion, 73
pragmatic clinical trial (PCT), 19, 27–28
PRECEDE-PROCEED Model, 45–47
preceptorships, 89, 94
precision medicine, 2, 8–9
pressure injury risk prediction in the emergency department, implementation of Braden Scale for, 144
programs of scholarship, 56, 62–65
Promoting Action on Research Implementation in Health Services (PARIHS), 43–45
psychological trauma mitigation in health care workers, 194–195
public and patient involvement and engagement, 184–185

Quadruple Aim framework, 168
quality and safety education for nurses and implementation science, 84
quality improvement, 5, 145, 147
quality improvement concepts, application of (coin-spinning exercise), 159–161
quality improvement tools, 151

RAND model of persuasive communication and diffusion of medical innovation, 42–43
randomized controlled trials, 27
RE-AIM (Reach, Effectiveness, Adoption, Implementation, Maintenance), 45–47
Registered Nurses' Association of Ontario, 78–79
research translation, 20–21
research-focused doctorate, 108, 112–121
residences, 89, 94
Rogers' diffusion of innovations model, 42–43
Rosswurm and Larrabee Model for Evidence-Based Practice Change, 24
run and control charts, application of, 156–158

scholarship, 56, 57–58
scholarship for academic nursing, 55–71
    alignment with implementation and dissemination sciences, 56

approaches to bringing scholarship of practice and teaching to life, 58–62

establishing, nurturing, and sustaining translational science scholarship, 62–65

exemplars

community health promotion project implementation, 70–71

knowledge discovery from electronic data, 68–69

possible research-focused and practice-focused questions for a translational science project, 60–61

scientific inquiry, scholarship for practice and teaching, and translational science, 57–58

scholarship of practice, 56, 57–62

scholarship of teaching, 56, 57–62

science of improvement, 146

service and patient outcomes, 182–183

simulation experiences, 89, 101–104, 121–122

sleep protocol, creation of, to limit sleep interruptions on a medical-surgical unit, 172–173

stakeholder involvement and engagement, 184

Stetler Model of Research Utilization to Facilitate Evidence-Based Practice, 24

strategic plan advancement in the clinical experience, 96–97

systems thinking, 134–136

taxonomy of dissemination and implementation outcomes, 10–11

teaching-learning strategies, 80–82

team and engagement sciences, 5, 134, 138–139

testing interventions, 26–28

testing methods of dissemination research, 30, 32–33

testing methods of implementation research, 28–30

theories, frameworks, and models for promoting evidence-based practice in nursing, 23–24

theories, frameworks, and models in implementation and decision science, 39–53

dissemination frameworks, 42–43

frameworks for either dissemination or implementation, 45–47

implementation frameworks, 43–45

Implementation Science Research Development tool and, 181

instruments, checklists, and methods associated with frameworks, 47–50

major theorists and scientists, 40–42

resource websites for translational science concept measurement, 49

theory, definition of, 40, 146

three-dimensional problem solving, 168–169

translational nursing, 2, 4, 13–15, 178

translational science, 4, 19, 39, 56, 108

translational science and doctor of nursing practice projects, 85

translational science and evaluation models (student assignment), 85

translational science competencies, 108, 112–127

translational science differentiated from implementation science and dissemination science, 22

translational science, historical perspective of, 20–22

Triple Aim framework, 8, 168

trust, 164–165

Type III error, 29

undergraduate nursing education, 89–106

accreditation, role of, 92–93

addressing barriers to ensure entry-level implementation science practices, 98–100

baccalaureate nursing curriculum, 92, 94–95

exemplars and assignments, 82–84, 106

implementation practices in the clinical setting

    advancing the placement site's strategic plan, 96–97

    congruency in vision, mission, and core values, 95

    exercises, 95, 97

    indicator performance practices in the clinical experience, 96–97

pathways to baccalaureate nursing, 90–92

simulation-based experiences, 101–104

    aspects of fidelity, 102

    simulation methodologies, 103

unintended consequences, 183

University of Iowa Hospitals and Clinics' framework, 75–78, 141

vision, mission, and core value congruence, 95

Printed in the United States
by Baker & Taylor Publisher Services